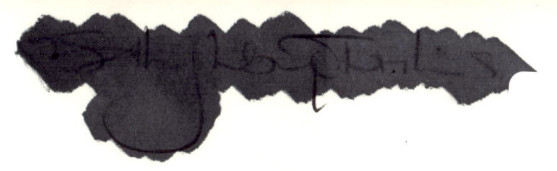

MEDICAL LIBRARY
WONFORD HOUSE HOSPITAL
DRYDEN ROAD
EXETER EX2 5AF

Methodology in evaluation of psychiatric treatment

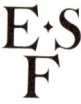

The European Science Foundation is an international non-governmental organization with its seat in Strasbourg (France). Members are Academies and Research Councils which are responsible for supporting scientific research at a national level, and which are funded largely from government sources. The term 'science' is used in its broadest sense to include the humanities, social sciences, biomedical sciences and the natural sciences with mathematics. The ESF has currently 48 members from 18 European countries.

The tasks of the ESF are to:

assist its Member Organizations to coordinate their research programmes and define their priorities;

identify areas in need of stimulation, particularly those of an interdisciplinary nature;

further cooperation between researchers by facilitating their movement between laboratories, holding workshops, managing support schemes approved by the Member Organizations, and arranging for the joint use of special equipment;

harmonize and assemble data needed by the Member Organizations;

foster the efficient dissemination of information;

respond to initiatives which are aimed at advancing European science;

maintain constructive relations with the European Communities and other relevant organizations.

The ESF is funded through a general budget to which all Member Organizations contribute (according to a scale assessed by country), and a series of special budgets covering Additional Activities not included in the main programme, to which only participating Organizations contribute. The programmes of the ESF are determined by the Assembly of all Member Organizations. Their implementation is supervised by an elected Executive Council, assisted by the Office of the Foundation which consists of an international staff directed by the Secretary General and located in Strasbourg.

European Medical Research Councils
a Standing Committee of the
European Science Foundation

Methodology in Evaluation of Psychiatric Treatment

Proceedings of a Workshop held in Vienna
10-13 June 1981

Edited by T. Helgason

In collaboration with
E.E. Anttinen
L.B. Cronholm
R. Daly
H. Hippius
E.A. Sand

CAMBRIDGE UNIVERSITY PRESS
Cambridge
London New York New Rochelle
Melbourne Sydney

Published by the Press Syndicate of the University of Cambridge
The Pitt Building, Trumpington Street, Cambridge CB2 1RP
32 East 57th Street, New York, NY 10022, USA
296 Beaconsfield Parade, Middle Park, Melbourne 3206, Australia

© Cambridge University Press 1983

First published 1983

Printed in Great Britain at the University Press, Cambridge

Library of Congress catalogue card number: 83-1782

British Library Cataloguing in Publication Data

Methodology in evaluation of psychiatric treatment
1. Mentally ill — Care and treatment
I. Helgason, T.   II. European Science Foundation
362.2'0425   RC454

ISBN 0 521 25592 9

Contents

Participants		xi
Foreword *H. Danielsson*		xv
Preface *T. Helgason*		xvi

INTRODUCTION   1

Evaluation of Psychiatric Treatment *B. Cronholm and R.J. Daly* 3
1. Introduction 3
2. Aims of psychiatric treatment 5
3. Terminology and definition of samples 6
4. Unsystematic observations, case reports 8
5. Systematic evaluation 9
   5.1 Introduction 9
   5.2 Rating scales 9
   5.3 Psychological methods 16
   5.4 Psychophysiological measures 19
   5.5 Projective tests 20
   5.6 Biochemical methods 21
6. Design and statistical problems 22
7. Cost-benefit analysis 25
8. Summary and discussion 27
9. Conclusions 28

The Aims of Psychiatric Treatment *Sir Martin Roth* 33
1. The scope and limitations of psychiatric treatment 33
2. Objectives in the treatment of depressive illness 34
3. Social models of depression and their implications for defining goals in treatment 36
4. Objectives in the social and medical treatment of schizophrenic illness 39
5. Setting aims in the treatment of neuroses 42
6. Psychosomatic disease and behavioural medicine 45

7	Treatment objectives in relation to personality disorder	47
8	Summary and conclusions	51
9	Some methodological issues	53

Evaluation in Mental Health Programmes *N. Sartorius* 59
1	Introduction	59
2	Specific issues in evaluation of mental health care	59
3	Preparation for evaluation and types of data necessary for it	61
4	WHO's contributions to the field of evaluation	63

I METHODS OF CLASSIFICATION 69

Principles of 'Multiaxial' Classification in Psychiatry as a Basis of Modern Methodology *P. Berner and H. Katschnig* 71
1	Introduction	71
2	The aims to be attained by so-called 'multiaxial' classifications	72
3	'Multi-area' classification (MAC)	74
4	The poly-diagnostic approach (PDA)	75

Standardized Methods of Classification of Mental Disorders
J.K. Wing 81
1	Introduction	81
2	Advantages of standardization	82
	2.1 Achieving comparability in clinical research	82
	2.2 Testing hypotheses	83
	2.3 Understanding clinical classifications	83
3	Methodological problems	85
	3.1 Algorithms	85
	3.2 Present clinical state	86
	3.3 Present episode	86
	3.4 Past episodes	87
	3.5 Pathology and aetiology	87
	3.6 Other clinical data	88
	3.7 A hierarchical element in classification	89
	3.8 Comprehensive versus specific instruments	90
4	Future developments	91

The Significance of Biological Factors in the Diagnosis of Depressions
H.M. van Praag 93
I	Biochemical variables	93
1	Biological factors of an aetiological and of a pathogenetic nature	93
2	Points of crystallization	94
3	Serotonin metabolism	94
	3.1 5-HIAA in cerebrospinal fluid (CSF)	94
	3.2 CSF 5-HIAA: therapeutic significance	95

	3.3 CSF 5-HIAA: prognostic significance	97
	3.4 Plasma tryptophan	98
4	Catecholamine metabolism	98
	4.1 Urinary MHPG	98
	4.2 Renal MHPG excretion: therapeutic significance	99
	4.3 Renal MHPG excretion: conclusions	100
	4.4 MHPG concentration in CSF	101
	4.5 HVA concentration in CSF	101
5	Discussion	102
6	Summary	103
II	Hormonal variables	107
1	The way to the anterior hypophyseal lobe	107
2	The dexamethasone suppression test (DST)	108
	2.1 The CRF/ACTH/cortisol 'axis' in depressions	108
	2.2 Changes in the DST in depressions	109
	2.3 Carroll's findings with the DST	110
	2.4 Therapeutic and prognostic value of the DST	111
	2.5 Conclusions	111
3	TSH response to TRH	112
	3.1 Changes in depressive patients	112
	3.2 Therapeutic and prognostic significance	114
	3.3 Conclusions	115
4	Growth hormone (GH) responses	115
	4.1 Changes in depressive patients	115
	4.2 Therapeutic and prognostic significance	116
	4.3 Conclusions	116
5	Discussion	117
6	Summary	117

II EVALUATION CRITERIA 121

Special Problems in Evaluation of Psychotherapy *R.J. Daly* 123

1	Introduction	123
2	Cost-benefit and cost-effectiveness studies	127
3	Cost-benefit studies	129
4	Accuracy of data	132
5	Self-monitoring	133
6	Conclusion	134

Special Problems in Evaluation of Milieu Therapy *O.S. Dalgard, S. Friis, T. Sørensen and P. Vaglum* 137

1	The need for evaluation of milieu therapy	137
2	Components of evaluation	137
3	Evaluation of effectiveness	138
	3.1 Design	139

		3.2 Characteristics of patients at admission	139
		3.3 Treatment variables	140
		3.4 Criteria of outcome	143
		3.5 Control groups	145
	4	Psycho-social problems in evaluation of milieu therapy	146

III RATING METHODS IN EVALUATION OF TREATMENT   149

The AMP Rating Methods   *B. Woggon*   151

1. Development of the AMP system — 151
2. Description of the AMDP assessment documents — 152
3. Training — 153
4. Instructions for raters — 153
5. Development of two second-order scales — 154
6. Comparison between the AMDP system and other well-known rating scales — 158
7. Summary — 160

The Comprehensive Psychopathological Rating Scale (CPRS)
B. Cronholm   163

The Use of Rating Scales for Affective Disorders   *P. Bech*   171

1. Introduction — 171
2. Quantitative rating scales for affective states — 171
   - 2.1 General considerations — 171
   - 2.2 The Hamilton Depression Scale (HDS) — 172
   - 2.3 The Bech-Rafaelsen Melancholia Scale (MES) — 173
   - 2.4 The Bech-Rafaelsen Mania Scale (MAS) — 174
   - 2.5 The Hamilton Anxiety Scale (HAS) — 174
   - 2.6 Error of Type II in clinical trials — 175
3. Qualitative rating scales for affective disorders — 175
   - 3.1 General considerations — 175
4. The combined use of qualitative and quantitative rating scales in endogenous depression — 177
   - 4.1 Hospitalized patients — 177
   - 4.2 Patients in general practice — 177
5. Conclusion and summary — 178

Self-Rating Scales in the Evaluation of Psychiatric Treatment
D. von Zerssen   183

1. Introduction — 183
2. General considerations — 183
3. Examples of scales — 187
   - 3.1 Survey — 187
   - 3.2 Scales from a psychiatric information system — 188

4	Examples of application	192
5	Conclusions	199

Methods for Measuring Social Adjustment *H. Katschnig*   205
1	Introduction	205
2	Terminological and theoretical issues	205
3	Research instruments	208
4	Conclusion	215

IV OTHER QUANTITATIVE METHODS OF EVALUATION OF TREATMENT   219

Psychophysiological Criteria *M. Lader*   221
1	Introduction	221
2	Psychophysiological techniques	222
	2.1 Peripheral autonomic	222
	2.2 Peripheral somatic	222
	2.3 Central measures	223
	2.4 Neuroendocrine measures	223
	2.5 Current developments	223
3	Psychophysiological measures and central state	223
4	Psychophysiological measures and treatment response	224
	4.1 Peripheral effects of psychotropic drugs	225
	4.2 Peripheral measures of central effects	226
	4.3 Central measures	227
5	Monitoring behavioural treatments	228
6	Prognostic indicators	229
7	Conclusions	229

Biological Quantitative Methods in the Evaluation of Psychiatric Treatment: Some Biochemical Criteria *P. Uytdenhoef, P. Linkowski and J. Mendlewicz*   231
1	Introduction	231
2	Response to tricyclic antidepressants	231
	2.1 3-Methoxy-4-hydroxyphenylglycol (MHPG) studies	231
	2.2 5-hydroxyindol acetic acid (5-HIAA) studies	233
	2.3 Red blood cell-catechol-O-methyltransferase (COMT) studies	235
	2.4 Sleep EEG studies	235
	2.5 Determination of optimal dosage by monitoring plasma levels of tricyclics	235
3	Response to MAO inhibitors	236
	3.1 Rate of acetylation	236
	3.2 Platelet MAO inhibition	237
4	Response to lithium	238
	4.1 Mania	238

	4.2 Depression	238
	4.3 Prophylactic treatment	239
5	Response to electroconvulsive therapy (ECT)	239
6	Biochemical predictors of antipsychotic treatment	240
	6.1 Biochemical variables	240
	6.2 Neuroendocrine studies	240
	6.3 Plasma levels studies	241
7	Conclusion	242

V   ETHICAL AND PRACTICAL PROBLEMS 249

Ethical and Practical Problems in Therapeutic Research in Psychiatry
H. Helmchen   251

1	Basic statements	251
	1.1 Therapy	252
	1.2 Therapeutic techniques and attitudes	252
	1.3 Psychiatric research	252
2	The basic problem	253
	2.1 Outline	253
	2.2 Solutions	254
	2.3 Comments	255
3	Psychiatric specifications	256
	3.1 Informed consent	256
	3.2 Controlled trials	257
	3.3 Confidentiality	258
4	Questions of control	259
	4.1 Levels of control	259
	4.2 Composition of ethical committees	260
	4.3 Access and competence	260
	4.4 Benefits and risks	260
	4.5 General control	261
	4.6 Task-oriented modes of control	261
	4.7 Education for ethical self-control	262
5	Conclusions	262

Index   265

Participants

Professor E.E. Anttinen
Faculty of Medicine
University of Tampere
Vuoleenkatu 11
P.O. Box 607
SF-33101 Tampere 10
Finland

Dr P. Bech
Psychochemistry Institute
Rigshospitalet
9, Blegdamsvej
DK-2100 Copenhagen Ø
Denmark

Professor P. Berner
Allgemeines Krankenhaus der
Stadt Wien
Psychiatrische Universitätsklinik
Währinger Gürtel 74-76
A-1097 Vienna
Austria

Professor Ph. Corten
Université Libre de Bruxelles
Laboratoire d'Epidémiologie et de
Medicine Sociale
Campus Erasme C.P. 590
Route de Lennick 808
B-1070 Brussels
Belgium

Professor B. Cronholm
Karolinska Hospital
Solnavägen 1
S-104 01 Stockholm
Sweden

Professor Dr Med. O.S. Dalgard
Dept of Psychiatry
Ulleval Sykehus
N-Oslo
Norway

Professor R.J. Daly
University College and
Regional Hospital
Wilton
Co. Cork
Ireland

Professor H. Danielsson
Secretary General
Swedish Medical Research Council
Box 6713
S-113 85 Stockholm
Sweden

Professore Dario de Martis
Clinica Psichiatrica
Università di Pavia
Ospedale Psichiatrico Provinciale
Viale Umberto, I, 88
27058 Voghera
Pavia
Italy

Dr Annette Gjerris
Psychochemistry Institute
Rigshospitalet
Blegdamsvej 9
DK-2100 Copenhagen Ø
Denmark

Participants

Professor T. Helgason
State Department of Education
Kleppsspitalinn
P.O. Box 1429
104-Reykjavik
Iceland

Professor H. Helmchen
Psychiatrische Klinik und Poliklinik
Freie Universität Berlin
Eschenallee 3
D-1000 Berlin 19
Federal Republic of Germany

Dr J.H. Henderson
Regional Officer for Mental Health
World Health Organisation
European Region
8 Scherfigsvej
DK-2100 Copenhagen Ø
Denmark

Professor H. Hippius
Ludwig Maximilians Universität
München
Psychiatric Clinic
Nussbaumstrasse 7
D-8000 Munich 2
Federal Republic of Germany

Professor H. Katschnig
Allgemeines Krankenhaus der
Stadt Wien
Psychiatrische Universitätsklinik
Währinger Gürtel 74-76
A-1097 Vienna
Austria

Professor M. Lader
Department of Pharmacology
Institute of Psychiatry
De Crespigny Park
Denmark Hill
London SE5 8AF
UK

Dr Pat Melia
St Finan's Hospital
Killarney
Ireland

Professor J. Mendlewicz
Université Libre de Bruxelles
Dept du Psychiatrie
Campus Erasme
Route de Lennik 808
B-1070 Brussels
Belgium

Dr P.V. Morozov
Division of Mental Health
World Health Organisation
CH-1211 Geneva 27
Switzerland

Professor Astrid Nöklebye Heiberg
Psychiatric Clinic
University of Oslo
N-Oslo
Norway

Sir Martin Roth
Department of Psychiatry
Clinical School
Addenbrooke's Hospital
Hills Road
Cambridge CB2 2QQ
UK

Dr R. Sadoun
Unité de Recherche sur
l'Epidémiologie des troubles Mentaux
Centre Paul Broca de l'Inserm
2 ter, rue d'Alésia
F-75014 Paris
France

Professor E. Sand
Ecole de Santé Publique
Campus Erasme
Route de Lennick 808
B-1070 Brussels
Belgium

Professor N. Sartorius
Director of the Mental Health
Division
World Health Organisation
CH-1211 Geneva 27
Switzerland

Participants

Professor M. Tansella
Clinica Psichiatrica
Università di Padova
Sede di Verona
Centro Ospidaliero Borgo Roma
I-37100 Verona
Italy

Professor Pekka Tienari
Oulun Yliopisto
Psikiatrian Klinikka
SF-90210 Oulu 10
Finland

Professor P. Vaglum
Dept of Psychiatry
Ulleval Sykehus
N-Oslo 1
Norway

Professor H.M. van Praag
Department of Psychiatry
University Hospital
P.O. Box 16250
3500 CG Utrecht
The Netherlands

Professor D. von Zerssen
Max-Planck-Institut für
Psychiatrie
Kraepelinstrasse 10
D-8000 Munich 40
Federal Republic of Germany

Professor J.K. Wing
MRC Social Psychiatry Unit
Institute of Psychiatry
De Crespigny Park
Denmark Hill
London SE5 8AF
UK

Dr B. Woggon
Psychiatrische Universitätsklinik
Zürich
Forschungsdirektion
Postfach 68
CH-8029 Zürich 8
Switzerland

Dr Stephanie Zobrist (Observer)
European Medical Research Councils
European Science Foundation
1 Quai Lezay-Marnésia
F-67000 Strasbourg
France

Foreword

The group of European Medical Research Councils (EMRC) was formed in 1971 and became a Standing Committee of the European Science Foundation in 1975. EMRC is an association of medical research councils or equivalent organizations in Western Europe. The National Institutes of Health and the European office of WHO are associated with EMRC and take an active part in the work of EMRC. Formally, these organizations have the status of observers. The main aims of EMRC are to exchange information on the research policies pursued by its Member Organizations and to initiate and stimulate international cooperation in biomedical research. Since biomedical research is highly international in itself, EMRC should concentrate its activities on furthering international cooperation in those fields where it can play a significant role as a complement to existing channels. Mental illness research is, in the opinion of EMRC, one such field.

After a survey of the activities of its Member Organizations in mental illness research, EMRC decided to set up a study group to analyse areas where EMRC could contribute. Several such areas were defined by the study group and it was decided that the first activity should deal with methodologies in evaluation of psychiatric treatment. The present volume contains the proceedings of an EMRC workshop on the subject, held in June 1981. EMRC hopes that this volume will contribute to further research and research cooperation on mental illnesses.

Henry Danielsson
Chairman of EMRC

Preface

This volume comprises the written-up versions of the presentations given at a workshop on Methodology in Evaluation of Psychiatric Treatment, organized by the European Medical Research Councils (EMRC). It is intended to be a source book for those research workers who are already established as well as for those contemplating research in this difficult field. It should also be of interest to others engaged in evaluating results of treatment, with regard to both patient management and health administration.

The EMRC decided in 1978 to set up a study group on mental illness research. This group was to study information which had already been collected by the Secretariat of the EMRC and point out research areas which might be promoted by the EMRC or its member organizations. The group was also to prepare a proposal to the EMRC on workshops in the field of mental illness research, especially with reference to the evaluation of treatment. The study group, which initially consisted of Professors E. Anttinen (Finland), B. Cronholm (Sweden), T. Helgason (Iceland; chairman), H. Hippius (Federal Republic of Germany) and E.A. Sand (Belgium) submitted its first report to the EMRC in 1979. At the same time Professor R. Daly (Ireland) joined the group.

Having discussed the report of the study group at its following meetings, the EMRC decided that effort should be concentrated on promoting research on evaluation of psychiatric treatment and, as a first step, a small workshop of research workers from the countries of the Member Organizations should be arranged. Before doing so, a background document briefly reviewing published research work in the area should be prepared and circulated to the national member research councils. Professor Cronholm agreed to write this document supported by the Swedish Medical Research Council and with Professor Daly produced a

Preface xvii

final paper, which was precirculated to the participants in the workshop. It appears as one of the introductory chapters to this volume.

The papers which were summarized at the workshop are arranged unabridged under five major headings in this book. The introductory part is composed of Cronholm's and Daly's background document, Sir Martin Roth's paper on the aims of psychiatric treatment and the contribution to the discussion of N. Sartorius, on evaluation in mental health programmes. As a necessary basis for treatment, Part I includes three papers on methods of classification of mental disorders, multiaxial classification, standardized methods of classification, and biological factors in the diagnosis of depression. Part II on criteria of evaluation comprises papers on special problems in evaluation of psychotherapy and milieu therapy. Part III includes papers on certain rating scales and their use in specific disorders, objective scales, self-rating scales, and methods for measuring social adjustment. Part IV considers psychophysiological and other biological methods of evaluation of psychiatric treatment. Finally, in Part V the ethical and practical problems of therapeutic research are discussed.

Wide areas pertaining to the methodology of evaluation of psychiatric treatment are thus reviewed in the book. Also, a number of suggestions for further research are presented. It is, therefore, hoped that the reader will agree with the organizers that this is an important and useful publication, as it will stimulate further research on the evaluation not only of psychiatric treatment but of medical treatment in general.

The volume would not have been put together without the support and interest of the representatives of the medical research councils in the thirteen countries constituting the EMRC. The enthusiasm and active interest of the Chairman, Professor H. Danielsson, Sweden, was crucial as was the hospitality of the Österreichischer Fond zur Förderung der Wissenschaftliche Forschung. It is a pleasure to express the study group's thanks and appreciation to the European Science Foundation and others who contributed to the success of the workshop. Particular thanks are due to the authors of the papers contained in this volume.

Reykjavik, July 1982 Tómas Helgason

INTRODUCTION

Evaluation of Psychiatric Treatment

B. CRONHOLM and R.J. DALY

1. Introduction

For several reasons, interest in the development and improvement of objective and, as far as possible, uniform methods for the evaluation of desired effects and undesired side-effects of various psychiatric methods of treatment has increased enormously during the past few decades. The introduction of highly potent psychotropic drugs such as the phenothiazines, butyrophenones, tricyclic antidepressants and lithium, has enormously improved the treatment of patients with schizophrenic, depressive, manic and other syndromes. Of course, there are still many problems. We know little about the mechanisms of action of all these drugs, and we do not know enough about possible specificity of different drugs for particular syndromes. There are also side-effects. Some of these, such as tardive dyskinesia with antipsychotic drugs are quite severe. In the public mind there has been great alarm about rather mild troubles and there has been a tendency to overlook the benefit of these drugs and to consider them only as harmful. This also holds true for other somatic treatments such as electroconvulsive therapy (ECT) and still more for different forms of psychosurgery.

In several countries there has been during recent decades very great interest in various forms of psychotherapy. Unfortunately, this term has been used with a great number of meanings. It has been used to denote particular methods or groups of methods but also in a much more general sense. One group of methods is founded on psychodynamic theories. Here belongs psychoanalysis in its classical sense, a highly time-consuming method with one-hour treatment sessions several times every week, quite often for years. The evaluation of the therapeutic outcome is based mainly on comprehensive case reports, describing in detail the therapeutic process. An objective evaluation of psychoanalysis as a therapeutic method is difficult, but in at least some cases of neurotic disorders, there seems to be conspicuous improvement. However, the relation between the costs (for the individual or for society) and possible benefit, also has to be considered. It seems evident that psychoanalysis always will have to be reserved for a few, highly selected cases. Perhaps it will be of most value as a useful experience during the training of psychotherapists.

There is now a growing tendency to apply a psychodynamic frame of reference in various, less time-consuming and, from a practical point of view, more useful ways. This holds true for various forms of so-called brief therapy, for group therapy and family therapy. There is also a great interest in crisis intervention and prevention of mental disorders as a reaction to somatic illness. There is an enormous literature in the field, often quite enthusiastic. Even if there seems to be little doubt that these therapies are useful in many cases, there is still too little objective evidence. Some seem to be accepted at their face value and not on the basis of any systematic and controlled study of their beneficial effects and possible side-effects. Such studies are fairly uncommon, mainly due to the considerable methodological difficulties. Whereas an experimental design is quite often possible in psychopharmacological studies, this has proved much more difficult in the field of psychotherapy. However, there has also been an uncritical denigration and unjustified scepticism about all forms of psychotherapy based on psychodynamic theories — for example as repeatedly presented by the excellent English psychologist Hans Eysenck. Both trends — uncritical acceptance and uncritical rejection — indicate the need for development of adequate evaluation methods.

One group of psychotherapeutic methods is based on learning theory and denoted 'behaviour therapy'. One such method is 'systematic desensitization' which may be exemplified in the following way. A phobic patient is in phantasy confronted with an anxiety-producing stimulus. At the same time, general relaxation is brought about, by means of hypnosis or in some other way which inhibits the anxiety. Another method is 'flooding'. A phobic patient may be confronted with an anxiety-producing stimulus or situation in imagination or in reality. When anxiety has reached its maximum, it will automatically decline. In this way the patient is expected to learn to endure being exposed to these threatening stimuli. As these methods aim at alleviating particular symptoms, an experimental study is less difficult to design than for methods based on psychodynamic theories. They have proved to be most successful in phobic and obsessive-compulsive disorders.

An interesting way of treating some neurotic and psychosomatic disorders is by means of 'biofeedback'. To a fairly large extent, patients may be able to learn ways of controlling autonomic functions in an experimental setting. They get visual or auditory information about, e.g., their blood pressure or muscular tension and thus learn manoeuvres to regulate them — perhaps without being able to describe the way in which they do it. They may then be able to exert the same control also in real life, outside the laboratory.

The problem is not whether psychotherapy (in a general sense) has any effect at all, since it is evident that all sorts of interactions between individuals have some influence on their behaviour and ideas. The problem should be formulated in other ways. For example, to what extent is the effect dependent on the particular method used, and on the personality of the therapist? And if the technique is of some importance, which technique is the best to use on which patients? In both these fields much research remains to be done.

2. Aims of psychiatric treatment

The aim of all therapy is to bring about or to restore 'health'. In the daily routine of their work, psychiatrists — like other doctors — seldom call in question its aim. Their implicit definition of health will as a rule be the old one: 'Freedom from illness'. However, during the past few decades there has been much discussion about what should be meant by 'health'. It is evident that 'health' means something to which a high degree of positive value is assigned, but this does not necessarily mean that there will be a unanimity of opinion on a more explicit definition of the concept. This holds true especially for 'mental health' — there are many different opinions about the relative value of different aspects.

The WHO (1958) definition may seem pretentious: "Health means more than freedom from disease, freedom from pain, freedom from untimely death. It means optimum physical, mental and social efficiency and well-being." However, considered as a counsel of perfection it may be useful. Restricted and applied to mental health, it points to the most important aspects to be evaluated as a result of psychiatric treatment — freedom from psychopathology and suffering, suicide prevention, cognitive efficiency, social adaptation, working capacity — and also to such more elusive aspects as 'self-actualization', 'individuation' and 'ego strength'. Of course, the concrete aim of psychiatric treatment is very different in different cases and situations. In a patient with chronic schizophrenia, it may be just a slight improvement of his social behaviour by means of pharmacotherapy and training in activities of daily living (ADL). In a patient with severe depression it may be total freedom from psychopathology and return to his premorbid personality by means of treatment with antidepressant drugs or ECT; in a young person with neurotic inhibitions, no uncertainty and worry about his future, anxiety, etc.; it may be relieving an addict from his dependence on alcohol or other drugs; it may also be maturation and development of his personality by means of psychotherapy. Psychiatric methods of treatment, and especially various psychotherapy methods, are also important aids within medical specialities other than just psychiatry. This holds true for endeavours to prevent or treat psychosomatic disorders such as essential hypertension, duodenal ulcer or low-back pain. There is also a growing awareness of the need for psychiatric aid in handling psychological complications with severe somatic injuries or diseases, not least incurable ones, and to improve motivation in rehabilitation of the handicapped. This incomplete enumeration illustrates that there is no therapeutic goal common to all cases. There will thus be no omnibus method, useful to evaluate the therapeutic effects in all disorders and situations.

It is very difficult to compare the effects of two methods if the treatments are based on different ideologies with widely different aims. Unfortunately this is not uncommon. An example is the difference, not only in ideology, theories and methodology but also in aims and evaluation of treatment, between behaviour therapists and psychodynamically orientated psychotherapists, especially those with hermeneutic-emancipatory ideals, even when treating the same syndrome. For instance, a behaviour therapist will be quite happy if he succeeds in relieving a patient of his phobic symptoms, whereas a psychoanalyst probably will be more interested in whether his patient has insight into the mechanisms behind his symptoms, and whether some maturation of his personality has taken place.

3. Terminology and definition of samples

In all research, and especially in multicentre studies, it is necessary to use a well-defined, consequent and communicable terminology. Unfortunately, psychiatric terminology as a rule does not fulfil these demands. Even within the same country — and still more so in different countries — terms may be used with widely different implications. And words in different languages apparently referring to the same concept, may on closer examination prove to be used with rather different meanings. All this holds true for signs and symptoms, syndromes, diagnoses and theoretical constructs.

In psychiatric research — not least in the evaluation of treatment methods — it is necessary that the patients included in the sample are defined in an exact and communicable way. As a rule, it is also desirable that the sample is homogeneous in many respects, unfortunately meaning that it will be rather small within a reasonable time limit — or that the collection of a series will be very time-consuming. However, such narrow definitions are necessary for the results of a study to become valid. For sampling of a material in psychiatric research, conventional diagnostic classification systems are for these reasons not very useful. They aim at covering the whole field of psychiatric disorders which results in vague and inconsequent definitions, using different types of criteria for different diagnostic categories. This holds true even for the ninth revision of the *International Classification of Diseases* (ICD-9) from 1977 (ICD 1980). These classifications may be useful for describing the panorama of psychiatric illness and its changes over time, but not when a more precise, communicable and often narrow delineation of a group is considered necessary. One method may be to use such a multiaxial classification system as was suggested by Essen-Möller as early as 1961, and which has been further developed by Ottosson & Perris (1973).

The third edition of the American Psychiatric Association's *Diagnostic and Statistical Manual of Mental Disorders* (DSM III) from 1980 gives very good descriptions and operational definitions. They are given in still more detail in the *Research Diagnostic Criteria* (RDC) by Spitzer *et al* (1978) with its complement, the *Schedule for Affective Disorders and Schizophrenia* (SADS) by Endicott & Spitzer (1978). The RDC is constructed with the deliberate purpose of ensuring as few 'false positives' as possible at the cost of a certain number of 'false negatives'. This means that a patient who is not for research purposes accepted as, e.g. suffering from a 'major depressive disorder' by the RDC, may all the same have to be accepted as such in clinical work and treated accordingly.

Another example of highly formalized classification is the diagnostic index for affective disorders designed by Martin Roth and his co-workers (see Gurney *et al* 1972). By means of a multiple regression analysis of anamnestic data, signs and symptoms in a group of patients with affective disorders, weighted data were computed and used to classify patients in two categories: depression and anxiety states. The anxiety states may be further divided into a 'phobic anxiety-depersonalisation syndrome' and others, the depressions into endogenous and neurotic types. The advantage of such a system is not that it should result in a 'truer' diagnostic classification than others, but that by means of strict formalization it is more communicable and replicable.

Only rarely will a classification based on biochemical data be possible. However, the development of highly sensitive and reliable chemical methods has started a new epoch in this field. An example is that among patients suffering from 'primary depressive illness' as defined by Feighner et al (1972), there is a bimodal distribution of 5-hydroxyindol acetic acid (5-HIAA) — the main metabolite of the important CNS transmitter serotonin — in the cerebrospinal fluid. This indicates a biochemical heterogeneity within this group of patients. Clinically, there is no conspicuous difference between the two groups except in one — very important — respect: suicidal attempts, and especially serious ones, are more frequent in the group with low 5-HIAA. Of course, it will be of paramount importance to study these two groups of depression separately in treatment evaluations — e.g. in a comparison of the effects of antidepressant drugs differing in respect of their uptake-inhibiting effects on serotonin and on norepinephrine. (Bertilsson et al 1974; Åsberg et al 1976a, 1976b; and Träskman et al 1979.)

The main conclusions as regards selection of a material in the evaluation of psychiatric methods of treatment will be: 1. It is necessary to use formalized methods with precisely defined criteria for both inclusion and exclusion of patients; 2. Conventional diagnostic classification will not be satisfactory; 3. There is no *one* correct classification system useful in all situations but the classification and selection of patients have to be adapted to the particular research problem.

4. Unsystematic observations, case reports

It is not uncommon for a new method of psychiatric treatment to be introduced as a result of casual observations in a series of cases. If the psychiatrist sees a regularity, some invariance in his observations, he may form a hypothesis and, going further, test it in a systematic way. There are many examples of this — and it is enlightening that the hypothesis may be fruitful even if it is soon disproved. One example is the introduction of convulsive treatment, another is the introduction of chlorpromazine as an antipsychotic drug (Swazey 1974; Jeste et al 1979).

Of course, all accidental or unsystematic observations have to be supplemented with systematic and controlled studies, especially for any generalization to be possible. But for innovation, both serendipity and the courage to form possibly false hypotheses may be necessary.

Single case reports (not identical with systematic 'single case studies': see section 6) may be very useful in some situations. This holds true, for example, in the description and evaluation of psychotherapeutic procedures, especially various types of 'insight therapy'. Detailed descriptions of intrapsychic processes and of the therapist/patient interaction may be highly instructive for other therapists. However, the richness and vividness of such a report is bought at the price of uncertainty as regards reliability and validity (see section 6). It will also be difficult to generalize from such descriptions of unique cases. All the same they may be highly influential — the most striking examples are Sigmund Freud's case reports.

Tape recording has brought about a considerable improvement in the research on case studies. Therapeutic sessions may be recorded and later on repeatedly listened to and possibly also seen by the therapist. This makes possible a much more careful study of the therapeutic process than if it were just stored in the memory, possibly supported by a few notes. It may also be studied by other therapists, making possible comparisons between their observations and evaluations.

5. Systematic evaluation
5.1 Introduction

Even if unsystematic observations by patients themselves, by their relatives, psychiatrists and others may often be informative, their reliability always has to be questioned. This holds true not least for statements about the effect of treatment methods — they may be old or new, biological or psychological. For that reason, systematic evaluation of most treatment methods is a necessary part of their scientific development.

What a patient says about his physical or mental state may be very difficult to understand merely because of linguistic problems and because of his 'unscientific' frames of reference. There are also many reasons for a patient to give distorted information, unconsciously or even consciously. One important factor is that of 'social desirability'. For example, in a Swedish study it was found that the alcohol consumption, estimated on the basis of a questionnaire, was far less than that estimated on the basis of reports from the 'Systembolaget' which has a monopoly on selling alcoholic beverages. This indicates a tendency to underestimate and embellish drinking habits in the population. Similar trends in embellishing have been found for information given about smoking habits. For example, Donovan (1977) found that there was a conspicuous under-reporting during pregnancy as was later revealed post partum. For that reason he recommends objective measurement, e.g. measures of expired carbon monoxide, if valid estimates are required.

5.2 Rating scales
5.2.1 Introduction

When there is a need for measuring the severity of a disorder and its possible changes during treatment, the use of a rating scale will often be the best way. However, too often a clear distinction is not made between diagnostic scales — aiming at separating patients with a specific syndrome from others (see section 3) — and scales aiming at measuring the severity of a syndrome and its changes as a result of treatment. Even if scales originally designed for diagnostic purposes may be useful also for measuring change, the requirements of the scales for the two purposes are different.

Rating may be defined as the transformation of signs or symptoms, behaviour or mental events to some sort of numerical measure. As a rule the scale is digital — i.e. with discrete steps from e.g. 0 (absence of the phenomenon) to 5 (very marked and/or frequent presence). The transformation into numerical measures may be made by an observer, e.g. a psychiatrist, a psychologist or a nurse, or by the patient himself. There are also analogue scales where the degree is marked on a line, ranging from, for example, 'absent' to 'most pronounced' and/or 'most frequent'. The score is the distance from 'absent'. (See also section 5.2.3.5.)

A rater may make an estimate of a patient's general degree of mental disorder or of isolated fragments, 'atoms', of behaviour — or of anything between these two extremes. Both extremes have their drawbacks. Global ratings are difficult to describe and to communicate. They are also fairly insensitive as the number of scale steps has to be restricted. Global ratings further tend to be made more light-heartedly than ratings of more specific, less comprehensive items. For that reason it is preferable to use the sum of the rated degree of severity in a number of separate variables ('items') to arrive at a measure of the severity of a psychiatric disorder. The more or less explicit hypothesis behind this procedure will be that the severity of all signs or symptoms rated will be in a linear and monotonic way related to the severity of an underlying illness. The illness may be conceptualized as a psychological construct only, but more often there is the idea of an underlying, definite but as a rule hypothetical or so far unknown biological disturbance. In any case, we think that we will be able to measure a 'nomothetic' variable, i.e. a variable that may be considered to be 'the same' in different individuals.

A complete list of 'atoms' of behaviour would become interminable and already for that reason useless in practice. It would also become pointless. The recognition of sadness or any other mental state in an individual is not based on a conscious summing of isolated, objective observations, e.g. number and depth of wrinkles on the forehead, number of words spoken per minute, loudness of voice, etc. A list of behavioural details does not communicate the image of a depressed patient. A sum of ratings of such items is unlikely to be strongly related to global severity, even if the individual signs are associated with the illness. The best way to arrive at a measure of the severity of a mental disorder seems to be the rating of a series of items in between global and 'atomic' estimates; and to use the sum of these ratings as an estimate of the severity.

Psychiatric rating scales are instruments used by people who not only observe, but also interact with the subjects they rate. The most valid and reliable ratings seem to be obtained when the items are so delineated and described that they correspond to the way people normally perceive each other's mood and behaviour. We seem to have inborn abilities to judge other persons' mood and attitudes to us — certainly quite useful abilities from the point of view of survival. Such abilities may, of course, improve as the result of training, e.g. during clinical work. An example is that the inter-rater consistency of observed 'Psychomotor retardation' was very low in a group of untrained raters but good among those who were well trained (Cronholm *et al* 1974).

Probably, many observations are primarily of a global character. The observation of 'sadness' in an individual appears to be an immediate perception, and only on reflection are we able to analyse our impression and register the details. On the other hand, several psychiatric signs and symptoms are complicated constructs, based on specific hypotheses and concepts, and their registration has to be the result of a deliberate synthesis of a number of discrete observations. This seems to hold true for such items as 'Lack of appropriate emotion' and 'Withdrawal'.

These considerations lead to the problem of how to describe the items and the scale steps in a manual. From what has been said earlier, it is evident that a mechanical enumeration of behaviour 'atoms' would be useless. What is needed is a text that communicates the essence of the variable in question. To quote Karl Popper, clarity rather than precision is the goal. To be really good, the description of signs and symptoms and of the scale steps in a rating scale must have certain literary qualities. Whether the scale text 'works' or not, i.e. whether it is communicable, should be tested empirically by means of inter-rater reliability studies (see section 6).

At first sight, construction of a rating scale may seem deceptively simple. In reality, it is a complicated procedure if the scale has to fulfil all requirements necessary for it to be useful.

A great number of psychiatric rating scales — probably too many — have been described. Here only a few examples will be mentioned. For a more comprehensive review see Pichot (1974).

5.2.2 Comprehensive psychiatric rating scales

Many rating scales have been designed with the purpose of covering as far as possible all psychopathological signs and symptoms.

Quite often, they also aim at being useful both for diagnostic purposes and for measuring the severity of a psychiatric disorder. This may make them less useful in both respects, and for that reason separate scales for these different purposes are preferable.

A few examples of comprehensive scales will be briefly mentioned.

One of the most ambitious is the *'AMDP-system'* (earlier AMP; AMDP = Arbeitsgemeinschaft für Methodik und Dokumentation in der Psychiatrie). It comprises 123 psychopathological and 58 somatic symptoms, rated from 0 (not present) to 3 (severe). The use of the scale is only possible for well trained raters, owing mainly to a lack of operational definitions of the four scale steps of each item. The data are recorded on sheets that can be read automatically and computerized. There are also sheets for the medication, and for the assessment of the efficacy of treatment. The AMDP has been extensively used in several research centres in continental Europe. For further information see Angst *et al* (1969); Scharfetter (1974); and Woggon (1979).

The *'Brief Psychiatric Rating Scale (BPRS)'* was originally designed to be used for the evaluation of treatment effects in clinical drug studies, and it has been extensively used for that purpose. However, it has also been used for classification of psychiatric disorders. It was originally described by Overall and Gorham (1962). The present version comprises 18 items, rated from 1 (not present) to 7 (extremely severe). The items — but not the scale steps — are described in detail. A general principle in designing the scale was to provide psychiatrists with a scale where the items correspond to their usual way of conceptualizing psychopathology (Overall 1974). This probably is one of the reasons for its popularity; another is that it is short and not very time-consuming. It seems to be most useful in the evaluation of drug effects on psychiatric in-patients.

A very popular scale is the *'Nurses' Observation Scale for In-patient Evaluation (NOSIE)'*. It comprises 30 items describing the patient's behaviour in the ward, rated from 0 (never) to 4 (always). It is very useful, at least as a complementary instrument for the evaluation of treatment effects in schizophrenic in-patients (Honigfeld 1974).

The *'Comprehensive Psychopathological Rating Scale (CPRS)'* was designed by a working team as a result of an initiative from the Swedish Medical Research Council. It comprises 65 items scoring from 0 to 3 (with half-steps allowed) and covers a great number of psychiatric signs and symptoms. It differs from most other rating scales, through having been conceived as a pool, from which a smaller number of items could be drawn for studies of particular psychiatric syndromes. Each item and its separate steps are described systematically and in detail; 0 always means absence of a sign or symptom; 1 that it is present but not more pronounced than it could apply both to a normal variant and to a pathological deviation; 2 that it could only exist in a pathological state; 3 that it represents an extreme degree of pathology (Åsberg et al 1978; Perris 1979). It has been used *inter alia* for development of subscales, designed to measure depressive, schizophrenic, obsessive-compulsive, and neurasthenic syndromes.

5.2.3 Psychiatric rating scales applicable to particular syndromes

As a rule, studies of the effect of a form of psychiatric treatment are restricted to one particular syndrome. To use a scale that includes, in addition to the relevant, a number of irrelevant signs and symptoms, will make the rating procedure unnecessarily time-consuming and — still worse — increase error variance and thus decrease reliability. For that reason a number of rating scales have been designed to measure the severity of particular syndromes and their change during treatment. A few examples will be described.

5.2.3.1 Depression scales

Several scales have turned out to be useful in studies of the effects of antidepressive drugs and of ECT. The internationally most well known depression scale is the Hamilton scale (Hamilton 1967) that has been used in a great number of studies on therapeutic outcome after antidepressive treatment. Another scale was designed by Cronholm & Ottosson (1960) and has been applied in several Scandinavian studies, for example by d'Elia (1970). A depression scale, specially designed to be sensitive to change, with as starting point the CPRS (see above), was recently published by Montgomery & Åsberg (1979).

The method of developing this scale is of general interest. In the study, 106 patients, all suffering from 'primary depressive illness', were rated with the whole of CPRS before and after treatment with various antidepressant drugs. The sum of scores in the 17 most common items (above zero in 70 per cent of the sample) was used as a preliminary estimate of the severity of illness. (This procedure does not guarantee that these signs or symptoms, such as 'inner tension', 'worrying over trifles', and 'reduced sleep' are common only in depression and not also in many other psychiatric disorders. However, this is of no importance when the aim of rating is not diagnostic but just measurement of severity. On the other hand, some 'typical' symptoms such as diurnal variation must not be used as it is evident that their relation to the general severity of illness is not monotonic.) To get an estimate of their sensitivity, the mean changes of scores in the 17 items after four weeks of treatment were calculated and ranked. Another estimate of sensitivity was the correlation between the change in each separate item and the overall change on the preliminary 17-item scale. These estimates reflect different aspects of sensitivity to change during treatment, and for that reason the summed ranks on both estimates was used to select 10 items for the final depression scale.

The 10-item scale proved to be valid for pharmacological treatment effects as estimated by computing the point-biserial correlation (0.70) between the sum of change scores and a clinical division in groups of responders and non-responders.

Schildkraut has designed a rating scale to be used by nurses. It is very useful because of the careful and detailed description of the signs and symptoms to be rated.

Among many clinicians there seems to be a somewhat unrealistic belief in the 'truth' of self-ratings. They have an apparent 'face validity' — it may seem evident that you are better able to describe yourself than other people are. However, this is highly questionable — there are at least as many difficulties in observation of yourself as in observation of others; prejudices and biases may be even more important. But self-rating certainly may be complementary to expert rating — different aspects may be observed and the sources of error different. Two self-rating depression scales have become rather popular, the Beck depression inventory (Beck *et al* 1961; Beck & Beamesderfer 1974), and the Zung scale (Zung 1965, 1974).

5.2.3.2 Schizophrenic syndromes

Only a few scales have been designed particularly to measure the severity of schizophrenic syndromes, and it seems far more difficult to design a useful rating scale for schizophrenic than for depressive syndromes. The symptomatology is much more variable between patients; and even in the same patient, many symptoms are elusive and difficult to observe and to record, and do not seem to have any simple, linear and monotonic relation to an underlying disease process.

The so-called S-scale was designed by Mårtens (1966) with the specific purpose of measuring possible improvement in schizophrenic patients treated with ceruloplasmin. The scale comprises 23 items, measuring severity of symptoms belonging to a schizophrenic syndrome. Two items are bipolar with 9 steps, the others are unipolar with 5 steps (from absence to high degree of a sign or a symptom). The separate items have a good inter-rater reliability as shown by Andersen *et al* (1974).

Scales based on items drawn from the CPRS and designed to measure various aspects of 'psychotic morbidity' have been used by Sedvall and his co-workers in studies of drug effects (Bjerkenstedt *et al* 1978; Wode-Helgodt *et al* 1978).

5.2.3.3 Anxiety

'Anxiety' is one of the most important but also most equivocal terms of psychiatry, and it may be used with rather varying meanings. From a phenomenological point of view, the core manifestations of anxiety are feelings introspectively characterized as uneasiness, distress, tenseness, nervousness, anguish, apprehension, panic or fright. It differs from 'fear' in its lack of clear, cognitive clues as to the source, and no interpretation is readily available. There are also physiological manifestations such as pallor, sweating and changes in pulse rate, and behavioural concomitants such as muscular tension, tremor and stereotype movements.

Basically, anxiety refers to a temporary, emotional state. In English, however, the term anxiety is also often used to denote habitual anxiousness or anxiety-proneness, i.e. the trait of anxiety. This has led to some confusion such as the use of the Taylor Manifest Anxiety Scale (MAS) — clearly an instrument for measuring trait anxiety — in studies of changes in state anxiety.

Several models of the genesis of anxiety assume an association with physiological 'over-arousal'. However, such a model is certainly an oversimplification and it has had to be modified and made more complicated. Without going into too much detail, an important distinction is that between 'autonomic' and 'cortical' arousal — the latter connected with the ascending reticular activating system, the former with the limbic system. A distinction has also been made between 'psychic' and 'somatic' anxiety, the latter assumed mainly to be related to 'autonomic' and the former also to 'cortical' arousal. 'Psychic' anxiety is characterized *inter alia* by anticipatory worrying, apprehension and rumination, whereas vague uneasiness and distress, feelings of inner tension, and panic attacks dominate in 'somatic' anxiety. (It should be pointed out that the terms 'psychic' and 'somatic' anxiety will be misleading if taken too literally.) This description of two main components of state anxiety has been made on the basis of factor analysis of results from clinical studies of ratings (Hamilton 1959, 1969; Buss 1962; de Bonis 1974).

The Buss anxiety rating scale (Buss *et al* 1955; Buss 1962) may be used to measure the degree of anxiety and its two components in the evaluation of psychiatric treatment aimed at a reduced anxiety level. Further studies indicate that it may be essential to separate a third component, 'muscular tension', from 'psychic anxiety' (Schalling *et al* 1975). Another instrument that may be useful for the same purpose is a set of items drawn from the CPRS.

5.2.3.4 'Guessing'

A particular way of rating, quite close to the common, clinical way of global assessment of improvement during treatment, may be called 'guessing'. It has been used in double-blind cross-over designs with a drug and placebo. An observer sees the patients during both periods — drug and placebo — and guesses which period was the one with the active substance. He need not report, and does not know perhaps, what clues he has used. If there is more than one observer, they may make correct guesses significantly more often than by chance, indicating some validity of the procedure. It is of interest that this may hold true even if the inter-rater reliability is rather low, indicating that the two observers have used different, but relevant clues (Mindus *et al* 1976; see section 6).

5.2.3.5 Rating of dominant symptoms

In some disorders, especially in schizophrenic and neurotic syndromes, one or more symptoms, not included in a general rating scale, are the dominant ones. In such cases they should be rated separately, in addition to a rating of psychopathology in general. There are of course many ways to do this. One way is to ask the patient — every day or every week — to mark the position of a dominant symptom on an analogue scale, e.g. on a 20 cm line ranging from 'none' to 'extremely severe'. The score of severity will be the distance in mm from 'none'. From these measures a curve may be designed, illustrating changes over time.

5.2.3.6 Hostility

Foulds (1965) described the development of a psychometric test to measure hostility or punitiveness in normal and psychiatrically ill populations. He described his concept of hostility as being an entity directed inward on the self or outward against other people or objects, and denoted this by the terms intropunitiveness and extrapunitiveness.

Hostility is a more pervasive and disabling category of emotional problem than many others and is very suitable for correlation with treatment factors (cf Daly 1969, 1970).

5.3 Psychological methods

5.3.1 Measurement of mental performance

Mental performance may be measured in order to study possible beneficial effects of treatment in patients where a lowering has been diagnosed or seems possible. In these cases, the lowering will most often be connected with a chronic, organic syndrome, due for example to a traumatic injury, to a more or less pronounced normal or pathological aging process or to some other degenerative disorder. Possible lowering of mental performance due to side effects may also be measured — e.g. in pharmacological treatment, ECT or psychosurgery. Measurements should preferably be made at least twice, before and after treatment. For this reason, parallel methods and methods with training effects that are negligible or reach an optimum after a short training period, are as a rule most useful. It is also important that the methods are adapted for use on patients — simply to take over methods designed for experiments on healthy students will as a rule lead to embarrassing disappointments.

5.3.1.1 Psychometric 'paper and pencil' tests

Most psychometric tests are designed to be diagnostic. This holds true both for 'intelligence tests' and so-called 'brain injury tests'. However, some of them may also be used to study change over time, be it improvement or decline.

Perceptual and perceptuo-motor tests may be very sensitive to various noxious influences on the brain. Many tests of this type have been designed and a few examples will be described. These tests, like some others, may be said to measure various aspects of mental efficiency. When they are called tests of more explicitly defined mental functions, this is as a rule an oversimplification and in some cases it may even be misleading. They are useful in studies of lowering of the level of consciousness due to the administration of drugs, whether this is an effect aimed at or an undesired side effect. They may also be used to study improvement in mental efficiency as a result of treatment with stimulating, 'nootropic' or other drugs in organic brain syndromes.

5.3.1.1.1 Cancellation tests

These tests are often called tests of 'attention', a rather wide concept. Typical examples are various forms of the Bourdon test where the task is, within a given time limit, to find and cross out one letter in a text that may be meaningless or meaningful (more difficult). The test may also be made more difficult by means of other modifications. One modification is the Bourdon-Wiersma test where dots are substituted for letters. These tests may be produced in an unlimited number of parallel versions.

5.3.1.1.2 The Digit Symbol Test

The Digit Symbol Test is a so-called code-learning test and a good example of those visuo-motor tests where speed is of great importance (Wechsler 1958). Typically, digits from 1 to 9 are paired with simple symbols. The task is, within a given time limit (e.g. 90 seconds), to write as many correct symbols as possible under a series of digits on a sheet of paper. A number of parallel versions have been designed. Several other tests have similar purposes, e.g. the Spoke Test (Reitan 1957).

5.3.1.1.3 The Benton Visual Retention Test

This test is an example of visual-constructive tests where the task is to reproduce geometric figures, most often from memory. It consists of 10 cards with drawings of one or more simple geometric figures. The task is to reproduce the drawings on each card from memory after an inspection period of 10 seconds. There are three parallel versions. Performance in these tests is lowered in various chronic organic syndromes. This sensitivity seems to be due to the fact that they require a great number of different functions to be intact: perception or apperception (gnosia), short-term memory, and motor abilities (praxia) (Benton 1955, 1962).

5.3.1.1.4 Memory tests

'Memory' is a broad and rather vague concept, and 'bad memory' is often used as a euphemism for general, cognitive decline, e.g. with aging ('Tout le monde se plaint de sa mémoire et personne ne se plaint de son jugement' — de la Rochefoucauld). Many 'memory' tests do also to a large extent measure the same mental abilities as the common, so-called intelligence tests. This holds true for, for example, the Wechsler Memory Scale (Wechsler 1945).

To elucidate some problems it may be useful or even necessary to get estimates both of short-term memory and retention over a longer period. For example, directly after presentation of material to be remembered, an 'immediate memory score' may be recorded and considered an estimate of 'registration'. If a 'delayed memory' is also recorded a few hours later, the difference between these two scores may be termed 'forgetting', the opposite of 'retention'. Such a test has been used to study the most important side-effect after ECT, the memory dysfunction (Cronholm 1969). Ottosson (1960) was able to show that impairment of 'retention' became more pronounced with supra-optimal electrical stimulation and d'Elia (1970) that it was less pronounced with unilateral instead of bilateral application of the electrodes.

5.3.1.2 Neuropsychological apparatus tests

Under this heading some tests will be described that measure mental efficiency but — in contrast to the 'paper-and-pencil tests' described above — demand rather complicated equipment.

A classical test of mental efficiency is measurement of Reaction Time — e.g. the time between presentation of a visual stimulus and pressing a button. Various modifications — more or less complicated choices between reactions to different stimuli — have been used in a great number of studies. Another classical test is measurement of the Critical Flicker Fusion Frequency (CFFF). The frequency of a flickering light has to be slower for the flicker to be perceived when mental efficiency is lowered for some reason. These tests may be considered routine methods in psychopharmacological studies. Another useful test, less well known among psychiatrists and pharmacologists, is the Krakau Visual Acuity Test (KVAT), originally designed by an ophthalmologist (Krakau 1967). Successive stimuli consisting of a line with either a small upward or downward deflection in the middle are shown on an oscilloscope screen. The patient is seated at a distance of four metres from the oscilloscope and the task is to respond by pressing one of two buttons, 'up' or 'down'. The direction of the deflection is varied at random, but the amplitude depends on previous reactions — increase after one incorrect, and decrease after three correct answers. The smaller the mean amplitude that is correctly recognized, the better the performance.

In all three tests there is a considerable variation between individuals and for that reason they are most useful in intra-individual studies. The tests have become far more useful since a computer has been used to give stimuli, record the responses and deliver a numerical value of the performance level (Levander & Lagergren 1973; Lagergren & Levander 1974, 1975; Mindus et al 1976).

5.4 Psychophysiological measures

Anxiety states and reactions are not only subjective phenomena but also imply various physiological and behaviour changes (see section 5.2.3.3).

There is a great number of studies of various parameters of the *'Galvanic Skin Resistance'* (GSR), such as spontaneous fluctuations and amplitude of reactions to various stimuli, such as pain stimuli or loud white noise. The parameters are related to various aspects of personality and of anxiety. The GSR may also be influenced by sedative and anxiolytic drugs, and has been used in a great number of studies of their effects (Lader & Wing 1966). Other physiological parameters related to anxiety are, e.g. heart rate, pulse volume, blood pressure, respiratory rate, and muscular tension as measured by means of electromyography. Psychophysiological measures may be useful in the evaluation of psychiatric treatment. However, their interrelations and their relations to various personality variables are very complicated, and interpretation of the results may be difficult. To get reliable measures, rather complicated equipment is necessary.

5.5 Projective tests

All normal and many pathological perceptions may be understood as the result of a central nervous integration and interpretation of afferent impulses, resulting from stimulation of sense organs in the periphery. However, the relative roles of the afferent impulse stream elicited by some object or event and the central interpretation may differ greatly. This is most easily described in psychological terms. As a rule we take it for granted that there is a good correspondence between our perceptions and the objects or events around us that have activated our sense organs. (We leave aside epistemological problems, not necessary for the present discussion.) However, sometimes we make 'mistakes' — our expectancies or fears have been strong enough to model our perception into a form which corresponds only badly or not at all to objective reality. In psychiatry this will be called an 'illusion'. One way of describing that same process is to say that owing to an unusually strong emotional loading, particular expectancies have been 'projected' on to the field of perceptions. Even when the emotional loading is not very pronounced, a similar interpretative activity may take place when the external stimulus is very poor or only loosely organized. As a commonplace example we may perceive faces, horses and other animals when looking at the clouds with a relaxed, non-critical attitude. And in the dark, a young girl may easily mistake an innocent juniper bush for a threatening, unknown man.

The perceptions of loosely organized visual stimuli have been utilized in some, so-called projective tests or methods. The idea is that different individuals will perceive highly ambiguous pictures in different ways. It is assumed and is supported by empirical findings that these different interpretations of the material will be highly idiosyncratic, reflecting particular personality traits, abilities, attitudes, inner conflicts, etc. As a rule, the subject is innocently unconscious about the mental processes that he will reveal in this way.

The most used and perhaps also most typical among all projective methods is the Rorschach test. It was designed as early as 1921 by a Swiss psychiatrist, Herman Rorschach, and the same test material is still being used. It is rather simple, consisting of ten tables, representing symmetrical ink-blots, six of them black and grey, four with some colours also. As a rule the test has been used for diagnostic purposes, most often applying a psychodynamic frame of reference. Formal traits of the perception such as seeing the whole or details, seeing movements, the use of form, colour and shades, play a great role in the psychological analysis of the subject's reports. The content of the perceptions — men, animals, anatomical details, more or less overt sexual symbols, etc. — is also considered. In the practical, diagnostic work, the analysis results in a free description of various personality traits, psychological mechanisms, etc. An enormous literature has grown up around these ten ink-blots. Attempts to substitute new and 'better' tables for the old ones have so far failed, and there is no really good parallel version. The Rorschach test may also be useful in the evaluation of psychiatric treatment. The examiner's report has to be strictly formalized. Rating of particular traits, attitudes or symptoms, etc., should then be based on a global evaluation of the qualities of the perceptions reported by the patient and on his behaviour during the test session. The rating system should, of course, also be strictly formalized. In many respects, it will be similar to that resulting from a clinical rating, based on an interview with a patient (see section 5.1). In some situations, it is preferable that this rating should be performed by a psychologist other than the examiner; it may thus be made blindly with respect especially to the position before or after treatment.

Another projective method is the Thematic Apperception Test (TAT), first described by Morgan and Murray in 1935. It consists of a series of pictures in black, figurative but with an ambiguous content. They are emotionally provocative but numerous and highly different interpretations will be possible. Attitudes to parents, friends, sex partners, etc., may be more or less unconsciously revealed and interpreted by the examiner. Both of these tests may be used in studying differences before and after a period of psychiatric treatment. A drawback is the lack of useful, parallel methods, and also the fact that both of them are fairly difficult to handle and require considerable training and experience. They are specialist methods for qualified psychologists and are useful when such experts are available.

5.6 Biochemical methods

During the last few decades there has been a rapid development of methods for measurement of minimal amounts of various important organic substances — mass fragmentography, radioimmunoassay (RIA), high pressure liquid chromatography (HPLC), etc. These methods have enabled studies of biochemical reactions during psychiatric treatment. Such studies are possible not only in animal experimentation but also in man. They are not restricted to pharmacological treatment, even if most studies have been made in that connection.

A few examples will be mentioned. It is now well established that one common effect of antipsychotic drugs such as the phenothiazines or butyrophenones is a blocking of dopamine receptors, resulting in an increase of the main metabolite of that transmitter, homovanillic acid (HVA) in the cerebrospinal fluid (CSF). The increase is most probably due to a feedback mechanism. It has also been possible to demonstrate that there is a relation between the plasma level of active substance(s) in the blood plasma and/or in the CSF, and the therapeutic effect on psychotic symptoms. As dopaminergic neurons in the hypothalamus inhibit prolactin secretion, increase of prolactin in plasma indicates the biological activity of drugs, blocking the inhibiting neurons. The rise of prolactin level in plasma is related to therapeutic effects.

It has also been shown that those tricyclic antidepressant drugs that inhibit reuptake of norepinephrine in presynaptic neurons will markedly lower the level of its main metabolite (hydroxymethoxyphenyl glycol, HMPG) in the CSF, whereas those which inhibit reuptake of serotonin will markedly lower the level of its main metabolite (5-hydroxyindol acetic acid, 5-HIAA). As with the effect of antipsychotic drugs on HVA, these effects are probably due to feedback mechanisms, working in the opposite direction.

It is now well known that there is a relation between the plasma level of antidepressant drugs and their therapeutic effect. Most interesting is perhaps the discovery that with some drugs such as nortriptyline, the relation is not linear and monotonic but the effect is optimal at a medium level; there is a 'therapeutic window' (Åsberg *et al* 1971; Cronholm 1979).

The development in the field briefly mentioned here is very rapid. References will soon be out of date, but for comprehensive reviews see Mendels (1975) and van Praag (1977).

The recent discovery of peptide transmitters in the CNS — especially the endorphins — has opened new areas of research on the mechanisms of action of various forms of psychiatric treatment. An interesting observation is, for example, that amelioration of pain induced by a placebo will be inhibited by naloxon, an opiate antagonist.

6. Design and statistical problems

The design of research projects aimed at the evaluation of psychiatric treatment does not differ in principle from the design of projects within other fields of science. The ideal is an experimental design isolating and studying one or a few factors at a time. However, compromises will be necessary for practical or ethical reasons just as in other fields of medicine. A few problems of particular relevance in the present context will be briefly discussed.

The starting point for the evaluation of psychiatric treatment has to be some sort of estimation of a difference in relevant variables before and after a treatment period. This requires that the measurements of these variables should be reliable and valid. Reliability may be defined in different logical or operational ways. Guilford (1950) gives a very precise definition: "The reliability of any set of measurements is logically defined as the proportion of their variance that is *true* variance". The remaining part is *error* variance. This proportion, the so-called reliability coefficient, may vary from 0 to 1. A simpler and less technical definition was given by Ekman (1952). He defines the reliability of an instrument as its preciseness in measuring that which it does in fact measure. There are several ways of estimating reliability, giving somewhat different information about the proportion of 'true' variance. For psychometric tests, split-half reliability is often used. This means the correlation between two halves of a test, corrected for its length. Retest reliability means the correlation between the results of the same or parallel tests at different sessions. The reliability of rating scales is most often estimated as the inter-rater reliability, i.e. the correlation between the ratings performed by two or more raters, of the same patients and at the same sessions.

Validity was defined by Ekman (1952) as the precision of a method in measuring that which it was meant to measure. There are several kinds of validity, estimated as validity coefficients by the use of different criteria. For example, the predictive validity of an 'intelligence' test may be given as the correlation between IQ and College success, its concurrent validity as the correlation with another intelligence test. 'Construct validity' is an interesting concept but much more difficult to define. Logically, it should mean the correlation between a series of measurements with a definite method, and a hypothetical, not directly observable variable. As this is, of course, impossible to estimate directly, other ways have to be used. One example is a method delineated by Campbell & Fiske (1959) in an article with the informative title 'Convergent and discriminative validation by the multitrait-multimethod matrix'. This means that a number of methods are used to measure at least two hypothetical variables. The validation consists in examining whether there are high positive correlations between those measurements assumed to be estimates of the same hypothetical variable, but low (or even negative) between those assumed to be estimates of different variables. This method has been used in several studies, *inter alia* to test the construct validity of memory test measures, some of them according to the hypothesis estimating 'registration', others 'retention'. Generally, the findings were in line with the assumed 'construct validity' of the test measures (Cronholm & Ottosson 1963).

The measures used in psychiatric research can often not be considered as ratio scales or even as interval scales but just as ordinal scales. In addition, their distribution is sometimes very uneven. This raises problems concerning which types of statistics may be used. There has for these reasons been much discussion whether parametric statistics may be used on ratings — they typically will form ordinal scales. However, means, t-tests, and parametric correlation are nevertheless often used; and in spite of theoretical criticism that can be raised against such procedures, they have proved to be useful from a pragmatic point of view. But in some situations non-parametric methods will certainly be preferable. It is wise to consult a statistician on concrete problems — but he has to be interested in the application of stochastic models to empirical data and not only in these models as abstract, mathematical constructs.

Data registered before and after treatment in a series of patients are as a rule highly correlated. For that reason, a test on possible significance may be best applied on a series of intra-individual differences, and not on the difference between means of measures before and after treatment. It is true that the degrees of freedom will be fewer, but the variance will be so much smaller that the efficiency of the test will be higher.

Group comparisons between two types of treatment may raise special problems. A usual design is to compare the effects in one group treated with a well-known and effective method, with the effects in another group treated with a new method. If a significant difference in effects does appear and the groups are comparable in other respects, it will be a reasonable conclusion that one method is better than the other. If there is no difference, this may of course be due to the possibility that the new method is just as effective as the old one. However, this conclusion is too often uncritically drawn. There may be a real difference, not appearing because the methods used have not been reliable or valid enough or the groups have been too small. Finally, the patients may have been selected in a way that introduced too much error variance — too many of them may have been either placebo responders or non-responders. Especially when it is important to settle the possible efficiency of a particular method and to expose as few patients as possible to any risk, a sequential analysis may be the best way. An example is the crucial experiment performed by Baastrup *et al* (1970), that demonstrated the prophylactic effect of lithium in manic-depressive and recurrent depressive disorders. They paired off patients on prophylactic lithium with respect to relevant variables and substituted placebo for lithium in one of the 'artificial twin' pairs. It was soon found that the placebo 'twins' relapsed before those on lithium. As a matter of fact, this held true within *all* pairs where one 'twin' relapsed before the level of significance had been arrived at. This experimental design minimized the number of patients exposed to the risk of a relapse, at the same time giving a conclusive answer.

In chronic disorders with slow or negligible changes over time, double-blind cross-over designs will often be most rewarding as intra-individual comparisons will be possible. An example is a study on the treatment of cognitive decline with aging (Mindus *et al* 1976).

When one form of treatment is given for a long time, and another treatment is tried in addition, a so-called single case study will be adequate. In one patient, some signs or symptoms are measured regularly. The treatment to be tried is given during some periods, but not during others. A regression line is then designed on the basis of all positions in the variables studied. If the positions during periods of treatment with the method to be tried significantly deviate from the regression line, this indicates that the treatment has been effective.

In all studies of the therapeutic efficacy of a method, it is desirable to use several measurements, all of them as valid as possible but with as low inter-correlations as possible. It is common that the last desideratum is difficult to realize, and then we have to be satisfied with a few methods; further additions will make only marginal increases in discriminative ability of the battery of methods.

7. Cost-benefit analysis

Cost-benefit analyses of psychiatric methods of treatment are far from simple, and for that reason they are too often neglected. However, the necessity of a realistic evaluation of the efficiency of different methods of treatment, not only in relation to each other but also in relation to their relative costs, is increasingly being realized. This holds true not only for developing but also for industrial countries. In the latter, the costs of medical care now have reached a level where no further increase may be tolerated. In a cost-benefit analysis of various methods of psychiatric treatment, a great number of factors have to be considered. It is difficult enough to evaluate direct and indirect costs of psychiatric disorders to the individual and to society and to relate them to possible gains from psychiatric treatment. First of all, these gains have to be weighed against the direct costs of medical care, plus the economic loss involved in the reduced working capacity of the patient and possibly also of other members of the family, etc. A realistic evaluation of the merely economic losses due to psychiatric disorders and possible gains due to treatment thus meets with great difficulties and experts of economic sciences have to be involved. However, non-economic values also have to be considered, and weighed against economic gains and losses. This holds true especially for the value of relieving suffering, and of improving living conditions for psychiatric patients, not least the chronic ones.

It is quite evident that effective treatment of severe mental disorders such as schizophrenia and manic-depressive disorder will lead to considerable economic gains and also have very high humanitarian value. Fairly high treatment costs will thus pay off both economically and in other ways. All the same, empirical studies may be needed. If two methods turn out to be just as effective but their costs differ considerably, the less expensive one should, of course, be preferred.

Cost-benefit analyses of psychotherapy meet with special difficulties. It may be held that the ratio between costs and benefits is unreasonably high when psychoanalysis for one or more years just aims at maturation and emancipation of the client's personality. However, the advantages of various forms of psychotherapy are easily under-estimated, and have to be empirically studied. This holds true especially for the treatment of neurotic disorders with more or less evident and disturbing symptoms. Adequate treatment may result in improved social adaptation, increase of working capacity and productivity. Home conditions may also improve, and mental deviation and even drug abuse and criminality in children may be prevented. Both such possible gains and the possibility of preventing psychosomatic disorders should be further studied and the gains of psychotherapy weighed against its costs. It should in this context be pointed out that psychotherapy is by no means always either very time-consuming or very expensive. Classical psychoanalysis will never become a method of widespread use; at present its main value seems to be as part of the training of psychotherapists. Crisis intervention and various forms of short-term psychotherapy applying a psychodynamic frame of reference, and possibly some forms of behaviour therapy, will probably be the methods of most practical importance in the future. A cost-benefit analysis within these fields will for that reason seem most rewarding. One way of measuring the effect of psychotherapeutic intervention is by studying the utilization of other medical services. Follett & Cummings (1967) in San Francisco found a considerable reduction of utilization in a group of psychiatric patients and in a group of high medical utilizers when studied for one year before and five years after psychotherapeutic intervention. The psychotherapy was not very time-consuming. One visit alone produced a 60 per cent reduction in utilization, while 2-8 visits produced a

75 per cent reduction. Goldberg *et al* (1970) in Washington, DC, found a 30 per cent reduction in utilization of medical services following psychotherapy. Jameson *et al* (1978) in Western Pennsylvania looked at monthly costs of medical services per patient, and by using psychotherapy reduced these by $9.41, from $16.47 to $7.06. In West Germany, Duehrssen & Jorswieck (1975) in a five-year study of 1000 consecutive psychoanalytic patients found a reduction of their average medical hospitalization from 5.3 hospital days per year to 0.78 days after psychotherapy (the general average for the population was 2.5 hospital days per year).

8. Summary and discussion

The survey has illustrated the existence of a number of research methods useful in the evaluation of various ways of treating psychiatric disorders. However, it is also evident that many methodological problems remain to be solved. A practical problem of great importance is the difficulty in finding a group of patients large enough for a particular project at one research centre and within a reasonable time. This leads to the need to organize multicentre studies which implies a number of further problems. Multicentre studies require uniformity and unanimity in a number of respects. First of all, a uniform terminology has to be used for communication between research centres, for comparison of their results and for combination of the materials. This is much more difficult than it may seem — difficult enough within the same country but, of course, still more so between centres in different countries with different traditions and literally different languages. Description of symptoms and classification of disorders may fairly easily be made to appear uniform. However, closer analysis may reveal that similar terms denote rather different concepts in different centres, and 'synonyms' in different languages differ in more or less important respects. For these reasons, before the start of a multicentre study, especially one planned to take place in several countries, terminology has to be carefully analysed and all terms as far as possible defined operationally.

Psychiatric examination and evaluation has to a very large extent to be formalized in rating scales. Synonymous descriptions of the signs and symptoms are necessary for a uniform rating in different countries. Translation of a rating scale is no easy task, and cross-linguistic inter-rater reliability studies have to be made before two versions of the same scale in two languages are considered parallel. Psychological tests quite often are based on verbal material or at least on verbal instructions. Translation thus meets with similar difficulties as the translation of rating scales. Of course, the examination of patients with non-verbal tests, and with neuropsychological or psychophysiological methods, has to be performed in identical ways at different centres. Even if a great number of methods for the evaluation of psychiatric treatment are already available, further improvements and innovations will be needed. Examples are the need for methods of rating for various aspects of psychosocial adaptation, and further development of methods for the measurement of biochemical variables which affect therapeutic outcome.

A problem is the heterogeneity of models used for describing and understanding mental disorders (medical, psychodynamic, learning models, etc.). These models often imply different attitudes to the choice of therapeutic methods, and also different formulations of therapeutic aims. (For a comprehensive review of models of mental disorders, see Siegler & Osmond 1974.) There will be great difficulties in finding common denominators for the aims of treating, for instance, a phobic or obsessive-compulsive syndrome with pharmacological methods, behaviour therapy, or with individual or group psychotherapy on the basis of psychodynamic theories. However, some such denominators have to be agreed on to allow any comparison between these different methods of treatment.

A number of difficulties have been listed above. This was not meant to give a pessimistic impression of the field. On the contrary, progress has been rapid and remaining methodological difficulties certainly can be largely overcome.

9. Conclusions

Many methods have been designed with the purpose of measuring psychological, physiological and also biochemical changes as a result of psychiatric treatment. However, greater uniformity in the application of methods would facilitate both comparison and combination of results from different research centres. The same holds true for terminology and classification that are neither uniform nor consistent at different centres in the same country and still less so in different countries. There is also a need to improve existing methods by making them more communicable and more reliable and valid. Finally, new methods should be designed.

In order to facilitate and stimulate multicentre studies in research on problems of psychiatric treatment and to improve and develop methods in the field, a workshop would be very useful. Investigators from different centres with different attitudes should meet in order to discuss the possibility of reaching agreement about aims of treatment, classification and methodology in general. It is especially important to establish a common and uniform terminology. The possibility of attaining these goals in spite of different ideas about models of psychiatric disorders should be

an interesting and certainly also fruitful topic of the discussions.
Time is now ripe for introducing on a wider scale all the technology that is now available for measuring the efficacy of *all* methods of treatment in psychiatry.

References

American Psychiatric Association (1980): DSM III: *Diagnostic and Statistical Manual of Mental Disorders*, 3rd ed. American Psychiatric Association, Washington, DC.

Andersen, K., Malm, U., Perris, C., Rapp, W. & Román, G. (1974): The Inter-rater Reliability of Scales for Rating Symptoms and Side-effects in Schizophrenic Patients during a Drug Trial. In Perris, C. (ed.): A Multicenter Multidimensional Study of some new Longacting Neuroleptic Drugs. *Acta Psychiatr. Scand., Suppl. 249*, 38-64.

Angst, J., Battegay, R., Bente, D., Berner, P., Broeren, W., Cornu, F., Dick, P., Engelmeier, M.-P., Heimann, H., Heinrich, K., Helmchen, H., Hippius, H., Poeldinger, W., Schmidlin, P., Schmitt, W. & Weise, P. (1969): Das Dokumentationssystem der Arbeitsgemeinschaft für Methodik und Dokumentation in der Psychiatrie. *Arzneimittel — Forsch., 19*, 339-405.

Åsberg, M., Cronholm, B., Sjöquist, F. & Tuck, D. (1971): Relationship between Plasma Level and Therapeutic Effect of Nortriptyline. *Br. Med. J., 3*, 331-334.

Åsberg, M., Thorén, P., Träskman, L., Bertilsson, L. & Ringberger, V. (1976a): 'Serotonin Depression' — A Biochemical Subgroup within the Affective Disorders? *Science, 191*, 478-480.

Åsberg, M., Träskman, L. & Thorén, P. (1976b): 5-HIAA in the Cerebrospinal Fluid — A Biochemical Suicide Predictor? *Arch. Gen. Psychiatry, 33*, 1193-1197.

Åsberg, M., Montgomery, S.A., Perris, C., Schalling, D. & Sedvall, G. (1978): A Comprehensive Psychopathological Rating Scale. *Acta Psychiatr. Scand., Suppl. 271*, 5-27.

Åsberg, M. & Schalling, D. (1979): Construction of a New Psychiatric Rating Instrument, the Comprehensive Psychopathological Rating Scale (CPRS). Proceedings of the XIth CINP Congress, Vienna 1978. *Prog. Neuropsychopharmacol. 3*, 405-412.

Baastrup, P.C., Poulsen, J.C., Schou, M., Thomsen, K. & Amdisen, A. (1970): Prophylactic Lithium: Double Blind Discontinuation in Manic-Depressive and Recurrent-Depressive Disorders. *Lancet, II*, 326-330.

Beck, A.T., Ward, C.H., Mendelson, M., Mock, J.E. & Erbaugh, J.K. (1961): An Inventory for Measuring Depression. *Arch. Gen. Psychiatry, 4*, 561-571.

Beck, A.T. & Beamesderfer, A. (1974): Assessment of Depression: The Depression Inventory. In Pichot (1974), 151-169.

Benton, A.L. (1955): *The Revised Visual Retention Test: Clinical and Experimental Applications*. The State University of Iowa, Iowa City.

Benton, A.L. (1962): The Visual Retention Test as a Constructional Praxis Task. *Conf. Neurol., 22*, 141-155.

Bertilsson, L., Asberg, M. & Thorén, P. (1974): Differential Effect of Chlorimipramine and Nortriptyline on Cerebrospinal Fluid Metabolites of Serotonin and Noradrenaline in Depression. *Eur. J. Clin. Pharmacol., 7*, 365-368.

Bjerkenstedt, L., Härnryd, Ch., Grimm, V., Gullberg, B. & Sedvall, G. (1978): A Double-Blind Comparison of Melperone and Thiothixene in Psychotic Women using a New Rating Scale, the CPRS. *Arch. Psychiatr. Nervenkr., 226*, 157-172.

Bonis, M. de (1974): Content Analysis of 27 Anxiety Inventories and Rating Scales. In Pichot (1974), 221-237.

Buss, A., Weiner, M., Durkee, A. & Baer, M. (1955): The Measurement of Anxiety in Clinical Situation. *J. Consult. Clin. Psychol., 19*, 125-129.

Buss, A. (1962): Two Anxiety Factors in Psychiatric Patients. *J. Abnorm. Soc. Psychol.*, 65, 426-427.
Campbell, D.T. & Fiske, D.W. (1959): Convergent and Discriminant Validation by the Multitrait-Multimethod Matrix. *Psychol. Bull.*, 56, 81-105.
Cronholm, B. & Ottosson, J.-O. (1960): Experimental Studies of the Therapeutic Action of Electroconvulsive Therapy in Endogenous Depression. In Ottosson, J.-O. (ed.): Experimental Studies of the Mode of Action of Electroconvulsive Therapy. *Acta Psychiatr. Scand. Suppl.*, 145, 69-102.
Cronholm, B. & Ottosson, J.-O. (1963): Reliability and Validity of a Memory Test Battery. *Acta Psychiatr. Scand.*, 39, 218-234.
Cronholm, B. (1969): Post-ECT Amnesia. In Talland, G. & Waugh, N. (eds.): *The Pathology of Memory*. Academic Press, New York, 81-89.
Cronholm, B., Schalling, D. & Åsberg, M. (1974): Development of a Rating Scale for Depressive Illness. In Pichot (1974), 139-150.
Cronholm, B. (1979): Utilisation des antidépresseurs. Bases pharmaco-konétiques. *L'Encéphale, V*, 605-615.
Daly, R.J. (1969): Hostility and Chronic Intermittent Haemodialysis. *J. Psychosom. Res.*, 13, 165-173.
Daly, R.J. (1970): *Measurement of Emotional Factors in Patients Maintained on Haemodialysis*. M.D. Thesis, University of Dublin.
Donovan, J.W. (1977): Randomised Controlled Trial of Anti-smoking Advice in Pregnancy. *Br. J. Prev. Soc. Med.*, 31, 6-12.
Duehrssen, A. & Jorswieck, E. (1975): An Empirical-statistical Investigation into the Efficacy of Psychoanalytic Therapy. *Der Nervenarzt*, 36, 166-169.
Ekman, G. (1952): *Differentiell Psykologi*. Hugo Gebers förlag, Stockholm.
d'Elia, G. (ed.) (1970): Unilateral Electroconvulsive Therapy. *Acta Psychiatr. Scand., Suppl. 215*.
Endicott, J. & Spitzer, R.L. (1978): A Diagnostic Interview: The Schedule for Affective Disorders and Schizophrenia. *Arch. Gen. Psychiatry*, 35, 837-844
Essen-Möller, E. (1961): On Classification of Mental Disorders. *Acta Psychiatr. Scand.*, 37, 119-126.
Feighner, J.P., Robins, E., Guze, S.B., Woodruff, R.A., Winokur, G. & Munoz, R. (1972): Diagnostic Criteria for Use in Psychiatric Research. *Arch. Gen. Psychiatry*, 26, 57-63.
Follett, E.W. & Cummings, N.A. (1967): Psychiatric Services and Medical Utilisation in a Prepaid Health Plan Setting. *Med. Care*, 5, 25.
Foulds, G.A. (1965): *Personality and Personal Illness*. Tavistock, London.
Goldberg, I.D., Krantz, G. & Locke, B.Z. (1970): Effect of a Short-term Out-patient Psychiatric Therapy Benefit on the Utilisation of Medical Services in a Prepaid Group Practice Medical Programme. *Med. Care*, 8, 419.
Guilford, J.P. (1950): *Fundamental Statistics in Psychology and Education*, 2nd ed. McGraw-Hill Inc., New York.
Gurney, C., Roth, M., Garside, R.F., Kerr, T.A. & Schapira, K. (1972): Studies in the Classification of Affective Disorder. The Relationship between Anxiety States and Depressive Illnesses — II. *Br. J. Psychiatry*, 121, 162-166.
Hamilton, M. (1959): The Assessment of Anxiety by Ratings. *Br. J. Med. Psychol.*, 32, 50-55.
Hamilton, M. (1967): Development of a Rating Scale for Primary Depressive Illness. *Br. J. Soc. Clin. Psychol.*, 6, 278-296.
Hamilton, M. (1969): Diagnosis and Ratings of Anxiety. In Lader, M. (ed.): Studies of Anxiety. *Br. J. Psychiatry, Special Publication*, 3. Headley Brothers, Ashford, Kent.
Honigfeld, G. (1974): NOSIE-30: History and Current Status of its Use in Pharmacopsychiatric Research. In Pichot (1974), 238-263.

ICD (1980): *International Classification of Diseases 9th revision, Clinical Modification*, 2nd ed. (ICD-9-CM). Department of Education, Health and Welfare, Washington, DC.
Jameson, M.A., Shuman, L.J. & Young, W.W. (1978): The Effects of Out-patient Psychiatric Utilisation on the Costs of providing 3rd Party Coverage. *Med. Care, 16,* 383.
Jeste, D., Gillin, Ch. & Wyatt, R.J. (1979): Serendipity in Psychiatry — a Myth? *Arch. Gen. Psychiatry, 36,* 1173-1178.
Krakau, C. (1967): An Automatic Apparatus for Time Series Analysis of Visual Acuity. *Vision Res., 7,* 99-105.
Lader, M. & Wing, L. (1966): *Physiological Measures, Sedative Drugs, and Morbid Anxiety.* Oxford Univ. Press, London.
Lagergren, K. & Levander, S. (1974): A Double-Blind Study on the Effects of Piracetam upon Perceptual and Psychomotor Performance at Varied Heart Rates in Patients Treated with Artificial Pacemakers. *Psychopharmacology* (Berlin), *39,* 97-104.
Lagergren, K. & Levander, S. (1975): Effects of Changes in Heart Rate in Different Body Positions upon Critical Flicker Fusion Threshold and Reaction Time Performance in Patients with Artificial Pacemakers. *J. Psychiatr. Res., 12,* 257-264.
Levander, S. & Lagergren, K. (1973). Four Vigilance Indicators for Use with a Minicomputer. *Rep. Psychol. Lab., University Stockholm,* No. 381.
Mårtens, S. (1966): *Effects of Exogenous Human Ceruloplasmin in the Schizophrenic Syndrome,* Dissert., Stockholm.
Mendels, J. (1975): *Psychobiology of Depression.* Halsted Press, New York.
Mindus, P., Cronholm, B., Levander, S. & Schalling, D. (1976): Piracetam-induced Improvement of Mental Performance. A Controlled Study on Normally Aging Individuals. *Acta Psychiatr. Scand., 54,* 150-160.
Montgomery, S. & Åsberg, M. (1979): A New Depression Scale Designed to be Sensitive to Change. *Br. J. Psychiatry, 134,* 382-389.
Morgan, C.D. & Murray, H.A. (1935): A Method for Investigating Fantasies: The Thematic Apperception Test. *Arch. Neurol. Psych., 34,* 189-306.
Ottosson, J.-O. (1960): Experimental Studies of Memory Impairment after Electroconvulsive Therapy. In Ottosson, J.-O. (ed.): Experimental Studies of the Mode of Action of Electroconvulsive Therapy. *Acta Psychiatr. Scand., Suppl. 145,* 103-131.
Ottosson, J.-O. & Perris, C. (1973): Multidimensional Classification of Mental Disorders. *Psychol. Med., 3,* 238-243.
Overall, J.E. & Gorham, D.R. (1962): The Brief Psychiatric Rating Scale. *Psychol. Rep., 10,* 799-812.
Overall, J.E. (1974): The Brief Psychiatric Rating Scale in Psychopharmacology Research. In Pichot (1974), 67-78.
Perris, C. (1979): Reliability and Validity Studies of the CPRS. Proceedings of the XIth CINP Congress, Vienna 1978. *Prog. Neuropsychopharmacology, 3,* 4.
Pichot, P. (ed.) (1974): *Psychological Measurements in Psychopharmacology.* Karger, Basel.
Praag, H. van (1977): *Depression and Schizophrenia. A Contribution to their Chemical Pathologies.* Spectrum Publications Inc., New York.
Reitan, R.M. (1957): The Comparative Effects of Placebo, Ultram and Meprobamate on Psychological Test Performances. *Antibiot. Med., 4,* 158-164.
Schalling, D., Cronholm, B. & Åsberg, M. (1975): Components of State and Trait Anxiety as Related to Personality and Arousal. In Levi, L. (ed.): *Emotions — Their Parameters and Measurement.* Raven Press, New York, 603-617.
Scharfetter, Ch. (1974): AMP System. Report on a System of Psychiatric Documentation Used in some Continental Countries. In Pichot (1974), 64-66.
Siegler, M. & Osmond, H. (1974). *Models of Madness, Models of Medicine.* Macmillan Publishing Co. Inc., New York.

Spitzer, R.L., Endicott, J. & Robins, E. (1978): Research Diagnostic Criteria: Rationale and Reliability. *Arch. Gen. Psychiatry, 35,* 773-782.

Swazey, J.P. (1974): *Chlorpromazine in Psychiatry.* The MIT Press, Cambridge, Mass.

Träskman, L., Åsberg, M., Bertilsson, L., Cronholm, B., Mellström, B., Neckers, L.M., Thorén, P. & Tybring, G. (1979): Plasma Levels of Chlorimipramine and its Demethyl Metabolite during Treatment of Depression. Differential Biochemical and Clinical Effects of the Two Compounds. *Clin. Pharmacol. Ther., 26,* 600-610.

Wechsler, D. (1945): A Standardized Memory Scale for Clinical Use. *J. Psychol., 19,* 87-95.

Wechsler, D. (1958): *The Measurement and Appraisal of Adult Intelligence.* William and Wilkins, Baltimore.

Wode-Helgodt, B., Borg, S., Fyrö, B. & Sedvall, G. (1978): Clinical Effects and Drug Concentrations in Plasma and Cerebrospinal Fluid in Psychotic Patients Treated with Fixed Doses of Chlorpromazine. *Acta Psychiatr. Scand., 58,* 149-173.

Woggon, B. (1979): Comparison between CPRS and AMDP System. Proceedings of the XIth CINP Congress, Vienna 1978. *Prog. Neuropsychopharmacology, 3,* 4.

Zung, W. (1965): A Self-rating Depression Rating Scale. *Arch. Gen. Psychiatry, 12,* 63-70.

Zung, W. (1974): The Measurements of Affects: Depression and Anxiety. In Pichot (1974), 170-188.

The Aims of Psychiatric Treatment

SIR MARTIN ROTH

1. The scope and limitations of psychiatric treatment

It is as well to examine both the scope and limitations of psychiatric treatment at the outset. The precepts in the constitution of the World Health Organization implicitly define the scope and purposes of health care in the following terms. "Health is a state of complete physical, mental and social well-being, and not merely the absence of disease or infirmity." The 1958 definition of 'health' aspires even higher. "Health means more than freedom from disease, freedom from pain, freedom from untimely death. It means optimum physical, mental and social efficiency and well-being."

In the attempts that have been made to define positive mental health, concepts such as 'ego strength', 'autonomy', 'individuation', 'positive self attitudes', 'integration', 'self-actualization' and 'perception of reality' have been employed by different authors (Jahoda 1958). This implies that there is some state of mental strength and integrity that can render individuals invulnerable to all forms of mental disorder whether it be schizophrenia, alcoholism, sadomasochistic sexuality, manic-depressive illness, anorexia nervosa, obsessional neurosis or senile dementia. If such a psychic state existed or could be envisaged, it might be regarded as the obverse of mental illness. However, insofar as knowledge has been acquired about their genetical and environmental antecedents, mental disorders differ from each other with little or nothing common to them. There is no foreseeable advance in knowledge that could provide the basis for the prevention of all mental disorders, nor any optimal state of mental well-being that could be expected to define the ultimate goal and end-point of all psychiatric treatment. Aims have to be set in distinct, specific and limited terms for each kind of psychiatric disorder.

Although there have been significant advances in the treatment of a number of forms of psychiatric disorder and some success in the prevention of relapse in some forms of illness, this is far from complete and predictions regarding the degree of control likely to be achieved in an individual case are far from reliable. The most serious forms of psychiatric disorder are liable to recur, to leave residual deficits, to become chronic or to be characterized in all these ways despite the improved methods of treatment available. Aims have, therefore, to be set for care over relatively long periods of time.

The central aim in the treatment of psychiatric illness has to be the realistic and modest one of bringing psychopathology under control and employing such specific treatments as are available in restoring the individual to his pre-morbid state of adaptation. This main objective applies universally in respect of the main forms of mental suffering known in all societies and cultures. None of the major psychiatric illnesses have survival or adaptive value in any culture that has been described nor are they regarded in any of these settings as other than maladies to be relieved. The theory that the definition and diagnosis of mental disorder depends heavily upon the cultural context in which it is manifest is upheld only in respect of the threshold at which some disorders are socially recognized as such and the tolerance with which they are treated.

There would have to be some qualification in respect of 'personality disorder'. But extremely aggressive, hostile, paranoid, egotistical personalities are treated as abnormal even in societies where there are no psychiatrists to affix any label upon them. The predatory aggressor or killer of strangers is repudiated and punished in all societies although he will be studied and treated by such means as are available to psychiatric and behavioural science in the countries with well-developed mental health services.

This paper will attempt to review the main areas in which recent developments have improved the prospects of effective psychiatric treatment and have called for a revision of aims. An attempt will be made to find areas in which research might fill gaps in knowledge and make possible a sharpening of objectives in the management of those who suffer from mental disorder. In the final section an attempt is made to examine some of the conceptual and methodological problems that need to be resolved to pave the way for enquiries into improved methods of care. The review is confined to general psychiatry with only brief reference to the special issues within child and geriatric psychiatry.

2. Objectives in the treatment of depressive illness

The psychopharmacological revolution which began in the 1950s and the more rigorous investigations of the social and familial factors that influence treatment response and outcome, have greatly expanded the available means for promoting recovery from psychiatric illness. But they have, not unexpectedly, brought a number of problems in their wake and have compelled the modern psychiatrist to balance the risks against the advantages when defining his goals in the management of patients. In the case of 'endogenous', 'autonomous' or 'major depressive' illness, approximately three-quarters of the cases can be expected to respond to tricyclic compounds and a rather higher proportion to electroconvulsive therapy. But this is not the treatment of first choice except in psychotic and seriously suicidal patients. In 'neurotic' depression, the disorders of highest prevalence, particularly in the community but also in clinical practice, a lower success rate of about 50 per cent can be expected. A central aim of treatment must be to apply these treatments in appropriate cases at an early stage.

Some recent studies (Weissmann *et al* 1979) have shown that optimal results were achieved in the treatment of out-patient depressives when drug treatment was combined with psychotherapy. There is other evidence in favour of such an additive effect between the treatments (Friedman 1975). However, psychotherapy alone affects neither the intensity of symptoms nor the rate of relapse.

Maintenance treatment with drugs has been shown to be indubitably effective (Mindham *et al* 1973) in averting relapse into depression. Here dilemmas and conflicting aims present themselves. In younger patients side effects are rarely troublesome and maintenance treatment presents few problems. In older subjects there is a greater need to protect against the risk of suicide. As against this, the hazard of complications from the long-term administration of tricyclic compounds, in the form of glaucoma, hypotension, and cardiac dysrhythmias, has to be weighed. There is no perfect resolution of such problems and a decision has to be made on the individual features and circumstances in each case.

There is, however, a more general issue which arises from the wide dissemination of antidepressant substances. The overgenerous prescription of psychotropic drugs has contributed to the epidemic of parasuicide witnessed in most developed countries in the past 15 years. And the free availability of antidepressant compounds has increased the number of seriously harmful and fatal suicide attempts. A number of recent observations have made a compelling case for redefining the aims and methods of treatment in certain depressive states and those encountered in the community in particular. There is evidence that a high proportion of those identified in community surveys as suffering from 'depression' do not satisfy the criterion of 'caseness' (Wing *et al* 1978). The majority of these individuals suffer from a condition with a different natural history and there is other evidence to suggest that this is likely to be qualitatively distinct from 'depressive illness' in the sense in which this term is understood and applied by psychiatrists. Although initial symptoms may be conspicuous, they are of limited range and usually prove transient having run their course within weeks.

Recent evidence has made it clear that, in the commonest depressive states in young people in particular, psychotherapy may be an acceptable alternative to drug treatment (Weissmann *et al* 1979). These observations related to patients diagnosed as being ill. But they reinforce the view that simple psychotherapy may provide the most appropriate treatment of first choice in disorders that appear to be understandable responses to social adversity. While some help should never be denied, once an approach to a doctor has been made, one aim in the management of depression in particular is to avoid medicalizing everyday familial and social problems.

3. Social models of depression and their implications for defining goals in treatment

In defining objectives in treatment there is a wide consensus among psychiatrists that account has to be taken of a wide range of factors including disharmony in interpersonal relationships and any adverse social circumstances that may have helped to initiate illness or may serve to impede recovery. This applies particularly to cases of suspected neurosis and depressive illness which are intuitively felt to have some measure of kinship with everyday emotional experience. But a diagnosis of depressive illness is judged appropriate only when there is emotional change that is inexplicable in terms of antecedent events and adverse social circumstances, and when the duration, severity and range of symptoms and abnormal patterns of behaviour, and their imperviousness to changes in the environment, demand it. The concept of 'understandability' and the criteria applied to test it are, of course, subjective. But as recent studies have shown (Wing *et al* 1974, 1977), some of these features can be reliably measured and others have withstood the test of time.

If the depressive disorders admitted or referred to psychiatric hospitals could be shown to be wholly determined by social vicissitudes, the psychiatric concept of depressive and related forms of illness would have to undergo radical revision. This would apply also to the methods of treatment generally employed to promote recovery.

A sociological model of depressive illness has been developed by Brown and his colleagues (Brown *et al* 1973a, 1973b, Brown *et al* 1975, Brown &

Harris 1978) from observations carried out in a community sample of 458 women and 114 female psychiatric patients. Considerable importance was attached to the contribution made to causation by significant life events or difficulties that impinged upon the individual affected. In an attempt to estimate the magnitude of the causative effect, Brown and his colleagues (1973b) developed the concept of 'brought forward time'. This referred to the average period by which the spontaneous onset of depressive illness had been advanced by life events. Using a mathematical formula which they have developed to calculate this period, they estimate that on average life threatening events hasten the onset of the depressive illness by about two years. In another estimate, Brown & Harris (1978) conclude that life events had caused the illness of more than 50 per cent of their depressed patients.

The severity of the stress imposed by life events is assessed in terms of their 'contextual threat', which entails bringing them into relationship with the social setting, the marital and occupational status and the social vicissitudes of the individual. As Tennant *et al* (1981) have pointed out, this has the effect of magnifying the contribution of life events. It also ignores the association between the social conflict and the premorbid personality patterns of those who suffer from the commonest forms of depression. Those so afflicted are not merely the passive victims of social circumstance; they create social vicissitudes as well as 'life events' through their life-long attitudes and behaviour patterns.

Brown and his colleagues have repeatedly stated that the conditions they studied were similar in character and severity to those treated in hospital. Recent evidence throws some doubt upon this claim. Depressive states identified in the course of community surveys have been found on followup (Wing *et al* 1978) to have resolved within about six weeks, suggesting that they were transient responses to adversity rather than 'autonomous' illnesses. A recent investigation of 74 out-patients from Camberwell (Bebbington 1980) made it possible to compare the severity of their symptoms with those of the community cases. It was found that whereas 87.8 per cent of out-patient cases reached an index of definition level (Wing *et al* 1977) of 5 + and 33.8 per cent a level of 7 and over, the corresponding figures for the community cases in Camberwell were 9 per cent scored at a level of 5 + and only 0.9 per cent at 7 +. It would seem that the depressions of those ascertained in community samples are on the whole of a different order of severity from those of hospital out-patients. And psychiatrists do not claim to have treatments or solutions at their disposal for dealing with the tide of ordinary unhappiness to be found in every society.

Another group of causal agents judged by Brown and his colleagues to be distinct from life events were the 'vulnerability factors'. These comprised having three or more children under the age of 14 years at home, lack of employment outside the home, parental loss before the age of 11 years and lack of an intimate relationship with a spouse or consort. These factors were not judged capable of provoking illness by themselves but to increase the chances of developing depression, should a significant life event or difficulty impinge upon the individual concerned. The effect of vulnerability factors was thought to be exerted through a 'cognitive set' which undermined self-esteem and feelings of mastery. Hence when life events interacted with vulnerability factors they cause a recrudescence of the early experiences of abandonment, failure and rejection engendered by the loss of a parent. Here the model of Brown and his colleagues has some affinities with the concept of depression developed by psychoanalysts such as Bibring (1965).

Interactions along the lines described were an integral part of the theory. However, Tennant & Bebbington (1978) were unable to find any evidence for overall interaction between life events or provoking agents on the one hand and vulnerability factors on the other. This poses a question as to whether they can be regarded as independent causal agents essentially similar in character to the life events as Tennant & Bebbington (1978) suggest or whether the facts can be interpreted along different lines. Longstanding personality difficulties are often found among those with the commonest forms of depression ('the self-pitying constellation', 'hostile depression', 'hysterical dysphoria', 'chronic characterological depression'). Those endowed in this manner are liable to experience difficulties in establishing close relationships with spouses or consorts, to behave in importunate ways, to exaggerate the severity of threats and vicissitudes, and to lack the independence and assertiveness required for pursuing employment outside the home.

The fact that all forms of vulnerability prove to be highly correlated with membership of an underprivileged social status completes the chain of causal agents that leads Brown and his colleagues to conceive of depressive illness in sociological terms. However, if the features subsumed under 'vulnerability' result primarily from personality factors rather than social deprivation, the findings cannot be regarded as consistent with a model that allocates the greater part of the variance in respect of depressive illness to socio-political factors.

The enquiries of this group of workers have made a significant contribution to greater precision in thought and scientific enquiry relating to the social and environmental contributory causes of depressive illness. In the multifactorial models which provide the basis for the pragmatic decisions in the management of affective disorders in clinical practice, social and familial adversity have to receive attention along with other factors that may contribute in causation. But one central purpose of scientific investigation in the future must be to lay factual foundations for methods of management that direct efforts to social, biological, familial and other factors that are proportionate to their importance in the causation of illness.

If the model erected by Brown and his school were to prove essentially correct, psychiatrists would have to recast their concepts and revise their goals in the treatment of affective illnesses, the commonest forms of psychiatric disorder in both psychiatric and general practice. Further investigations in new populations are needed. But the recent critique and reappraisal of Brown's data suggests that alternative explanations to those he has advanced can account for the facts. It is possible that in respect of some vulnerability factors and some life events the direction of causation is in an opposite sense from that conceived by Brown. The social vicissitudes and the disorders of many of the depressions studied may to a considerable measure have stemmed from the life-long personality traits shaped in the formative years by genetical factors in interaction with environmental influences. Comparative studies of the prevalence of 'life events' and of 'vulnerability factors' in patients with affective disorder during periods of remission in control subjects should help resolve some of the outstanding problems in this field.

4. Objectives in the social and medical treatment of schizophrenic illness

It has been obvious for some decades that the rehabilitation of schizophrenic illness demands expert medical and pharmacological treatment as well as a systematically planned approach to the social and environmental aspects of the disorder, both in its acute and chronic stages. The polarization between medical and sociological approaches that was evident about 15 years ago has been replaced by a more balanced approach which seeks to accommodate all relevant dimensions of illness. This has been due in considerable measure to the work of social psychiatrists such as Wing and his colleagues. In their studies of the contribution of social environment to the course and outcome of schizophrenic illness they have included painstaking analyses of the effects of biological treatment and their interactions with familial and environmental influences. The situation remains in flux and the facts required for a balanced scientifically based perspective in the management of schizophrenic illness in all its phases are lacking. Here, too, further scientific exploration will be likely to pave the way not only for clearer goals and for more effective methods of treatment of schizophrenia but a sharper definition of the scope and limitation of psychiatric practice.

The value of neuroleptic drugs in the prevention of relapse is now firmly established. In a comprehensive review of 24 controlled studies, Davis (1976) demonstrated that the mean rate of relapse in patients treated with drugs was less than half that observed in control subjects. The rapidity with which drugs can be relied upon to bring about remission from symptoms within a relatively short time and the valuable contribution made by depot medication to deal with the problem of non-compliance in treatment has made it possible to discharge many patients after short periods of hospital stay.

As might have been expected, the benefits have not been achieved without cost. There is a hazard of developing lasting extrapyramidal complications such as tardive dyskinesia as a result of long-term medication with neuroleptic drugs. Increased receptor supersensitivity of dopaminergic neurones which underlies tardive dyskinesia is lasting and measures to avert it as often as possible should be among the objectives of treatment. But having regard to the benefits of depot medication in the prevention of relapse, the complications that may arise in some cases deserve only limited weight. The risks of treatment in the long term have to be accepted in patients with illnesses of early insidious onset, those with 'negative' features or a precarious premorbid social adjustment and others judged as being at high risk of relapse.

However, to establish every case of schizophrenic illness on neuroleptic medication for a period of years would be undesirable. The need for continuing with treatment has to be kept under constant review after six to twelve months. Unfortunately, there is no prognostic index of proven value to provide reliable guidance in deciding which patients should be maintained on treatment for months rather than years. To place excessive weight upon indices such as the presence of stressful live events before onset, strong affective colouring, good premorbid personality and the absence of autism and negative features would be misconceived. It has become clear that some of the most valuable results are achieved in 'schizoaffective' and related cases with a tendency for frequent relapse and in whom depot medication may prove of critical importance in promoting stable and effective social adaptation.

Specific goals must be set for the programme of rehabilitation that follows recovery from the acute illness and subsequent discharge from hospital. Deficits often remain after the disappearance of positive psychotic symptoms. A systematic attempt needs to be made to equip patients with the new skills required for coping with social and personal interactions so as to enable them to return to a role in society as close as possible to that occupied before illness.

Recent evidence regarding the interaction between the effects of drugs and of the familial environment has provided useful guidance regarding the planning of rehabilitation and after-care. The work of Vaughan & Leff (1976) has shown that among those who return to a familial environment in which there is a high level of expressed emotion (EE) with exposure for more than 35 hours per week, the rate of relapse in those not receiving maintenance neuroleptics is 92 per cent as against 53 per cent among those on drugs. In contrast, among those who live in families with low EE scores maintenance on drugs made little difference to relapse rates.

However, a two-year follow-up study of the original (Leff & Vaughan 1981) shows the situation in a different light. Among those in high EE environments the prophylactic effect of maintenance neuroleptics was no longer in evidence. In contrast, drugs exerted a highly significant effect in averting relapse among those in low EE environments. As the authors point out, one of the questions posed relates to the direction of causality. The possibility arises that the high EE environment was in part a reflection of the emotional stresses created within families by patients with refractory forms of illness. Forty-three per cent of the hospital sample of schizophrenics not living alone were in low EE environments. It may be that it is in those with a relatively neutral environment (due in some cases to the non-provoking effect of a remission of good quality) that neuroleptics achieve some of the best results in the long term. The problem is of great practical importance and further investigations are needed to tease out the many factors involved and the manner of their interaction.

There is urgent need for a reappraisal of the programme of de-institutionalization of psychiatric patients that has been in progress in many countries during the past twenty years. After short periods of care in a hospital for their acute illness, large numbers of schizophrenic patients with residual and chronic disabilities have been discharged into communities without adequate services or medical supervision to make their lives as tolerable, secure and productive as they were in the best-run psychiatric hospitals of the past. 'Community Care' has in many countries become no more than a pious hope, a rigid doctrine, an unrealistic policy without factual basis or all of these. Of the 60,000 people living in the streets of New York, approximately half have a previous history of serious mental illness and they live under conditions of misery and deprivation. The role of the psychiatric hospital in the future and its relationship to the community, hostel and day centres in respect of medical supervision and after-care is in urgent need of reappraisal, to make it possible for medical and social services to arrive at informed decisions regarding rehabilitation and long-term management of those with chronic schizophrenic illness.

5. Setting aims in the treatment of neuroses

The aims set in the management of neurotic disorders will vary according to the conceptual framework employed by the psychiatrist in question. Those who take their inspiration from behavioural methods of treatment will place the manifest symptoms at the focus of therapeutic concern, holding that the symptoms are the disease. There are organic psychiatrists who employ drugs alone and many abandon effort when these prove unhelpful. For the psychiatrist who draws his inspiration from the psychodynamic and psychoanalytic approaches, symptoms are symbolic defences against unconscious conflicts. The goals of treatment must be to lay bare their unconscious origins, their relationships to the storms and vicissitudes of the early formative years. For those who view neurosis in sociological terms, life events, deprivations associated with the onset of symptoms and their roots in familial and social deprivation are placed at the centre of therapeutic concern. It is the narrow and restrictive character of each of these approaches that limits the success they achieve unaided in the management of neurotic illness.

However, these different philosophies are frequently all incorporated within a single formulation in the course of everyday clinical work in many contemporary centres of psychiatry. The fact that there is insufficient factual observation to give such formulations scientific precision or validity deprives them neither of their practical nor their heuristic value.

Each has recent achievements to its credit. Behaviour modification therapy has applied the methods of experimental and social psychology as well as principles derived from learning theory to the treatment of psychiatric disorders. Although the extravagant hopes expressed after the appearance of Wolpe's seminal work (Wolpe 1958) have not been fulfilled, the new therapeutic weapons forged have radically modified the manner in which a substantial proportion of practising psychiatrists approach the treatment of neurotic illness. The systematic objective, quantitative analysis of the symptoms that cause distress and limit achievement and effectiveness in the different spheres of the patient's life is perhaps the most valuable single contribution. The environmental settings in which anxious, phobic or obsessional symptoms are present are carefully explored. The consequences of neurotic behaviour in the patient's personal and physical environment have to be evaluated in that they may serve to reinforce or reward the neurotic symptoms. But they can also be exploited for the purpose of reshaping behaviour. Techniques such as flooding, graded exposure, and behavioural modelling can sometimes achieve valuable results. But there are failures in severely disabled patients and many relapses, not all of them responding to booster courses of treatment. That the results are neither as consistent nor as sustained as the more enthusiastic exponents of the methods sometimes claim stems in part from lack of knowledge of the nature and origins of neurotic illness.

The conflicts between the concepts and methods of behavioural treatment and those of psychotherapists which derive some of their inspiration from psychoanalysts have been productive and have some important consequences for the management of neurotic patients. Behavioural therapists maintain that the symptoms constitute the disease and that exploration of their supposed historical origins and early development can be misleading as well as superfluous and unhelpful. On the other hand, psychoanalysts criticize the attention devoted to manifest symptoms and the omission from consideration of their causes in the personality and its vicissitudes in early development. And the recognition that this is the case has brought about rapprochement between the many exponents of the two types of approach. Yet neurosis commonly commences in stepwise fashion with the entry of qualitatively distinct patterns of behaviour and adaptation.

It is difficult for psychodynamic accounts of neurosis to accommodate such breaks in continuity. Moreover, psychoanalytic treatment may expand insight without making any impression upon the severe disabilities associated with a phobic or obsessional neurosis. Psychodynamic therapists may also unwittingly shape the maladaptive conduct of their neurotic patients towards more adaptive patterns by means that have a kinship with behaviour therapy. In recent years some have adopted such measures in more deliberate and explicit ways. On the other hand, the many behavioural therapists achieve part of their success through insight, empathy and the establishment of a relationship of trust and understanding with their patients and there has been increasing recognition of the common elements between different forms of psychotherapy (Sloane *et al* 1975).

Clinical analysis of the phenomenology and historical development of neurotic symptoms will generally reveal them to be an extension or parody of mildly disabling personality traits which have been present over a long period prior to breakdown. Agoraphobia usually arises in anxious, dependent, individuals in some cases with mild circumscribed phobias they have previously been able to circumvent. This will generally come to light only after skilful exploration, for there is a reluctance to reveal them and a more or less conscious effort to camouflage such traits as dependence and helplessness. The presence of such kindred personality traits before illness also holds true for social phobias and anxiety states with fears of non-existent disease and, with some qualification, for obsessive-compulsive states.

There are three interrelated components of neurotic disorder that need to be defined as a precondition for the understanding and management of neurotic disorders. The first comprises the symptoms which incapacitate the patient, perhaps confining her helplessly in her home or needing the presence of some supportive person if she is to move more than yards from it; or excluding her from the company of others; or imposing a crippling set of rituals. As already mentioned, transient and circumscribed forms of such symptoms are often present prior to illness.

The second is the adverse life event that precedes the first appearance of severe neurotic symptoms in the majority of patients. This may be a bereavement or failure, a move to an unfamiliar environment or to a higher responsibility which poses new challenges or some threat to physical health and well-being, the latter particularly in men. The nature of this stressful circumstance often provides insight into the individual's Achilles' heel. Only in the rare instances of natural disasters will such a life event prove to be a sufficient cause of neurotic breakdown. Its effects may be regarded as additive to those of the third component.

This is made up of the premorbid personality and those aspects of it in particular which render the individual vulnerable through dependence upon others, inflexibility, suspicion and incapacity for trust, hostility manifest in resentment, jealousy and anxiety in personal relationships, inadequate self-esteem through real, imagined or exaggerated deficits.

The knowledge gained from the exploration of these components of neurosis and their interactions can be utilized to deepen the insight into those aspects of personality that render the neurotically ill person vulnerable. This may provide him with some measure of protection in the event of re-exposure to the situations that have precipitated the current disorder, by impinging upon the weak points in the armour of his personality.

Assessment of the results of treatment in neurosis is notoriously difficult. But it is an integral part of the professional responsibility of psychiatrists to provide specialized forms of care for the most common forms of disorder in clinical practice. It follows that they must be prepared to use psychological measures and to set specific goals to be attained with their aid.

One of the principal questions for research is to determine whether methods entailing frequent sessions extended over years achieve results that are superior to brief periods of treatment that entail a far smaller investment in time and effort. The burgeoning of interest in psychotherapy manifest in the last ten to fifteen years is reflected in the inclusion of courses of training in the relevant skills in the curricula of schools of psychiatry that formerly ignored psychodynamics and psychotherapy. But to derive the greatest possible benefit from this development, stringent methods of evaluation will have to be fostered. Otherwise the next few decades will see a further proliferation of rival schools of conflicting and unsubstantiated claims for different methods of treatment.

6. Psychosomatic disease and behavioural medicine

Only a few selected areas in which recent advances have created fresh opportunities for psychiatric intervention and have made it possible to define specific aims in treatment can be mentioned. A number of studies have adduced evidence that there is a substantial measure of overlap between psychiatric and somatic disease (Roth & Kay 1956, Shepherd *et al* 1966, Kerr *et al* 1969). The relationships are complex and the direction of causality is not the same in all cases. Physical disease and disablement have emotional implications and the special meaning they carry for the patient gives rise to responses that range from understandable anxiety and depression to grave psychiatric illness. On the other hand, a recurrent emotional disorder makes, at the least, some contribution to the causation of physical maladies. It has, for example, been shown to contribute to the causation of arterial hypertension (Sainsbury *et al* 1974).

The psychological aspects of physical illness, the patient's strategies for coping with disability and the behaviour elicited by its meaning for him whether in the form of despair and inertia or a determination to prevail are an integral part of all varieties of disease. There is a growing body of evidence that concomitant emotional disorder exerts a powerful and independent influence upon the course and outcome of those diseases that enter a chronic stage or leave residual defects in particular.

It is noteworthy that it is the affective disorders of middle and late life that are associated with a diminished life expectation (Kay & Bergmann 1966, Kerr *et al* 1969). One contributory factor is that depressive or neurotic disorder may be the first harbinger of later physical disease including malignant disease. Mortality from carcinoma has been found to have been in excess of normal expectation in cohorts of patients with affective disorder (Kerr *et al* 1969, Whitlock 1977). In a proportion of the cases in the study by Kerr *et al,* the malignancy was discovered at post-mortem and could not, therefore, have been the primary cause of the emotional illness. This is yet one more argument for setting goals within a holistic framework within psychiatric as well as medical departments.

The last group of observations raises questions about the contribution of emotional disorder to rates of mortality in somatic disease. Does the complication of serious physical disease by depressive illness increase the chances of a fatal outcome? There is some evidence that it may do so. Among elderly, depressed people who 'give up' and turn their faces to the wall, death may follow with little in the way of definable physical cause to explain their demise. Death induced by cursing or sorcery among aboriginal peoples is a well-attested observation (Cannon 1942). It has become known among anaesthetists and surgeons that those who exhibit severe and sustained anxiety or a conviction that they may die under the anaesthetic, are at some risk; steps have been taken to give them adequate emotional support and sedation. Neuro-radiologists who have wide experience of intra-carotid injection for the purpose of cerebral angiography have come to similar conclusions (Hawkins 1981).

Recent developments in cardiovascular disease have provided some particularly clear examples of the interdependence and interplay of psychic and somatic ill health.

In an investigation of 117 patients who had experienced life-threatening ventricular arrhythmias, 62 of them with one or more episodes of ventricular fibrillation, Lown *et al* (1980) concluded that three sets of conditions contributed to the recurrence of malignant ventricular arrhythmias. The first was the presence of proven ischaemic heart disease. The second was the presence of a lasting state of depression, "or a sense of psychological entrapment without possible exit." The third condition was some immediate life event which acted as a psychological trigger for ventricular arrhythmia. The cardiac and emotional disorders appeared to be correlated in a clear and orderly fashion. In the presence of extreme electrical instability of the myocardium, a stressful event of a minimum nature would suffice to provoke arrhythmia even where no sustained background of affective disturbance was present. At the other extreme of the spectrum where myocardial derangement was absent, fibrillation could not be precipitated irrespective of the magnitude of the psychological trigger. In the intermediate position, minor stresses potentiated by a background of depression might precipitate ventricular fibrillation. Twenty patients who showed more than one ventricular ectopic beat were taught a meditative state involving relaxation (Lown & Graboys 1977). In a follow-up study they were found to have a diminished mortality as compared with controls who had not received such treatment.

In the burgeoning of behavioural medicine (Pomerleau & Brady 1979) that began two decades ago, far-reaching claims were made for the efficacy of bio-feedback techniques in the treatment of many medical conditions. As further evidence has accumulated, the claims advanced have become more modest. In a recent report by Whitehead (1979), bio-feedback techniques were judged to have been satisfactorily, though not conclusively, established for the following groups of conditions:

(1) Raynaud's disease treated by means of hand temperature feedback.

(2) Faecal incontinence in cases where complication arose in the course of rectal surgery treated by means of anal sphincter feedback.

(3) Migraine headaches treated by means of hand temperature feedback or temporal artery pulse amplitude feedback among other techniques.

(4) Muscle contraction headaches treated by means of EMG feedback.

(5) Hemiplegia, spasmodic torticolis and some types of back pain.

(6) Cerebral palsy, treated by means of head position and limb position monitors.

In these, and other conditions, there is need for collaborative work by psychiatrists trained in behavioural techniques and physicians so that goals can be defined in management in respect of all aspects of illness. In particular, there is clamant need for more systematic clinical trials to evaluate the results of such joint endeavours and estimate their costs and benefits.

7. Treatment objectives in relation to personality disorder

In the conditions described in the ninth edition of *WHO's International Classification of Disease* as "deeply-ingrained maladaptive patterns of behaviour generally recognisable by the time of adolescence or earlier and continuing through most of adult life," neither psychological nor biological nor social methods of treatment have achieved successful results. This reflects a serious limitation in the practice of psychiatry. Approximately 10 per cent of psychiatric admissions in the UK are described as suffering from 'personality and behavioural disorders'. But this is an underestimate in that it refers only to those disorders in which difficulties in adjustment or persistently impulsive and anti-social conducts are at the forefront in the presenting problem. There are many forms of psychiatric illness in which long-lasting maladaptation or frank personality disorder constitutes an underlying basis and often an important causal agent in the development of illness. In a relatively high proportion of patients with chronic or relapsing neuroses, the diagnosis of personality disorder as well as a specific neurosis is appropriate. This is one reason why the distinction between neurosis and a personality disorder was not recognized in classical European psychiatry, both being subsumed within the concept of 'psychopathy' (Schneider 1958). This ignores the periodic and transient emotional disorders which often punctuate the lives of many of those with long-lasting personality difficulties and cause them to seek psychiatric help. The treatment of such an illness is a realistic goal and may be followed by a long quiescent interval. But there are no known remedies (social or medical) for the lasting disorder of maladjustment.

The contemporary psychiatrist often has to deal with cases of personality disorder who have been referred from the Courts of Law: chronic alcoholics and those who abuse drugs and a mounting tide of patients with attempted self-poisoning or suicide. Such features as a broken parental home, a disorganized marriage, poor parental care, frequent separation from parents and a high prevalence of alcoholism and criminality in the family have recently been found in a high proportion of such patients, those with self-poisoning as well as those with recurring forms of delinquent, criminal and destructive behaviour. Personality disorder is the most frequent diagnosis made in such patients and numerous studies (Hawks *et al* 1969, Bejerot 1970, Backhouse & James 1969, Drapkin & Landau 1966) have shown that this is also true for those who suffer from the more serious forms of drug dependence.

There is a sufficient consistency within and between the different forms of consistently impulsive, aggressive and anti-social behaviour to regard them as off-shoots of a single syndrome of which these different disorders are varying manifestations. "For there is a well-defined age of onset, a family history covering a range of disorders mainly affecting personality, typical sex distribution, a course predictable within limits, a number of definable hazards, an increased rate of mortality, and a clinical picture in which hostility, anxiety, immaturity and impulsiveness and low frustration tolerance are combined, and to which the presenting disturbances (aggressive, violent or self-destructive acts and a quest for oblivion-promoting or confidence-boosting substances) can be meaningfully related." (Roth 1972). The exception in respect of sex distribution is presented by self-poisoning or attempted suicide in which females predominate; it is among the male first-degree relatives that criminal record, alcoholism and violent behaviour are found in excess.

Although the results achieved by treatment are disappointing, management aimed at the limited goal of tiding patients over crises and emotional decompensation is helpful. It requires special therapeutic skills.

In a recent practical paper Egdell (1981) has pointed out that behavioural analysis is an essential precondition for success. A number of questions have to be posed. What initiated and what factors continued to provoke the unwanted behaviour? What factors were associated with previous good spells? How can desirable patterns be reinforced? In setting goals he points out that priorities set by the patient such as finance, housing or police problems need to be dealt with as a first step. Triggers to outbursts of disturbed behaviour — real or imagined criticism, rejections or losses, failures in particular social situations — have to be defined and insight imparted as far as possible into the link between such 'sensitivity spots' and bouts of drinking, aggression or behaviour that elicits rejection. Impulsiveness needs to be analysed and situations helping or hindering self-control can be realistically transferred to the patient. Another objective is to try to help the patient by psychotherapeutic or behavioural means to live with feelings instead of acting them out through intolerance of any form of emotional distress, whether anger or anxiety, which provokes thoughtless behaviour.

Such measures, though helpful in the management of acute disturbances, have little effect upon the unfavourable course followed by most subjects in the long term. The reasons for this may be connected with the origins of these conditions in the early formative years. The patterns of behaviour then shaped through the operation of both genetical and familial-environmental factors are liable to become firmly ingrained.

Evidence regarding heredity has been recently derived from Danish-American investigations. One hundred and forty-three individuals with criminal records were investigated together with matched controls and also the psychological status of biological and adoptive parents. The three most powerful predictors of criminality in the index case proved to be criminality in at least one biological parent, a similar state in at least one adoptive parent and a psychiatric diagnosis in a biological mother. Antisocial adaptation in the adoptee had the highest correlation with a history of criminality in the biological father. In the studies of Robins (1966, Robins & Lewis 1966), neither living in a slum, low social class nor a broken home proved to have a clear influence on the subsequent fate of children referred for anti-social behaviour.

However, the evidence that social factors make a substantial contribution comes from a number of sources and is well established. Affectionless psychopathy has an association with multiple separation experiences and institutional care in early childhood, not so much on account of the disruption of bonds but because firm bonds fail to develop (Rutter 1966). It is plain that while low socio-economic status will be conducive to the creation of such circumstances, the adverse psychological influences in question may prevail in the homes of the affluent as well as the underprivileged.

Nor are the effects confined to those who are convicted of crimes or come into contact with psychiatric services. In a recent investigation by

West (personal communication) those who had been submitted to repeated separations, poor quality of parental care and long periods of residence in institutions, had not always come into conflict with the law. But even those who were law abiding were often living isolated, friendless and relatively unproductive, dependent lives.

Neither treatment programmes nor efforts at prevention devoted to improving the early environment of children at risk have succeeded in making a significant impression on the problem.

The largest venture undertaken to date was the Cambridge-Somerville study of which there has been a recent follow-up report (McCord 1978). A comparison of 253 men who had been in the treatment programme with 253 controls yielded a very disappointing result. Not a single one of the 57 comparisons made showed preventive treatment to have improved the chances of those at risk avoiding alcoholism, mental illness, poor occupational achievement or a relatively high mortality. Paradoxically, the treatment group appeared to have fared even worse than the controls. No method of intervention that can favourably influence the emotional development of children so as to avert the development of personality disorders has been discovered for the present.

Nor has secondary prevention achieved better results. There is no known form of treatment that can be relied upon to influence the course of chronic alcoholism, drug dependence or habitually aggressive and violent behaviour.

In relation to self-poisoning, an enquiry by Gibbons *et al* (1978) found no difference in the rate of recurrence of self-poisoning in a group of subjects who had received intensive community care in comparison with a group which had not been given such help.

These and other failures have led workers such as Lee Robins to view with pessimism the possibilities of any form of preventive intervention whether they be psychotherapy, improved education or Head Start programmes in the United States which have sought to enrich the educational environment of underprivileged children. These, too, have failed to place any successes on record.

Yet there can be little doubt that the efforts of investigators such as Bowlby, Rutter, Graham West and Lee Robins who have in recent years undertaken intensive enquiries into the familial settings in which delinquency and 'conduct' disorders are now known to be the early progenitors of later social maladjustment, made a significant contribution to the delineation of the early formative stages, subsequent course and also the socio-familial setting and childhood of many forms of serious personality maladjustment in adult life. Rutter's recent investigations (Rutter *et al*

1975, Berger *et al* 1975, Rutter *et al* 1974) have shown that disturbed children both in inner London and on the Isle of Wight were drawn from disruptive, disturbed and disharmonious homes. The higher prevalence of these forms of disorder in inner London stemmed from the higher rate of prevalence of homes of this nature among school children there than in the Isle of Wight. A comparison of the papers published on the subjects of delinquency and other forms of maladjustment and their psychological, familial, and social origin in early childhood with the publications of the last five to ten years makes it clear that significant advances in knowledge have been achieved through a combination of clinical and epidemiological research. They have served to redefine aims and goals in relation to a whole range of disorders encountered by child psychiatrists.

There is, therefore, a compelling need for fostering programmes of enquiry to be undertaken by clinical psychiatrists in collaboration with epidemiologists and social and behavioural scientists into disorders that constitute the major social and medical problems of our time. The fact that efforts at prevention have met with no success for the present, should not be construed to mean that endeavour in this field is futile. The contribution of psychiatrists to the indubitable advances of knowledge in this field for the past 20 years have laid a firm factual foundation for the clinical practice and preventive experiments of the future. It would be no more logical to abandon such efforts than it would be to give up attempts to solve the problems of disseminated sclerosis, virus diseases, many forms of cancer, and the problems of dementia in middle and late life.

8. Summary and conclusions

The social importance of mental disorders derives from their high prevalence and the amount of personal disability, social dislocation, and unavoidable loss of life they cause. In those forms of disorder that enter a chronic phase or leave residual defects there are reciprocal interactions between the sick person and the family often with adverse effects on both.

The advances achieved during the past two to three decades have made it possible to aim at more ambitious goals in treatment and secondary prevention in several forms of major psychiatric illness. In the case of each group of disorders further investigations will be needed to define aims more precisely so that treatment can exert an optimal effect.

In the case of depressive illness, the value of antidepressive drugs is firmly established. There is now evidence to indicate that maintenance treatment is of value in protection against recrudescence of symptoms and in preventing or attenuating relapse. However, the length of time for which long term treatment should be sustained remains unclear. The figures for relapse rates in studies of long-term treatment vary widely and there is no consistent evidence that maintenance of antidepressant drug treatment beyond a period of six to twelve months remains effective in prevention. In bipolar forms of illness long-term treatment with tricyclic and related compounds is contra-indicated.

In the milder forms of neurotic depression recent evidence suggests that the first aim should be to control symptoms by simple psychotherapeutic measures. The finding that in neurotic depression and those treated on an out-patient basis, psychotherapy and drugs potentiate each other's effects, is important. But further observations are needed to provide a firm, factual foundation for certain aims and decisions in this field: (a) the optimal duration of maintenance treatment with antidepressive drugs, (b) the precise indications for psychological rather than pharmacological methods of treatment, (c) the comparative results achieved by different forms of psychotherapy (psychodynamic, behavioural, group techniques and support and reassurance).

The recent observations which have adduced evidence in favour of a sociological model of depressive illnesses have been important in stimulating precise enquiries into their social and familial associations. But the direction of causation remains unclear. It remains uncertain how far adverse social circumstances function as independent causes and to what extent they reflect difficulties in adaptation that stem from life-long personality traits. One beneficial effect of these controversies has been to direct attention to a wider range of psycho-social features in defining aims in the treatment of depressive and related states. It has also led to more stringent enquiries in an attempt to establish criteria of demarcation, such as the 'Index of Definition' (Wing *et al* 1978), between ordinary distress on the one hand and psychiatric illness that calls for treatment, on the other.

Neuroleptic drugs have improved the outcome of schizophrenic illness, though they have made little impression upon negative features and residual defects. The aims of treatment have been to encompass the rehabilitation of the patient and his resettlement in the community. The relatively poor prognosis of cases of insidious onset makes it imperative that more effort should be devoted to the early recognition of schizophrenic illness. This is of particular importance in relation to those forms of illness that commence in the second decade and are manifest in occupational and social decline before disturbed behaviour becomes socially conspicuous. Further progress in the field of 'high risk' research will be needed to make the achievement of such aims feasible in more than a minority of cases.

Pharmacological remedies have in recent years come to play a significant role in the treatment of depressive, anxious and obsessive neuroses. But perhaps the most important single contribution in this area has been that of behaviour therapy which demands a systematic analysis of the patterns of behaviour from which neurotic suffering emanates. This in turn makes it possible to define specific goals in treatment and to plan systematically the steps to be taken in re-shaping disordered conduct. The alliance between the methods of behavioural and psychodynamic psychiatry which has taken shape in recent years is a significant new development. But for its full exploitation more intensive therapeutic trials to evaluate the results achieved and refine the methods used will have to be undertaken.

It is in relation to deeply ingrained forms of maladaptation or 'personality disorder' that progress has been most disappointing during the past half-century. These conditions have become increasingly prominent in the practice of hospital and community psychiatry in recent decades. But we remain almost as helpless in the face of serious drug dependence, alcoholism, persistently vile, aggressive and anti-social conduct as we were half a century ago. Some ambitious attempts at prevention have not for the present succeeded in registering any result. This does not signify that skills in clinical management have not been gained. Psychiatry cannot avoid this challenge and the observations made by the epidemiological studies of child psychiatrists and sociologists such as Rutter, Graham, Wing, and Lee Robins have begun to lay factual foundations for new approaches to the problem.

9. Some methodological issues

The aims that can be realistically set in the management of mental suffering have thus been transformed by contributions that have come from clinical and neurobiological research.

Controlled therapeutic trials have become established as the most reliable means for evaluating the results of treatment. And to an increasing extent changes in psychopathology are recorded with the aid of special measures applied at regular intervals so that the results can be expressed in quantitative terms.

Rating scales for measuring severity and assessing progress such as the Hamilton Anxiety and Hamilton Depression Scales (Hamilton 1959, 1960) and scales for measuring phobic states (Gelder & Marx 1966), scales for diagnostic discrimination such as the Newcastle Anxiety Depression Scale (Gurney *et al* 1972) and comprehensive rating scales such as the CPRS (Åsberg *et al* 1978) from which sub-scales for measurement of a wide range of psychiatric syndromes can be derived, have played an important role in the development of psychiatric research in recent decades. It is desirable that a number of different parameters of behaviour and adaptation should be measured in addition to the symptom profile; for significant improvements may be recorded along a rating scale in the course of a therapeutic trial with little in the way of corresponding improvement in the ability of patients to lead ordinary lives.

In the course of psychiatric research, the criteria that have been employed to arrive at a diagnosis have to be made explicit in terms as clear and precise as possible and rules have to be laid down for using the criteria to arrive at a diagnosis. The development of such operational criteria for scientific purposes has been advanced to a considerable extent by standardizing the examination of the present mental state notably in the Present State Examination (PSE) of Wing and his colleagues (Wing *et al* 1974). The Research Diagnostic Criteria (Spitzer *et al* 1978) and the criteria proposed in DSM III (American Psychiatric Association 1980) have provided research workers with reliable instruments for standardizing clinical diagnoses, so enabling them to communicate the results so that others can attempt to replicate them.

It has to be made clear that these instruments cannot of their nature be employed as an alternative for the diagnostic process in clinical practice. Only a limited part of the process of conducting a psychiatric examination has been standardized. And a psychiatric diagnosis entails bringing findings derived from the examination of the present mental state into relationship with different kinds of historical, developmental and social findings and often observations on behaviour conducted before and after examination.

There is yet a further reason why many sets of operational criteria that have been developed in recent years should not be allowed to replace full psychiatric assessment and diagnosis in setting aims for treatment. There is an arbitrariness about the assembly of items being brought together under different diagnostic headings. Their high overall reliability arises in part, from the fact that groups of investigators have agreed to use certain rubrics with their associated operational definitions. But the diagnostic and discriminating value of the features incorporated in the criteria has not been established with the aid of systematic enquiries. Multivariate statistical techniques such as principal components and multiple regression analysis which have been important in the last two to three decades in refining classification and diagnosis in certain areas of psychiatry could improve on this situation by assigning numerical weights to the different items proportionate to their value in the delineation of syndromes and in discrimination between them.

Multiaxial schemes of classification and diagnosis such as those originally suggested by Essen-Möller (1961) replicate the process of clinical diagnosis more closely than other reference classifications; and there are arguments in favour of conducting exploratory experiments with such schemes at the present stage. Among other considerations more information is needed to determine the criteria by which physical and psycho-social factors should be judged as having aetiological importance for the presenting illness, so that a greater measure of consistency in the use of this axis is achieved. It is essential also that improved means of defining personality and deriving a 'personality diagnosis' should be developed.

In the meantime all such components of the clinical picture have to be delineated as systematically as possible with the aid of clinical observation and incorporated alongside other findings. It is a clinical formulation along these lines that has to provide a basis for plans of management of psychiatric illness and the objectives set within such plans. There can be little doubt that the precision, clarity and reliability of clinical diagnosis and of clinical practice in general have also benefited greatly from the various sets of operational definition of psychiatric disorder originally introduced for use in psychiatric research.

References

American Psychiatric Association (1980): DSM III: *Diagnostic and Statistical Manual of Mental Disorders*. 3rd ed. APA, Washington, DC.

Åsberg, M., Perris, C., Schalling, D. & Sedvall, G. (1978): The CPRS — development and applications of a psychiatric rating scale. *Acta Psychiatr. Scand., Suppl. 271*.

Backhouse, C.I. & James, I.P. (1969): The relationship and prevalence of smoking, drinking and drug-taking in adolescent boys. *Br. J. Addict., 64*, 75-79.

Bebbington, P. (1980): Causal models and logical inference in epidemiological psychiatry. *Br. J. Psychiatry, 136*, 317-325.

Bejerot, N. (1970): *Addiction and Society*. Charles C. Thomas, Springfield, Ill.

Berger, M., Yule, W. & Rutter, M. (1975): Attainment and adjustment in two geographical areas. II — The prevalence of specific reading retardation. *Br. J. Psychiatry, 126*, 510-519.

Bibring, E. (1965): The mechanism of depression. In Greenacre, P. (ed.): *Affective Disorders*. Int. Universities Press, New York, pp.13-48.

Brown, G.W., Sklair, F., Harris, T. & Birley, J.L.T. (1973a): Life events and psychiatric disorders. Part I: Some methodological issues. *Psychol. Med., 3*, 74-87.

Brown, G.W., Harris, T.O. & Peto, J. (1973b): Life events and psychiatric disorders. Part II: Nature of causal link. *Psychol. Med., 3*, 159-176.

Brown, G.W., Ni Bhrolchain, M. & Harris, T.O. (1975): Social class and psychiatric disturbance among women in an urban population. *Sociology, 9*, 225-254.

Brown, G.W. & Harris, T. (1978): *The Social Origins of Depression*. Tavistock, London.

Cannon, W.B. (1942): Voodoo Death. *Am. Anthropol., 44*, 2.

Davis, J.M. (1976): Overview: Maintenance therapy in psychiatry. II. Affective disorders. *Am. J. Psychiatry, 133*, 1-13.

Drapkin, I. & Landau, S.F. (1966): Drug offenders in Israel: a survey. *Br. J. Criminology, 6*, 376-390.

Egdell, H. (1981): Problem personalities — recognition and management. *Medicine: Psychiatric Disorders, 35,* 1, 1789-1793.
Essen-Möller, E. (1961): On classification of mental disorders. *Acta Psychiatr. Scand., 37,* 119-126.
Friedman, A.S. (1975): Interaction of drug therapy with marital therapy in depressive patients. *Arch. Gen. Psychiatry, 32,* 619-637.
Gelder, M.G. & Marx, I.M. (1966): Severe agoraphobia: a controlled prospective trial of behaviour therapy. *Br. J. Psychiatry, 122,* 309.
Gibbons, J.S., Buller, J., Unwin, P. & Gibbons, J.L. (1978): Evaluation of a social work service for self-poisoning patients. *Br. J. Psychiatry, 133,* 111-118.
Gurney, C., Roth, M., Garside, F.F., Kerr, T.A. & Schapiro, K. (1972): Studies in the classification of affective disorders. The relationship between anxiety states and depressive illness — II. *Br. J. Psychiatry, 121,* 162-166.
Hamilton, M. (1959): The assessment of anxiety states by rating. *Br. J. Med. Psychol., 32,* 50-55.
Hamilton, M. (1960): A rating scale for depression. *J. Neurol. Neurosurg. Psychiatry, 23,* 56-61.
Hamilton, M. (1967): Development of a rating scale for primary depressive illness. *Br. J. Soc. Clin. Psychol., 6,* 278-296.
Hawkins, T.D. (1981): Personal communication.
Hawks, D.V., Mitcheson, M., Ogsbourne, A. *et al* (1969): Abuse of methylamphetamine. *Br. Med. J., 2,* 715-721.
Jahoda, M. (1958): Criteria for Positive Mental Health. In: *Current Concepts of Positive Mental Health.* Basic Books Inc., New York.
Kay, D.W.K. & Bergmann, K. (1966): Physical disability and mental health in old age. *J. Psychosom. Res., 10,* 3.
Kerr, T.A., Schapiro, K. & Roth, M. (1969): The relationship between premature death and affective disorders. *Br. J. Psychiatry, 115,* 1277-1282.
Leff, J. & Vaughan, C. (1981): The role of maintenance therapy and relatives' expressed emotion in relapse of schizophrenia: a two-year follow-up. *Br. J. Psychiatry, 139,* 102-104.
Lown, B. & Graboys, T.B. (1977): Management of patients with malignant ventricular arrhythmias. *Am. J. Cardiol., 32,* 910-918.
Lown, B., DeSilva, R.A., Reich, P. & Murawski, B.J. (1980): Psychophysiologic factors in cardiac death. *Am. J. Psychiatry, 137,* 1325-1335.
McCord, J. (1978): A thirty-year follow-up of treatment effects. *Am. Psychol., 33,* 284-289.
Mindham, R.H.S., Howl, C. & Shepherd, M. (1973): An evaluation of continuation therapy with tricyclic antidepressants in depressive illness. *Psychol. Med., 3,* 5-17.
Pomerleau, O.F. & Brady, J.P. (eds.) (1979): *Behavioural Medicine: Theory and Practice.* Williams and Wilkins, Baltimore.
Robins, L.N. (1966): *Deviant Children Grown Up.* Willams & Wilkins Co., New York.
Robins, L.N. & Lewis, R.G. (1966): The role of the antisocial family in school completion and delinquency: a three-generation study. *Sociol. Quarterly, 7,* 500-514.
Roth, M. & Kay, D.W.K. (1956): Affective disorders arising in the senium. II — Physical disability as an aetiological factor. *J. Ment. Sci., 102* (246), 141-150.
Roth, M. (1972): Human violence as viewed from the psychiatric clinic. The Adolf Meyer Lecture. *Am. J. Psychiatry, 128,* 1043-1056.
Rutter, M. (1966): *Children of Sick Parents: An Environmental and Psychiatric Study. Maudsley Monogr. No. 16.* Oxford University Press.
Rutter, M., Yule, B., Quinton, D., Rowlands, O., Yule, W. & Berger, M. (1974): Attainment and adjustment in two geographical areas: III. Some factors accounting for area differences. *Br. J. Psychiatry, 125,* 520-533.

Rutter, M., Cox, A., Tupling, C., Berger, M. & Yule, W. (1975): Attainment and adjustment in two geographical areas: I. The prevalence of psychiatric disorder. *Br. J. Psychiatry, 126,* 493-509.

Sainsbury, P. (1964): Neuroticism and hypertension in an out-patient population. *J. Psychosom. Res., 8,* 235-238.

Schneider, K. (1958): *Psychopathic Personalities.* Cassell & Company, London.

Shepherd, M., Cooper, B., Brown, A.C. & Kalton, G.W. (1966): *Psychiatric Illness in General Practice.* Oxford University Press, London.

Sloane, R.B., Staples, F.R., Cristol, A.H., Yorkston, N.J. & Whipple, K. (1975): *Psychotherapy Versus Behaviour Therapy.* Harvard University Press, Cambridge, Mass.

Spitzer, R.L., Endicott, J. & Robins, E. (1978): Research diagnostic criteria. *Arch. Gen. Psychiatry, 35,* 773-782.

Tennant, C. & Bebbington, P. (1978): The social causation of depression: a critique of the work of Brown and his colleagues. *Psychol. Med., 8,* 565-575.

Tennant, C., Bebbington, P. & Hurry, J. (1981): The role of life events in depressive illness: is there a substantial causal relation? *Psychol. Med., 11,* 379-389.

Vaughan, C. & Leff, J.P. (1976): The influence of family and social factors on the course of psychiatric illness. *Br. J. Psychiatry, 129,* 125-137.

Weissmann, M.M., Prusoff, B.A., Di Mascio, A., Neu, C., Gohlaney, M. & Klerman, G.L. (1979): The efficacy of drugs and psychotherapy in the treatment of acute depressive episodes. *Am. J. Psychiatry, 136,* 555-558.

Whitehead, W.E. (1979): Biofeedback and health care. *Behav. Med. Update, 3,* 7.

Whitlock, F.A. (1978): Suicide, cancer and depression. *Br. J. Psychiatry, 132,* 269-274.

Wing, J.K., Cooper, J.E. & Sartorius, N. (1974): *The Measurement and Classification of Psychiatric Symptoms.* Cambridge University Press, London.

Wing, J.K., Nixon, J.M., Mann, S.A. & Leff, J.P. (1977): Reliability of the PSE (Ninth Edition) used in a population study. *Psychol. Med., 7,* 505-516.

Wing, J.K., Mann, S.A., Leff, J.P. & Nixon, J.M. (1978): The concept of a 'case' in psychiatric population surveys. *Psychol. Med., 8,* 203-217.

Wing, J.K., (1980): At the research front. Standardizing clinical diagnostic judgement. The PSE-Catego system. *Aust. NZ. J. Psychiatry, 14,* 17-20.

Wolpe, J. (1958): *Psychotherapy by Reciprocal Inhibition* Stanford University Press, Stanford.

Evaluation in Mental Health Programmes

N. SARTORIUS

1. Introduction

Evaluation at its best is a systematic way of learning from experience and using the lessons learned to improve both current and future action. At its worst, it is an activity used to justify the selection of a scapegoat for past failures.

There are several ways of increasing the probability that evaluation will be useful and not destructive. These include:

(a) making evaluation a continuing process rather than an isolated, short-lasting activity;

(b) ensuring that those who are responsible for the work in question actively participate in its evaluation;

(c) evaluating both quality and quantity of performance and using indicators in which this dual approach will be included (e.g. the number of home visits which were useful and were seen as such by those visited and those visiting);

(d) validating information which will be used in evaluations; and

(e) expressing the results of evaluation in a language which can be understood by those involved in a programme and ensuring that the results are seen as valid by all involved (or, alternatively, that the reasons and nature of disagreements are noted).

2. Specific issues in evaluation of mental health care

Principles governing the evaluation of health services in general all apply to the evaluation of mental health services. In addition, however, there are certain specific features of mental health problems which require additional attention. These include the following:

1. Only a minor proportion of all those with mental disorders are treated in mental health services, out of which two groups can be distinguished: the

first spends only a small proportion of the total time of illness in contact with the facility; the second spends most of the total time of illness — and life — in the facility.

2. Much of mental morbidity is handled outside the mental health services either at primary care level by general practitioners, community nurses, etc., or by specialists of other disciplines (e.g. internists, paediatricians, geriatricians). The role of school medical services, occupational health services and prison medical services may also be considerable in providing mental health care. This implies the need for a broad data base in evaluating mental health care to identify both what *is* being done by services outside specialized mental health services and what *is not* being done.

3. Other community agents — e.g. police, probation officers, social workers and teachers — are frequently closely involved in the care of the mentally ill. Their contributions, therefore, need to be monitored if a global evaluation is to be carried out. Such data may be particularly useful in the assessment of care for people with psychosocial problems such as those related to alcohol and drug abuse (Jones & Vischi 1979).

4. Many 'physical' diseases and disabilities have a significant 'mental' component. Evaluation of mental health care should, therefore, cover mental health care for physically-disabled persons and their families and establish whether mental health factors are taken into account in the rehabilitation of patients with myocardial infarction, cerebrovascular disorders and other common conditions.

5. Mental health programmes can make significant contributions to the functioning of other services: for example, by drawing attention to and providing advice on the dangers of institutionalization and the psychological effects of health care in general on individuals and communities. Evaluation of the activities necessary to influence other services should, therefore, be given the importance it merits.

6. Some individuals afflicted by mental disorders are subject to legal restrictions of their civil rights, being judged unable to make responsible decisions about their own health, their families and other matters, and being deprived of liberty which is consequent upon the involuntary commitment of mentally ill people to mental hospitals.

A number of possible mechanisms for the continuous evaluation of these issues have been suggested, including (a) statutory commissions; (b) ministerial bodies; (c) professional groups and associations; (d) lay associations and pressure groups; (e) academic institutions; (f) courts and tribunals.

7. The diagnosis of mental disorders when no damage to the central

nervous system can be demonstrated depends to a large degree on the existence of standardized instruments for psychological and psychiatric assessment. Since these are often not available, serious problems may arise in the evaluation of the care provided.

8. The standards of normality concerning the behaviour of individuals are more culture- (and time-) dependent than the standards of normality applied to physiological characteristics (although sensitivity to alcohol or pharmacological agents, for example, seems to vary considerably between people living in different parts of the world). Problems that may arise out of cultural variation are considerable, but can be overcome.

9. Mental disorders have a stigmatizing effect on individuals who suffer from them, as well as their families, and whilst this is true to a lesser degree for certain other disorders, mental disorders are the only conditions that stigmatize descendants over several generations. Such is not the case for leprosy, venereal disease and some other diseases carrying a stigma.

The reporting of mental disorders is, therefore, often incomplete and evaluation is made more difficult.

10. The boundaries between mental disorder, personality type and personality disorders are difficult to define in many instances and long-term observation has often to precede diagnostic decisions and subsequent action.

11. In the field of psychiatry — perhaps more than in almost any other field — treatment methods and possibilities have developed rapidly over the past two decades. Health planners (and indeed the general public) therefore need continuous education concerning the appropriateness of various forms of treatment such as psychotherapy, behaviour therapy, psychopharmacological treatments, electroconvulsive treatment, as well as training in social skills. Such knowledge is an essential prerequisite to the interpretation of evaluative data concerning mental health services.

3. Preparation for evaluation and types of data necessary for it

In the light of the above, it appears that evaluation of mental health care must be preceded by a systematic examination of the following questions:

(a) Will the evaluation concern the mental health programme or mental health services; in other words, will the evaluation concentrate on services/care for the mentally ill or also encompass the achievement of such objectives as the promotion of mental health, prevention of mental diseases, optimization of community (and individual) behaviour concerning mental health care, etc.?

(b) Is the evaluation going to concern itself with *structure* (e.g. quality of institution, staffing, distance between the patients' homes and institution, etc.), *processes* (e.g. treatment of patients, relations between patients and staff, and relations within the staff), or *outcome* in terms of objectives such as those mentioned under (a) above?

(c) Will the evaluation be summative (i.e. serve as a basis for decisions about services) or formative (i.e. mainly serve to help the service introduce improvements in its work)?

(d) Will the evaluation become part of the programme, with defined mechanisms to carry it out in an 'integrated' manner (i.e. planning and implementing it together with service development) or is it a single or sporadic event? The answer to this question may also help to answer questions about the meaningfulness of case registers, expenditure on evaluation, etc.

(e) In what way will the community, the patients and the service agents be involved in the evaluation process? What will be their role in the process of collecting data, making assessments, etc.?

The answers to these questions may then allow decisions to be made about the manner in which the evaluation will take place; more importantly, however, they will also provide information on how much has been left out in the evaluation process and to what extent (and how) this is likely to affect the validity of the evaluation and the ability to generalize its findings.

Despite the important role of non-numerical approaches in evaluating mental health services, there is much to be gained from the development and utilization of systematic data collection. If such information is to aid in the planning of more effective mental health care, it should include the following elements:

1. Data which can be used to estimate current needs and predict future trends in mental morbidity, e.g. prevalence and incidence of mental disorders; levels of health; rates of alcohol consumption; epidemiology and geography of drug dependence; indices of psychosocial dysfunction, e.g. rates of family breakdown, juvenile delinquency, educational failure, and rates of attempted and completed suicide.

2. Data concerning in-patient populations in mental health services of various kinds, e.g. mental hospitals, psychogeriatric, forensic, adolescent and child mental health institutions.

3. Data concerning out-patient services, e.g. rates of referral by source, attendance rates, data from specialized services (Kramer 1969).

4. Data indicating interaction with related or parallel services, e.g. social and medical services for the elderly, hostels and homes for the homeless and unattached, psychosocial problems encountered in prisons, school

Evaluation in mental health programmes 63

health services, etc.

5. Data concerning mental health legislation, e.g. availability of laws, procedures, ways of updating them, and so on.

6. Data about type and amount of mental health care provided by non-specialist services, i.e. primary health care, general medical services, school health services, etc.

7. Data about cost of care — at least concerning services and, where possible, with estimates of cost of other contributors to care, e.g. social welfare agencies.

The above types of data will have to be sought and obtained from a variety of sources, including health service providers, other social services, surveys of population opinion, socioeconomic planning agencies, and so on.

Two further issues deserve special attention in this respect (Sand & Baro 1981). The first concerns the possibility of assessment of the mental state and social functioning in such a way that comparison from service to service or country to country becomes possible; the second concerns the models which will be used in service evaluation.

4. WHO's contributions to the field of evaluation

WHO has made a contribution to this field. Over the past ten years a series of studies have taken place aimed at developing a common language in the field of mental health (Sartorius 1980). This work has concentrated on instruments for use in multicentric and collaborative studies, but also for use in service and teaching activities. WHO's efforts were directed to reaching an agreement on terms used in the description of mental and neurological functioning and pathology (including diagnosis); indicators of mental, neurological and psychosocial problems (e.g. those related to alcohol and drug dependence) and of the success of measures undertaken for their solution; terms referring to environmental factors or situations relevant in mental health investigations; and methods of investigation (e.g. how biological samples are obtained, sent to other centres, etc.).

After some ten years of work, WHO produced a classification of mental disorders, now included in the ninth revision of the *International Classification of Diseases* (WHO 1978). The methods used to achieve this included a series of case-history exercises, reviews of the literature and diagnostic practices in many countries, and intensive discussions between mental health experts and statisticians from some 30 countries on the most acceptable categorization of mental disorder (Sartorius 1976).

To ensure agreement on the content of categories included in the classification, a glossary with definitions of categories of mental disorders listed in the classification was developed in collaboration with experts in more than 60 countries. In addition, work has been undertaken on standardization of terms in relation to epilepsy and cerebrovascular disorders, in collaboration with experts from different countries and centres collaborating in neuroscience projects. The next phase of this programme concentrates on the development of (i) a nomenclature of mental disorders in which each of the terms will have a dictionary definition noting main differences between psychiatric schools and practice in different countries; (ii) a classification of disability; and (iii) a classification of mental disorders and psychosocial problems for use by primary health care workers.

In a series of projects undertaken over the years and still continuing, instruments have been adapted or developed for a standardized description of mental states and other characteristics of a patient's condition. The most widely used of these instruments is a description of the patient's present mental state (PSE: Wing *et al* 1974). This instrument, first developed in English by J.K. Wing and his colleagues, has been extensively tested in some twenty countries and fifteen languages; the fact that its application closely resembles a clinical interview is an important feature because reliable data on the mental state of a patient is acquired in a manner that is familiar and acceptable to both him and the research worker.

A shortened version of the PSE has been used with success as a screening instrument in non-patient populations and by investigators in WHO-co-ordinated studies on the extension of mental health care in Colombia, India, Senegal and Sudan, and on the psychosomatic sequelae of female sterilization in Colombia, India, Nigeria, the Philippines and the UK (Harding 1978).

The PSE was used in a major international study on schizophrenia. In this investigation some 1200 patients were examined to establish whether similar cases of schizophrenia exist in different cultures, with a view to developing the instruments needed to obtain comparable clinical and social data which would allow transcultural mental health studies (WHO 1975, 1979a).

Several other instruments standardizing the assessment of relevant facts have been developed in the course of this and subsequent studies. These include screening methods to identify patients with functional psychoses, as well as instruments to assess the psychiatric history and social condition of the patient and others. More recently, the centres involved in the schizophrenia study set out to examine reasons for differences in outcome of schizophrenia between developing and developed countries, and a whole set of new instruments is being tested in this work: they deal with the assessment of impairment and disabilities; the perception of mental illness by families in different cultures; the recording of life events, of follow-up information and of other facts relevant to the investigation of the origin, course and outcome of mental disorders. In view of the importance of data on the course and outcome of mental disorders over time, WHO has also undertaken a survey of longitudinal studies on psychiatric conditions and a publication summarizing the main findings of these studies has been prepared (Baert & Mednick 1981).

Instruments for the assessment of specific conditions have also been developed. So, for example, an instrument for the assessment of depressive disorders resulted from a multinational study of depression (Sartorius *et al* 1980). This instrument has now been tested in nine countries and exists in Bulgarian, Danish, English, French, German, Hindi, Japanese, Persian and Polish versions. It covers the clinical state, psychiatric history and sociodemographic data and was found to be applicable and acceptable in the populations studied. Instruments for the assessment of alcohol- and drug-related problems are being developed within the framework of projects on community response to alcohol-related problems and in the research and reporting programme on drug dependence.

In the study concerned with psychosomatic changes occurring in women after tubal ligation, instruments for the assessment of reproductive life and history were developed, based upon experience obtained previously with suitable additions for the case in point. This strategy has been used elsewhere; the first drafts of assessment instruments usually contain modules tested in the context of other schedules in a variety of cultures. As a result, the developmental lag in studies for which new instruments are needed can be substantially shortened.

Instruments for the assessment of impairments, handicaps and associated disabilities in psychiatric patients are being tested in eight countries in Europe and in the Sudan. Disability in patients with schizophrenic disorders is being assessed first; later, disability assessments will be carried out in other groups of patients suffering from mental and physical disorders. The present versions of the Psychological Impairments Rating Schedule (PIRS) and the Disability Assessment Schedule (DAS) are designed for use in conjunction with the Present State Examination (PSE). The PIRS covers impairments manifested in psychomotor behaviour and in losses of specific social skills, while the DAS allows recording and rating of disturbances in more global areas of social functioning. Data from initial trials suggest that the two instruments (available in Arabic,

Bulgarian, Czech, English, German, Serbo-Croat, Spanish and Turkish language translations) can be used in a comparable and reliable manner by research workers in several different cultures.

In addition to developing instruments for the assessment of mental states of individuals, the Organization has also undertaken to develop methods for evaluating the mental health needs and resources of communities and countries. These include a first stage screening procedure for the detection of psychiatric cases in primary health care settings (for both adults and children), an interview schedule for use with key informants, to assess their attitudes and obtain help in case identification, and a method for the assessment of the effects of psychiatric illness on the immediate family. These instruments have been shown to be applicable and acceptable in a number of developing countries. Equivalent versions of the whole set of instruments exist in Arabic, English, French, Hindi, Filipino, Portuguese and Spanish. In a study concerned with alcohol-related problems a method has been designed to assess their prevalence in the general population and among the clients of a number of health and non-health agencies.

A project co-ordinated by the European Regional Office brought together investigators from most European countries to define methods for the description of needs and resources for mental health care in defined catchment areas. In each of these areas teams of workers have carried out a census of patients and facilities providing care and proceeded to study pathways of patients in the services (WHO 1977). Routinely available data were used in this investigation, which has resulted in several publications. In another study, data available at national level are being examined to define a minimal set of information necessary to monitor mental health needs for purposes of planning and evaluation of national programmes concerned with mental health (WHO 1979b).

The importance of social and cultural factors in mental health care has been widely recognized but there is little agreement on what data should be collected in community mental health studies and how this should be done. Similarly, the response of communities to major psychosocial problems — such as those related to alcohol consumption — needs careful assessment prior to intervention programmes. A study on community responses to alcohol-related problems is in progress in Mexico, Scotland and Zambia, and preliminary reports indicate how this issue can be approached and what problems are likely to arise in collecting and interpreting such data.

WHO could carry out this work because of the interest in these matters in many quarters and because of the support these activities received from individuals, institutions, and governments of a large number of countries.

This support and the achievements that have resulted also demonstrate the feasibility of joint work in the field of mental health research and its usefulness. Nowhere will collaboration, sharing of knowledge, pooling of experience and mutual help and respect be of greater importance than in this area which is so complex — the evaluation of mental health programmes.

References

Baert, A.E. & Mednick, S.A. (1981): *Prospective longitudinal research: an empirical basis for the primary prevention of psychosocial disorders.* WHO/EURO, Copenhagen. Oxford University Press.

Harding, T.W. (1978): Psychiatry in rural societies. *Psychiat. Annals, 8,* 74-84.

Jones, K.K. & Vischi, T.R. (1979): Impact of alcohol, drug abuse and mental health treatment on medical care utilization. A review of the research literature. Supplement to *Medical Care, 17 (12),* 82.

Kramer, M. (1969): *Applications of mental health statistics: uses in mental health programmes of statistics derived from psychiatric services and selected vital and morbidity records.* WHO, Geneva.

Sand, E.A. & Baro, F. (eds.) (1981): *Evaluation et soins de santé mentale.* Troisième séminaire européen sur les politiques de santé (Luxembourg, 26-28 March 1980). Commission des Communautés européennes, Brussels.

Sartorius, N. (1976): Classification: an international perspective. *Psychiat. Annals, 4,* 359-367.

Sartorius, N. (1980): The research component of the WHO Mental Health Programme. *Psychol. Med., 10,* 175-185.

Sartorius, N., Jablensky, A., Gulbinat, W., & Ernberg, G. (1980): WHO collaborative study: assessment of depressive disorders (preliminary communication). *Psychol. Med. 10,* 743-749.

Wing, J.K., Cooper, J.E. & Sartorius, N. (1974): *The measurement and classification of psychiatric symptoms.* Cambridge University Press, London.

World Health Organization (1975): *Schizophrenia: a multinational study. Public Health Paper No. 63.* WHO, Geneva.

World Health Organization Regional Office for Europe (1977): *Report of a Conference on Mental Health Services in Pilot Study Areas, Lysebu, 1977.* Copenhagen (ICP/MNH/007).

World Health Organization (1978): *Mental disorders: glossary and guide to their classification in accordance with the ninth revision of the International Classification of Diseases.* WHO, Geneva.

World Health Organization (1979a): *Schizophrenia: an international follow-up study.* John Wiley & Sons, Chichester.

World Health Organization (1979b): Report of Third Meeting of Investigators Collaborating in the Project on Monitoring of Mental Health Needs. New Delhi, 1978. Unpublished document, WHO, Geneva.

I: METHODS OF CLASSIFICATION

Principles of 'Multiaxial' Classification in Psychiatry as a Basis of Modern Methodology

P. BERNER and H. KATSCHNIG

1. Introduction

In all branches of medicine, the establishment of a clinical diagnosis generally proceeds in the following way: the *first step* consists in the unbiased collection of the abnormal phenomena which the individual patient exhibits at present (examination data) or has previously shown (anamnestic data). In the *second step* the examiner will screen the identified symptoms in order to choose those which point, independently or in a characteristic combination, to a nosological entity or, more frequently, to several nosological entities. In the latter case, a *third step* becomes necessary in which the differential diagnosis is established by utilizing additional sources of information such as laboratory findings, anamnestic data of exposure to toxic substances, etc.

In psychiatry, the problems involved in the *first step* do not differ essentially from those encountered in other fields of medicine. They concern mainly efficient means of avoiding a biased selective registration of the abnormal phenomena by developing appropriate systems of standardized data recording. During the *second step* toward diagnosis however, psychiatry faces difficulties much less frequently encountered in most of the other medical disciplines, in which the choice of those symptoms to which a diagnostic significance can be attributed is reached on the basis of a *savoir médical* (Debray 1969), a knowledge acquired by medical science on the basis of proven relations between certain symptoms or syndromes and specific aetiologies or pathogeneses. In the case of many mental abnormalities, the significance attributed to symptoms or syndromes cannot be controlled by aetiological or pathogenetic references. The choice of significant symptoms in this step depends on hypothetical nosological entities which vary considerably from school to school. Some of them content themselves with using arbitrarily chosen symptoms or syndromes as hypothetical nosological entities as long as aetiological and pathogenetic research does not provide conflicting evidence. Others attempt meanwhile to find some confirmation of their hypotheses in other areas, such as onset, natural course and outcome, response to different types of treatment, genetic findings, etc. It is obvious that the shortcomings of the second diagnostic step weaken the *third one*. If a psychopathological syndrome is identified by means of a hypothetical nosological entity without the possibility of positive aetiological proof, only the evidence of an aetiology other than the supposed one retains a differential diagnostic value. As aetiology can be asserted in a convincing manner nearly exclusively by somatic findings, differential diagnosis is reduced to the statement that the syndrome stands for the assigned diagnosis except when a plausible causal relation with an organic disturbance is revealed.

This particular situation with regard to diagnosis attributes to 'multi-axial' classification systems in psychiatry a role different from the one they assume in many other medical disciplines, where diagnosis is frequently made on the aetiological 'axis', while other 'axes' may contribute to the clarification of pathoplastic problems, as for instance, whether, how, and to what degree, constitutional or social factors determine the quantity or quality of the symptomatology, the disease course, etc. In psychiatry most of the so-called 'multiaxial' systems are — as Helmchen (1980) points out very clearly — "not a classification of diagnosis in the customary sense, but rather a classification of the elements of diagnosis." Compared with the important role 'multiaxial' classifications play in arriving at psychiatric diagnosis, the coding of pathoplastic influences is, in our discipline, generally relegated to the background.

Experience finally suggests that many illnesses stem from multiple origins, each of which may affect the manifestation, symptomatological shape, severity, natural course of the disorder and therapeutic strategy. Such multiple origins seem to be more frequent in psychiatric disturbances than in many diseases pertaining to other branches of medicine. In our discipline, these origins may additionally belong to different types of influences, which in some systems can be recorded on different 'axes', but may be mutually exclusive in other diagnostic systems, thus leading to the loss of information.

2. The aims to be attained by so-called 'multiaxial' classifications

The classification systems on hand serve — more or less explicitly and to different extents — several, and sometimes even divergent, purposes such as:

— *classification of diagnoses*
— *diagnosis attainment* by classifying necessary elements
— *classification of possible pathoplastic influences* in the broadest sense (not only those which may have an effect on the symptomatology and the natural course of the disorder, but also those which may either quantitatively or qualitatively co-determine the response to therapeutic strategies)
— *recording of possible causal factors* in the case of multiple origins of the disturbance

All these aims are important not only for practical use but also for research and should enable the researcher to *form homogenous populations*.

Helmchen (1980) has instructively reviewed the 'axes' employed by the most frequently used systems in order to cope with these various purposes and the principal difficulties confronting them. According to Helmchen, the *minimal requirement* met in all reviewed classifications would be the utilization of at least two independent 'axes', one for clinical descriptive symptomatology and the other for aetiology. *Problems* arise concerning the clinical validity and practicability (diagnosis versus elements of diagnosis: "The more differentiated the system and the more explicit the rules of assignment, the less it is a classification in the customary sense, but rather a classification of the elements of a diagnosis.") and the coding of time-dependency (state versus trait), of severity (qualitative versus quantitative criteria) and of certainty. Furthermore, the author stresses problematic issues in strategy, for instance: which of the various proposed axes are meaningful for the majority of cases, or whether a free combination of syndromes and aetiologies will lead to an undesirable confusion in international, nosological diagnostic customs. Helmchen completes his review by defining six major directions to be observed in *developing and improving the* actual *'multiaxial' approaches* (Strauss & Helmchen, unpublished manuscript):

1. Improving reliability
2. Improving validity
3. The management of multiple 'axes' in terms of their relative importance, and data processing generally
4. Maximizing cross-national acceptability
5. Developing new 'axes' to represent areas of importance not previously covered
6. Developing the conceptual implications of 'multiaxial' diagnosis.

It is not possible in a short introductory statement to discuss all these issues and develop them extensively with regard to research. We shall, therefore, limit our considerations to some aspects of primary importance, namely to a *critical evaluation of the logical consistency of the systems* presently used and to the problem of achieving diagnosis, which is closely linked to that of the formation of homogenous populations.

3. 'Multi-area' classification (MAC)

Up to now we have used the expression 'so-called multiaxial classification' because, as a matter of fact, only very few of the many proposed or used 'axes' actually merit this name as they do not represent real dimensions (Helmchen 1980). They are not even categories in the strict sense of the term, in that they designate the most general form to which a given fact or object logically pertains. A rough survey of the systems under discussion easily proves this point. Most of these are mere 'fields', or better, 'spheres' or 'areas', out of which information is filtered, and which the inventor of the system considers relevant and of importance for the purpose the classification is to serve.

We would, therefore, advocate the abandonment of the incorrect terms 'multiaxial', 'multidimensional' and 'multicategorical' and their replacement by the term *multi-area classification (MAC).*

The argument raised against such a change of nomenclature, namely that in the meantime, the term 'multiaxial' has become widely used, does not seem a very convincing one. Apart from the fact that many authors already prefer the term 'multidimensional systems' there is no merit in perpetuating inappropriate and misleading terms only because they were once introduced without sufficient reflection as to their meaning.

As the attainment of diagnosis is only one aspect of the systems on hand, we would suggest the general use of the all-inclusive term of 'classification' instead. To speak of a 'multi-area diagnosis' seems justified only if this diagnosis relies on information stemming from two or more different areas, as is the case for example in the utilization of the St. Louis Diagnostic Criteria (Feighner *et al* 1972), which for the diagnosis of a primary affective disorder requires a combination of certain symptoms on the psychopathological, somatic and biorhythmical level and a certain duration of the disturbance.

It has become apparent that many of the so-called 'multiaxial' systems in use mainly represent combinations of 'areas' and seldom contain true 'axes', such as the intelligence quotient when covering the field of general intelligence (see Fig. 1). The same can be said for the subdivision of the areas constituting the elements of the system. Some of them do contain dimensions of various attributes, but the number and graduation of these frequently differ in the separate subdivisions, ranging from very rough scalings such as mild, medium or severe to quite subtle ones. Others are composed of 'sub-fields' which again vary in number from one area to another and are sometimes used in an additive manner where, for example, five out of eight items must be present — or are mutually exclusive when, for instance, only one item may be recorded.

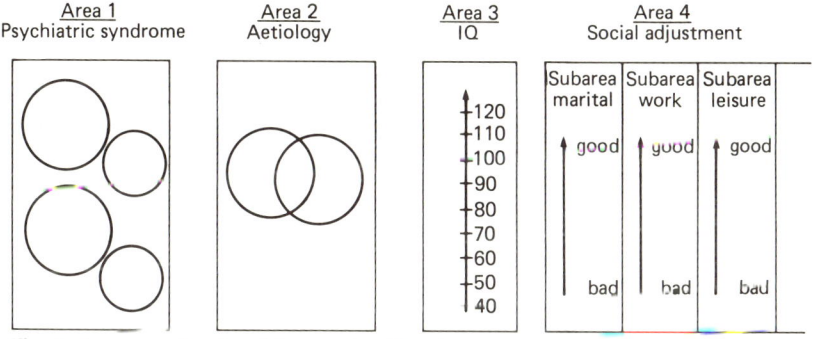

Fig. 1. An example of multi-area classification.

It is obvious that such inconsistencies are inherent in the complexity of the problems we have to face, but we should not lose sight of the fact illustrated by the described discrepancies that coding in one area might be quite different from that in another. Efforts to balance the statements deduced from the codings should, therefore, be more systematic.

4. The poly-diagnostic approach (PDA)

In the classical method still frequently employed in the attainment of diagnosis, which proceeds without the use of rating scales, the first step, namely the unbiased compilation of anamnestic and examination data, is practically always neglected. In his search for significant symptoms and syndromes, the examiner generally begins immediately by screening the abnormal phenomena exhibited by the individual patient. The selection of symptoms underlying this process depends on the *savoir médical* of the examiner. Selection is thus swayed by the entry, in an uncontrolled manner, of certain unclearly reflected criteria and the results remain inexplicit in many aspects.

Whereas rating scales, constituting the first step towards diagnosis, eliminate a biased attitude from the very beginning of the interview, modern diagnostic classifications attempt to reach a more explicit and uniform procedure in the second step by setting out the criteria requested for the establishment of diagnosis. The relevant criteria are contained either in glossaries (ICD 9) or in the diagnostic manuals themselves (DSM III). These criteria encompass information from different sources and different kinds of present and previous psychopathology, duration of the abnormalities, quantitative considerations, somatic findings, psychic and somatic influences and conditions determining the diagnostic choice (such as psycho-social stress or intoxication, etc.), time relations (for instance between psychic and somatic pathology or stress and pathology) — and so forth.

A considerable amount of time and effort has been devoted to the task of achieving an agreement on these criteria and thus an approach to conformity in diagnosis. The introduction of various diagnostic systems, however, emphasizes the fact that such an agreement is possible only on the basis of compromise, calling upon the many collaborators involved in this enterprise to sacrifice some of the elements of their own diagnostic models. The need to attain conformity for statistical purposes on a worldwide scale cannot be denied and strongly encourages such a compromise.

Different research workers or schools may, however, at any time feel the need for certain modifications of the diagnostic criteria imposed by the established classification system, because the necessity to change diagnostic customs in accordance with new scientific insights, regardless of whether they be right or wrong, must not be neglected. Reviews of broadly used classifications nevertheless take a considerable amount of time and involve compromises which engaged researchers would not willingly accept. The assurance therefore, that their arguments will be considered in the next version of an established classification pattern does not alleviate matters, so that it cannot be very surprising that they introduce their own systems for the time being. In order to overcome these difficulties we would propose, for research purposes, the replacement of the 'compromise procedure' by a *poly-diagnostic approach (PDA)*.

As many schools rely on different elements in order to reach diagnosis and as these elements stem from different 'fields', those can be included as 'areas' in 'multi-area classifications'. In other words: a research worker interested in comparing his results with the findings attained by one or several others should introduce the primary information from which those researchers draw the elements of their diagnoses as areas in his own multi-area classification, thus enlarging it to a tool capable of producing diagnoses based on different modes of attainment.

In our research programme on the Course and Classification of Endogenous Psychoses (Berner, Gabriel, Katschnig, Küfferle and Lenz), we use a poly-diagnostic approach in order to reach comparability between various methods of diagnosis, as in the study of Brockington *et al* (1978). Our purpose is to test their underlying hypotheses and would provide an appropriate example. All patients are rated with an extended version of the Present State Examination (Wing *et al* 1974) and the Süllwold Scale for schizophrenic basic symptoms (Süllwold 1977). In addition, the presence or absence of criteria for schizophrenia according to Bleuler ("basic symptoms", Bleuler 1911), to Schneider ("first rank symptoms", 1959), to the St. Louis Criteria (Feighner *et al* 1972), to the Research Diagnostic Criteria (Spitzer *et al* 1978), and to our own classification system ("schizophrenic axial syndrome", Berner 1979) is recorded. For the identification of differently formulated affective syndromes our method contains rating possibilities for Feighner's diagnostic criteria for depression and mania (1972) as well as for our own criteria ("cyclothymic axial syndrome", Berner 1979). Additionally it encompasses the elements needed to establish an ICD-diagnosis.

Table 1 presents by way of example the first 21 patients examined in the

Table 1.

Case code	Bleuler (basic symptoms)	Schneider (first-rank symptoms)	Feighner	RDC	Berner (Schizophrenic axial syndrome)	Berner (cyclothymic axial syndrome)
K 001	X	X		X	X	
K 006	X	X	X	X	X	
K 012	X					
K 013	X	X	X	X	X	
K 023	X	X		X	X	
K 040	X	X				
S 002	X	X	X	X		
S 007	X	X	X	X	X	
S 009	X	X	X	X		
S 010	X	X	X	X		
S 011	X	X	X	X	X	
S 012	X	X	X			
S 018	X	X	X	X	X	
S 020	X	X	X	X	X	
S 024	X	X	X	X	X	
S 026	X	X	X			X
S 030	X	X	X	X		
S 042	X	X		X		X
S 043	X	X	X	X		
S 053	X	X	X		X	
S 059	X	X				
n = 21	21	20	15	14	10	2

above-mentioned research programme who belong to the ICD-category 295.3 (schizophrenic psychoses, paranoid type). Without any attempt at interpretation, which would be beyond the scope of this paper, it demonstrates how a poly-diagnostic approach illustrates the differences and concordances of the compared diagnostic systems.

The need for such a poly-diagnostic approach is based on several reasons: the comparability of results obtained in different research centres by differing diagnostic systems would be increased, making it thus possible to replicate or refute results from previous studies; new diagnostic approaches might thus facilitate the identification of groups more homogenous with regard to course, outcome, treatment response, genetic or biochemical findings, etc., than the classical diagnostic categories.

A typical example of this is the hierarchical use of certain symptoms. In classically Schneider-orientated psychiatric schools (Schneider 1959) first rank symptoms override affective ones and determine the diagnosis and often the treatment as well, especially the application of lithium. Other authors, however (for instance, Pope & Lipinski 1978), claim that there are no known pathognomonic symptoms for schizophrenia, whereas some affective symptoms seem to possess some specificity in differential diagnosis and should thus be dominant in the diagnostic hierarchy. A third tendency postulates that, should first rank symptoms and affective criteria be present at the same time, the state should be labelled 'schizoaffective disorder' (e.g. American Psychiatric Association 1980). Only a systematic comparison will help to decide which of these positions — if any — is right.

Finally a poly-diagnostic approach represents a kind of 'mental exercise' by obliging the diagnosing psychiatrist to think simultaneously in different diagnostic systems, thus enhancing the precision of his thinking and imposing rigour in the definition of psychopathological and other important criteria. This 'mental exercise' reveals the weak points of the different diagnostic systems and shows clearly that many of them are very loosely or insufficiently defined and retain their frequently unquestioned prestige only by linkage with the name of a psychiatrist of high repute. Even in systems boasting well defined diagnostic criteria in one field, definition is frequently not adequate in other areas from which additional elements for the diagnosis are extracted — a fact which often leads to fatal illusions of exactitude.

These considerations lead us to the formulation of two guiding principles for diagnostic procedure:

1. The method of data gathering should be made as 'operational' — which means as precisely described — as possible, in order to be replicable in *each area*.

2. For each diagnostic system it must be clearly defined which elements are obligatory, tolerated and excluded.

Precautions analogous to those formulated for the diagnostic process should, of course, be applied to data methodology in other areas of psychiatric research as well, in order to *form homogenous groups* in a reliable way. For prognosis and outcome research for instance, where other criteria such as social position and treatment modalities play such an important role, the same principles apply.

In practising the poly-diagnostic approach as above proposed, we should have to deal with both the existing explicit multi-area classifications and the much more frequent implicit ones in which information from different areas is utilized for a single diagnosis without allowing either for the reconstruction of the elements or for the way in which the diagnosis in question is reached. Our aim for the future should be to make explicit those elements of diagnosis which are now implicit; and gradually to eliminate any 'diagnosis attainment' which does not lend itself to this process.

References

American Psychiatric Association (1980): DSM III: *Diagnostic and Statistical Manual of Mental Disorders.* 3rd ed., APA, Washington, DC.

Berner, P. (1979): *Psychiatrische Systematik.* Huber Verlag, Bern.

Bleuler, E. (1911): Dementia Praecox oder die Gruppe der Schizophrenien. In Aschaffenburg, G. (ed.): *Handbuch der Psychiatrie.* Deuticke, Leipzig.

Brockington, J.F., Kendell, R.E. & Leff, J.P. (1978): Definitions of schizophrenia: concordance and prediction of outcome. *Psychol. Med., 8,* 387-398.

Debray, H.R. (1969): Echelles d'appréciation: controle et comparaison des diagnostics psychiatriques à l'aide d'ordinateurs. *Confrontations psychiatriques, 4,* 73-86.

Feighner, J.P., Robins, E., Guze, S.B., Woodruff, R.A., Winokur. G. & Munoz, R. (1972): Diagnostic criteria for use in psychiatric research. *Arch. Gen. Psychiatry, 26,* 57-63.

Helmchen, H. (1980): Multiaxial systems of classification. *Acta Psychiatr. Scand., 61,* 43-55.

Pope, H.G. & Lipinski, F. (1978): Diagnosis in schizophrenia and manic depressive illness. *Arch. Gen. Psychiatry, 35,* 811-828.

Rutter, M., Shaffer, D. & Shepherd, M. (1973): An evaluation of proposal for multiaxial classification of child psychiatric disorders. *Psychol. Med., 3,* 244-250.

Schneider, K. (1959): *Clinical Psychopathology.* Grune & Stratton, New York.

Spitzer, R., Endicott, J. & Robins, E. (1978): Research diagnostic criteria: rationale and reliability. *Arch. Gen. Psychiatry, 35,* 773-782.

Strauss, J. & Helmchen, H.: Working paper on multiaxial diagnosis (unpublished manuscript).

Süllwold, L. (1977): *Symptome schizophrener Erkrankungen. Uncharakteristische Basisstörungen.* Springer Verlag, Berlin.

Wing, J.K., Cooper, J.E. & Sartorius, N. (1974): *Measurement and Classification of Psychiatric Symptoms.* An Instruction Manual for the PSE and Catego Programme. Cambridge University Press, London.

World Health Organization (1978): *Mental Disorders: Glossary and Guide to their Classification in Accordance with the Ninth Revision of the International Classification of Diseases.* WHO, Geneva.

Standardized Methods of Classification of Mental Disorders

J. K. WING

1. Introduction

This paper is chiefly concerned with the advantages of introducing a degree of standardization into the processes of psychiatric diagnosis. The term 'diagnosis' refers both to a particular category within a nosological system and to the means whereby a decision is reached that a particular category is the one most appropriate for describing the patient's condition. I shall be concerned mainly with the second of these usages, i.e. with methods of standardizing the processes whereby a clinician collects information from and about patients and then classifies it, using the categories of some established system such as the International Classification of Diseases (WHO, 1978). However, any attempt at operationalization reveals hitherto unsuspected gaps where new categories may be needed, overlaps between categories previously thought to be discrete and, above all, a lack of clarity and precision in the definitions used by clinicians in daily practice. Constructing an operational system that simulates the processes of diagnosis, whatever the nosological classification, therefore requires its designers to use their own clinical judgement whenever there is any doubt. From a clinical point of view, the 'standard' system will have many of the characteristics, both good and bad, of the clinical system it is simulating. There is no way out of this; all that can be claimed is that the designers' judgements are made within the spirit of a given school, and that they are specific, public and amenable to test by others. This claim, however, is a large and important one and lies at the heart of all scientific enquiry.

There is no possibility at the moment of standardizing all the elements in any diagnostic system, nor even of altogether standardizing any one of them. There will always be unforeseen contingencies, complex modifying circumstances, and large gaps in knowledge, particularly in the absence of highly discriminating laboratory tests. In the face of uncertainty, the clinician's judgement, fallible though it is, must be paramount. The techniques I shall discuss are of great value to research workers, but any tendency to use them as substitutes for clinical practice (except through their increasing role in education) is greatly to be deplored.

A final caveat so far as this symposium is concerned: Although my brief is to deal only with matters related to diagnosis, this is only one of the factors, and not always the most important, involved in evaluating the effects of treatment. Some of the instruments I shall mention are useful for measuring change in the type, severity and number of symptoms under various conditions of treatment, as well as providing a data-set on the basis of which standardized classifying rules can operate.

2. Advantages of standardization

The main advantages of standardization for scientific research are that it increases our ability to make comparisons between samples, allows more rigorous testing of biological, psychological and social hypotheses, and provides opportunities to analyse the way that clinical diagnoses are made. There are also advantages for clinical education and practice, but these do not come within the scope of the present symposium. Discussion of any particular technique of standardization is pointless without consideration of the particular purposes for which it was constructed. By the same token, any instrument which is used outside these limits loses its advantages.

2.1 Achieving comparability in clinical research

Clinical research, like any other branch of science, depends on replication. Unless the criteria for diagnosis are stated with sufficient clarity and precision to allow at least approximate reproducibility, it is impossible to be sure whether the results of a study by one group of workers have been confirmed or falsified by results obtained elsewhere. This is true whether the studies are descriptive, epidemiological or experimental. Many of the controversies in psychiatry arise and are perpetuated because of comparisons arising out of non-comparable results. This is true of all the elements in the research procedure, but we are particularly concerned with the description and classification of clinical disorders. The problem will not be solved simply by showing overall reliability between the members of one small research team, who may belong to the same clinical school and share each other's clinical concepts and practices or acquire those of the team leader. It is necessary for workers from a different psychiatric 'subculture' to be able to replicate, as closely as is currently feasible, the diagnostic procedures of the first group. For the purposes of scientific work, it is necessary to try to see through the eyes of the original workers. This requires both training and a willingness to be trained.

2.2 Testing hypotheses

The chief advantage of standardizing the description and classification of clinical disorders is that hypotheses can be subjected to more rigorous tests. In clinical research, these hypotheses are chiefly concerned with the pathology, causes, precipitation, prevention, treatment and prognosis of named disorders. Whether studies are focussed on brain tomography in alcoholics, the genetics of early childhood autism, the precipitation of depressive disorders by environmental events or circumstances, the treatment or prevention of attacks of schizophrenia by medication, or the epidemiology of 'minor neurotic disorders' in people who have not been referred to specialist services, the scientific community will be better able to replicate the procedures and evaluate the results in proportion to the extent that the clinical phenomena measured, including the diagnosis, are reproducible.

This statement is based on a particular view of what has come to be known as 'the medical model', one that avoids inflexibility and makes explicit the advantages of disease theories in elucidating and helping to ameliorate some of the miseries of mankind (Wing 1978).

2.3 Understanding clinical classifications

There are several ways in which current clinical nosologies can be better understood, and potentially, therefore, can be improved, by using standardized systems, apart from the simple but vital fact that specifying some of the rules lays them open to inspection and criticism. Some of these advantages can be illustrated by reference to recent investigations:

(a) Comparing the diagnoses made by a clinician and the 'reference classification' derived by applying a set of standardized procedures can give rise to interesting questions when trying to explain discrepancies. There are several examples in chapter 11 of the first volume of the report on the *International Pilot Study of Schizophrenia* (WHO 1973). One illustrates the possibility that new categories might be needed that are not at present available in the ICD.

Another intriguing observation was that there was general agreement between the reference classification and diagnosis of schizophrenic and paranoid psychoses made in seven of the nine participating centres, while in the other two (Moscow and Washington) there was a substantial discrepancy, a clinical diagnosis of schizophrenia often being made when the reference classification suggested some other condition. The similar observation made in the USA-UK Diagnostic Project (Cooper *et al* 1972) indicates that the discrepancy must be taken seriously and, indeed, it is fair to say that studies of this type have contributed to recent changes in diagnostic practice in the United States, particularly to the construction of the third edition of the *Diagnostic and Statistical Manual* (DSM III) of the American Psychiatric Association (1980).

(b) Other studies using standardized systems have emphasized the problems involved when making single versus double diagnoses. What, for example, are the advantages and disadvantages of classifying anxiety and depressive symptoms, when they occur together, as one disorder (e.g. 'neurotic depression') compared with allocating two classes? This issue has arisen in recent population surveys using standardized as well as clinical classifications (Finlay-Jones *et al* 1981; Wing *et al* 1981) and has not yet been resolved. An analogous question concerns the classification of disorders characterized by schizophrenic as well as severe depressive or manic symptoms. Only by further specification of alternative methods of classification can the questions of validity be adequately investigated. Attempts to study such problems without following these principles only muddle the issues further.

(c) A further, though possibly somewhat in-bred, opportunity created by the construction of different standardized systems is that they can be compared with each other. The reason why such an exercise might be profitable is that some of the systems represent very different clinical schools of thought and the reasons for discrepancies between the results of applying them to the same clinical material are precisely identifiable. There have been no serious studies of this type so far although the time is now ripe for them. The USA-UK Diagnostic Project employed a standardized examination based on two instruments, one European, the other American (the latter now obsolescent), both designed to elicit and record clinical symptoms. One comparative exercise was published (Fleiss *et al* 1971) but there was no detailed comparison between classifications.

Eventually, it will be possible to compare operationalized nosologies, like DSM III, and operationalized versions of the ICD, perhaps in its tenth revision. The results would be of great value when future systems come to be constructed.

(d) Because standardized systems must include specific definitions of disorders, it should be possible for them also to delineate 'non-disorders'. In fact, this possibility has not been deliberately investigated, except in one system (Wing 1976; Wing *et al* 1981) in which threshold points are drawn, below which the numbers or types of symptoms are inadequate to allow classification. Investigation of the sub-threshold area is of particular interest, particularly for liaison psychiatry and for primary medical care.

(e) Finally, standardized systems can be used to investigate the hierarchical element, or other structure, in various nosologies. This interesting possibility will be explored in a later section.

3. Methodological problems

In order to exploit the advantages of standardization it is necessary to accept certain limitations. Only within these limits can the advantages be gained and it is, therefore, necessary to specify them whenever an instrument is constructed. This principle is readily accepted in the case of a telescope or micrometer. It is often ignored in our own field. Many instruments, each with its own specification, are required if all the elements in the process of diagnosis are to be given a degree of standardization.

3.1 Algorithms

The most obvious feature of a standardized classification is an algorithm or set of pre-determined rules laid down with such precision that they can be incorporated into a computer program. Some limited progress has been made in the Glossary to ICD 9 towards supplying definitions for the diagnoses included (WHO 1978) but these can hardly be called operational. The criteria specified by Feighner and his colleagues (1972), subsequently modified and expanded into the Research Diagnostic Criteria (RDC) of Spitzer *et al* (1978) and then, with further elaboration and input from many sources, developed into DSM III (American Psychiatric Association 1980), provide better examples. These criteria may, however, be used in two quite different ways. DSM III, for example, is an official clinical nosology designed to be used by clinicians in the same way as ICD 9 (into which its categories are said to be convertible). The guidance given in DSM III is more fully operationalized, but clinicians can allocate disorders to its various categories without the aid of any further standardization. Indeed, this is how it will ordinarily be used. Very little information is yet available on the reliability with which the rules can be used in the varying circumstances of practice in different parts of the world. There ought to be some advantage over the ICD 9 Glossary, even if small, but this remains to be demonstrated.

However, the rules in DSM III are explicit enough to be applied to a database collected in a much more specific and standardized way. Several attempts have been made to standardize the collection of a reliable data set that will be sufficient, when algorithms are applied, to allocate each case to one or more 'diagnostic' classes.

As we have seen, such attempts cannot possibly cover all contingencies. Each of the elements in the process needs separate attention before we can consider what progress has been made toward standardizing the multidimensional systems discussed by Berner and Katschnig.

3.2 Present clinical state

Most advance has been made in standardizing the collection and recording of symptoms shown at interview with a patient in an acute episode of psychiatric disorder. Two of the best-known instruments are described by Woggon (AMDP) and Cronholm (CPRS). Others are the Present State Examination (Wing *et al* 1974) and the Diagnostic Interview Schedule (Robins *et al* 1981). All have been widely used and it is important that the experience gained should be pooled so that further advances can be made.

I shall not consider here single-category scales such as the Beck or Hamilton, although they are very useful for their purpose, since they do not incorporate standard criteria for a differential classification, but require a particular category of cases to be selected before they are applied.

The most completely standardized system requires:

(a) A glossary of differential definitions of symptoms — itself a miniature classification;

(b) A standardized procedure for conducting the interview, with guidance on how to proceed if various contingencies arise;

(c) A decision on the time period to be covered;

(d) Ratings of the adequacy of the interview;

(e) Rules for coding the symptoms present and their severity.

Data have been given showing the reliability of the various systems. As would be expected, this is reasonably high, between trained interviewers, for groups of symptoms, but can be quite low for individual items. In particular, behaviour and speech are more difficult to rate during the relatively brief time sample afforded by an interview. Observations over a longer period using behaviour rating scales, or techniques specifically devised to measure abnormalities of speech, may be used as a supplement.

Repeated interviews may be necessary if the first one is inadequate and information from other sources (e.g. case-records and other informants) may need to be collected in the same format. Then it is necessary to devise rules for combining the information from several interviews.

3.3 Present episode

If the present episode of disorder extends beyond the period covered by the 'present state' examination, a judgement is required as to whether symptoms have occurred that affect the current classification. Case-records and other informants may have to be consulted. The PSE-CATEGO system allows for this by providing a Syndrome Check List (SCL), derived from the PSE symptom list, which can be used as input to the same computer algorithms. In the IPSS, a narrative case-history supplied for each patient was used to rate relevant symptoms in the present episode with a fair degree of reliability.

3.4 Past episodes

The same considerations apply to past episodes of disorder, with the additional problem that the date of onset and offset of each episode may have to be specified. Unless good case-records are available, the further back in time the disorder stretches, the more doubtful both dates and content become and the more difficult it is to decide how much to include in an overall classification. This is particularly true of the neuroses; indeed the threshold problem may be impossible to overcome on the basis of a subjective account.

3.5 Pathology and aetiology

The standardization of data concerned with possible pathology and aetiology will not be considered here. A coding problem, however, is very relevant. For example, in the case of 'alcoholic hallucinosis' (ICD 291.3), a schizophrenic or paranoid state otherwise classifiable as such is converted to the diagnosis by a clinical judgement that alcohol is somehow causal. If it is not, alcohol abuse may be coded as a second diagnosis. Simply making this judgement explicit reduces much coding error. However, very specific criteria can be laid down, as in DSM III, where alcoholic hallucinosis may only be diagnosed if the hallucinosis follows, within three days, withdrawal from alcohol by someone already dependent.

Even without this degree of specificity, however, the clinician can be presented with the necessity to make the judgement as to whether the alcohol intake or withdrawal caused the hallucinosis, and this, in itself, removes some very common coding errors. In the PSE-CATEGO system, the Aetiology Schedule presents a number of forced choices of this kind, applicable to symptoms rated in the present state (PSE) or, separately, in each previous episode (SCL).

These principles apply also to psychological and social causes of symptomatic episodes. There are techniques of rating the presence, for example, of recent adverse life events, which might be regarded as contributing to causation. There is no reason, in principle, why a set of rules should not be laid down defining how they are to be taken into account in classification. The fact that, in practice, it might be difficult to find wide agreement as to how this should be done, does not detract from the value for research purposes of such an exercise if the research worker wishes to test hypotheses regarding such a classification compared with others.

3.6 Other clinical data

In addition to the elements discussed so far, clinicians take many other factors into account when reaching a diagnosis.

One of the most important is the nature and degree of any chronic impairment that persists between more clear-cut symptomatic episodes. There are two quite different kinds of measurement problem. One is the specification of standards of social behaviour when opportunities and expectations vary markedly from one society or social group to another. The other is the differentiation of what, in relatively 'poor' social performance, is due to specific psychological impairments, such as, for example, the cognitive slowness or thought disorder common in schizophrenia. These two problems are further confounded when we consider the evidence that environmental factors may influence the severity and duration of impairments. Thus the same individual may appear relatively unimpaired in one setting, but quite severely impaired in another. One of the most obvious examples can occur when social performance in structured day centres is compared with that of the same individual in a less structured setting such as a hostel.

Some progress has been made in constructing methods of measuring hypothetical impairments or vulnerability to particular social or psychological pressures. For example, the negative 'symptoms' often associated with chronic schizophrenia have been shown, in certain studies, to have some predictive value over quite long periods of time and to be useful in assessing the outcome of different forms of treatment or care. This progress is important for the theme of this symposium, but it has not so far proved very helpful in making a diagnosis when more discriminating symptoms are absent. This is less important in a multiaxial system since such factors can be recorded independently.

Other factors in diagnosis that raise somewhat similar problems are personality disorders and intellectual level. It is always important, because of the large gaps left by standardized procedures, to write a clinical narrative covering the history and course of the condition.

In discussing these elements of the diagnostic process we have also considered very briefly most of the factors likely to be used in a multiaxial system. Several difficult problems are solved if it is decided to deal with each factor separately without trying to reach an overall classification. For example, there is considerable diversity of practice as to how to diagnose a patient who no longer has active schizophrenic symptoms but who is not performing as well socially as before. Is this still 'schizophrenia' or not? Placing present symptomatic state on one axis, past symptomatic states on a second, and changed social performance on a third provides all the relevant information and avoids confusion, but it also avoids a decision. Alternative hypotheses can be tested, but without knowledge of the clinician's view. It may, therefore, be necessary to make both a multiaxial assessment and an overall diagnosis.

Much depends on the purpose of the investigation. In the first case, separate algorithms need to be provided for the standardized data collected on each axis and a 'diagnosis' becomes a profile of classes rather than a single class. Certainly, when evaluating the effects of methods of rehabilitation or care on chronic conditions, the clinical classification of the initial episode is of less interest than longer-term impairments, social performance and environmental circumstances.

3.7 A hierarchical element in classification

Most experience has been gained with rules for classifying symptomatic episodes, particularly, of course, the present episode, but here too there is the question of how many classes to aim at. This raises the further question of whether there is a natural hierarchy according to which symptoms should be placed in order of diagnostic precedence. Many clinicians do use such weightings although there is some difference as to the actual order. Sensorial changes are usually placed at the top, but some clinicians would place characteristic schizophrenic symptoms next, while others would give psychotic affective symptoms higher precedence. Either way, an algorithm can be constructed to simulate the practice and study its concomitants. So far, research workers have tended to concentrate on one system of weights only, but there is no reason, in principle, why more than one set of algorithms should not be constructed so long as the data-base is adequate.

At the lower end of the hierarchy, it is generally agreed that symptoms such as worrying or irritability are non-specific. At a slightly higher level, the mixture of depressed mood (without features such as subjective anergia, pathological guilt or retardation) and anxiety, found quite frequently in people who have not contacted specialist services, can less obviously be grouped within one class. Once again there is no reason why both a combined and a double classification should not be derived and tested.

This latter example can be used also to illustrate the way that algorithms must depend on the data they work upon. Some anxiety symptoms may cause depression, as when an individual housebound by phobias becomes depressed by the concomitant limitation of activities. On the other hand, some depressive symptoms, such as waking early in the morning dreading what the day will bring, take the form of anxiety. Unless such symptoms are carefully defined and recorded, no set of rules can take them into account. This principle holds true throughout the whole field of standardization dealt with in this paper.

The possibility that a natural hierarchy may exist even within the symptoms found in general population samples is suggested by a recent study in London in which rare symptoms such as pathological guilt were found to be associated with a much higher total symptom count than common 'symptoms' such as worrying (Sturt 1981).

3.8 Comprehensive versus specific instruments

It is not necessary, in every investigation, to use a comprehensive battery of standardized instruments, even if such a battery had been constructed and shown to be feasible, reliable in trained hands and useful. The simplest instrument that will do the job is the one to use. In a study of phobias of flying, or noise sensitivity, or anorexia nervosa, it may not be necessary to try to generalize the results beyond the immediate series.

However, where a differential diagnosis is important and where it would be useful to indicate that the results might have applicability within centres where diagnostic practices are known to be different, and at the least deserve replication, it is important to use methods that can be readily understood and copied elsewhere. It may then be convenient to adopt a procedure which standardizes several elements of the diagnostic process, since this not only provides a greater standardization, but also gives symptom profiles and scores.

For example, a study of the effects of pharmacotherapy in schizophrenia requires (a) a selection of patients according to specific criteria including diagnosis, (b) a standard classification, (c) comparison of clinical and reference classifications. This third step can take the form of matching clinical to reference class and also of comparing symptom profiles. The purpose is not to decide which is 'right' — that is not a useful question to ask in such a context — but to compare the clinical diagnoses with those made in other centres where the reference procedure has been used.

The Present State Examination, with its associated Glossary of differential symptom definitions, its Syndrome Check List for previous episodes and Aetiology Schedule, together with its computer programs — the Index of Definition and CATEGO — is one such package (Wing *et al* 1974; Wing & Sturt 1978), one moreover which has had extensive use throughout the world (Wing 1980). The Diagnostic Interview Schedule (Robins *et al* 1981) is another, more recent, introduction, aimed chiefly at deriving lifetime DSM III diagnoses.

It is, of course, feasible to add modules to a set of instruments which need be used only in studies with a particular focus, each covering, for example, an area of symptomatology such as phobias, obsessions, psychosomatic symptoms, thought disorder, symptoms occurring mainly in certain sub-cultures, sensorial changes, etc. The common core of the instrument would contain some items relevant to each of these areas, but with an optional cut-off point. Several instruments currently used already adopt this format in part.

However, I should re-emphasize that I do not think any set of techniques can ever cover all the contingencies likely to occur in clinical practice or substitute for clinical responsibility.

4. Future developments

I have not attempted to compare and contrast the various techniques now available for structuring and making more comparable the processes involved in clinical diagnoses. Several of these are promising and have been used sufficiently widely to demonstrate their uses and limitations. There is much to be gained from a plurality of further developments since there are many problems yet to be solved and the diversity of clinical practice throughout the world will not tolerate the imposition of a single solution, no matter how comprehensive. Moreover, fresh approaches, such as that recently proposed by Scharfetter (1981), might indicate new avenues for progress in future.

However, the exercise now being undertaken by the World Health Organization, in which instruments, algorithms and local sub-sections of diagnostic systems are being brought together and considered by a multinational group, should provide a new impetus to instrument development. Eventually, of course, we shall be able to rely far more than we can now on laboratory investigations and psychological tests that probe more deeply than a descriptive approach can do. But even these much-needed advances will depend to a considerable degree on the clarity with which we can state and therefore test hypotheses concerning the causation and treatment of clinical syndromes. That is the case for further work on standardization.

References

American Psychiatric Association (1980): DSM III: *Diagnostic and Statistical Manual of Mental Disorders*. 3rd ed. APA, Washington, DC.

Cooper, J.E., Kendell, R.E., Gurland, B.J., Sharpe, L., Copeland, J.R.M. & Simon, R. (1972): *Psychiatric Disorder in New York and London*. Oxford University Press, London.

Feighner, J.P., Robins, E., Guze, S.B., Woodruff, R.A., Winokur, G. & Munoz, R. (1972): Diagnostic criteria for use in psychiatric research. *Arch. Gen. Psychiatry, 26,* 57-63.

Finlay-Jones, R., Brown, G.W., Duncan-Jones, P., Harris, T., Murphy, E. & Prudo, R. (1981): Depression and anxiety in the community: replicating the diagnosis of a case. *Psychol. Med., 10,* 445-454.

Fleiss, J.L., Gurland, B.J. & Cooper, J.E. (1971): Some contributions to the measurement of psychopathology. *Br. J. Psychiatry, 119,* 647-656.

Robins, L.N., Helzer, J.E., Croughan, J.L. & Ratcliff, K. (1981): The NIMH Diagnostic Interview Schedule: its history, characteristics and validity. In Wing, J.K., Bebbington, P., Robins, L.N. (eds.): *'What is a Case?' The Problem of Definition in Community Psychiatric Surveys*. Grant McIntyre, London.

Scharfetter, C. (1981): Subdividing the functional psychoses: a family hereditary approach. *Psychol. Med., 11,* 637-640.

Spitzer, R.L., Endicott, J. & Robins, E. (1978): Research Diagnostic Criteria: rationale and reliability. *Arch. Gen. Psychiatry, 35,* 773-782.

Sturt, E. (1981): Hierarchical patterns in the distribution of psychiatric symptoms. *Psychol. Med., 11,* 783-794.

WHO (1973): *The International Pilot Study of Schizophrenia*. WHO, Geneva.

WHO (1978): *Mental Disorders: Glossary and Guide to their Classification in Accordance with ICD 9*. WHO, Geneva.

Wing, J.K., Cooper, J.E. & Sartorius, N. (1974): *Measurement and Classification of Psychiatric Symptoms*. Cambridge University Press, London.

Wing, J.K. (1976): A technique for studying psychiatric morbidity in in-patient and out-patient series and in general population samples. *Psychol. Med., 6,* 665-671.

Wing, J.K. (1978): *Reasoning about Madness*. Oxford University Press, London.

Wing, J.K., Mann, S.A., Leff, J.P. & Nixon, J.N. (1978): The concept of a 'case' in psychiatric population surveys. *Psychol. Med., 8,* 203-217.

Wing, J.K. & Sturt, E. (1978): *The PSE-ID-CATEGO System: Supplementary Manual*. Institute of Psychiatry, London.

Wing, J.K. (1980): Methodological issues in psychiatric case-identification. *Psychol. Med., 10,* 5-10.

Wing, J.K., Bebbington, P., Hurry, J. & Tennant, C. (1981): The prevalence in the general population of disorders familiar to psychiatrists in hospital practice. In Wing, J.K., Bebbington, P., Robins, L.N. (eds.): *'What is a Case?' The Problem of Definition in Community Psychiatric Surveys*. Grant McIntyre, London.

The Significance of Biological Factors in the Diagnosis of Depressions

H.M. VAN PRAAG

I. Biochemical Variables

1. Biological factors of an aetiological and of a pathogenetic nature

Diagnosis is the sensible classification of disease symptoms and their causes. I emphasize 'sensible'. A sensible classification is one that leads to more or less reliable conclusions about the type of treatment to be instituted and about the prognosis of the disease.

Do we know of biological factors of significance in the diagnosis of depressions? The answer to this question is a cautious 'yes', adding that prospects seem promising. Before I elucidate this, a few remarks may be made about the restrictions I impose upon myself.

Biological factors can contribute to the development of behaviour disorders in two fundamentally different ways. To begin with, they may be part of what I call the *pathogenesis* of a given syndrome. I define pathogenesis as the complex of cerebral prerequisites for the development of disturbed behaviour: in other words, as the constellation of cerebral functional disturbances which make disturbed behaviour instrumentally possible (van Praag 1969, 1971). Causative factors of a pathogenetic nature are, therefore, biological factors by definition.

Secondly, biological factors can contribute to the development of the pathogenetic process. Examples are: a traumatic head injury; a primarily extracerebral disease with a secondary influence on certain cerebral functions; a primordially marginal enzyme system. The factors that give rise to the pathogenetic process are what I call *aetiological* factors. They are of heterogeneous 'substance', and may be of a biological as well as of a psychological or psychosocial nature.

I do not intend to discuss biological factors of an aetiological nature, for their diagnostic significance is self-evident. In a case of hyperaesthetic-emotional symptoms it is important to know whether there is a history of head injury; in a case of depressiveness and apathy we want to know whether the thyroid is hypofunctional. These are two examples among many. I confine myself to biological variables of (suspected) pathogenetic significance.

A second restriction is that I confine myself to chemical variables, leaving physiological variables undiscussed. This paper focusses on biochemical variables, while hormonal variables will be discussed in part II.

2. Points of crystallization

Until now the central monoamine (MA) metabolism has been the focus of research into biochemical determinants of depressive behaviour. The reason is that the traditional antidepressants — tricyclic compounds as well as monoamine oxidase (MAO) inhibitors — increase the availability of MA at the central neuronal receptors. Since MAs function as neurotransmitters, the neuronal activity in MA-ergic systems should thus be enhanced. This led to the so-called MA hypothesis, which holds that a functional *deficiency* of one or several MAs plays a role in the pathogenesis of the type of depression susceptible to treatment with agents of this kind. Generally speaking, this type of depression is the vital depression — a *syndrome* usually described in Anglo-American literature under the heading 'endogenous depression' or 'primary depression' (van Praag 1976). Most members of the so-called second generation of antidepressants also potentiate central MA. The influence of antidepressants on postsynaptic MA receptors has received much attention in the past few years. However, it has remained uncertain whether the effects observed are primary effects or a result of increased availability of MA in the synaptic cleft.

The MA hypothesis generated the momentum for research into biochemical variables of possible significance in the diagnosis of depressions. The three principal MAs in the brain are serotonin (5-hydroxytryptamine, 5-HT), noradrenaline (NA) and dopamine (DA). Their principal metabolites are 5-hydroxyindol acetic acid (5-HIAA), 3-methoxy-4-hydroxyphenyl glycol (MHPG) and homovanillic acid (HVA), respectively. I shall discuss these three metabolic systems separately, always from a diagnostic point of view.

3. Serotonin metabolism
3.1 5-HIAA in cerebrospinal fluid (CSF)

Both in the brain and in the periphery, 5-HIAA is the principal metabolite of 5-HT. Transport of 5-HIAA from the blood to the CNS is virtually zero. The 5-HIAA concentration in the CNS, including the CSF, is therefore a function of 5-HT metabolism in the CNS. Some 5-HIAA is transported to the blood stream directly, and some via the CSF. Probenecid inhibits the transport of 5-HIAA from the CNS to the blood stream, and consequently 5-HIAA accumulates in the CNS. The 5-HIAA concentration in CSF after probenecid adminstration reflects the 5-HT metabolism in the CNS more faithfully than does the baseline concentration. The procedure of the so-called probenecid test has been described in detail elsewhere (van Praag 1977a).

In 1971, van Praag and Korf reported that the group of vital depressions includes a subgroup of patients in whom post-probenecid 5-HIAA accumulation is diminished. This phenomenon indicates reduced 5-HT turnover in the CNS. On this ground they postulated the existence of two pathogenetically different categories of vital depression: one category (subgroup) with, and one without, demonstrable disorders of central 5-H1 metabolism. This observation has meanwhile been corroborated by Åsberg et al (1976a) and Goodwin et al (1978). Jori et al (1975) and Berger et al (1980) found no differences between (small groups of) depressive patients and controls. They compared mean group values. A diminished 5-HIAA concentration in CSF, however, is not a group phenomenon but a subgroup phenomenon. If (subgroup) differences had existed, then the procedure used would have obscured them.

Are disorders of central 5-HT metabolism of significance for the treatment to be instituted and for the prognosis of the depression?

3.2 CSF 5-HIAA: therapeutic significance

5-HT precursors. If central 5-HT disorders are of importance in the pathogenesis of vital depressions, then enhancement of 5-HT availability in the brain can be expected to have a therapeutic effect. This contention prompted us to test 1-5-HTP therapeutically in vital depressions (van Praag et al 1972, 1974; van Praag 1979). 5-HTP is a 5-HT precursor rapidly converted to 5-HT in the CNS. This substance was given in combination with a peripheral decarboxylase inhibitor in order to suppress peripheral conversion of 5-HTP to 5-HT, thus enlarging the 5-HTP supply to the brain. It was established that 5-HTP has an antidepressant potency and that this effect is most pronounced in the subgroup with low CSF 5-HIAA values. The former observation has been repeatedly corroborated (for review: van Praag 1981), but the latter remains to be confirmed.

Tricyclic antidepressants. Within the group of tricyclic antidepressants, nortriptyline is the strongest NA potentiator, while clomipramine (Anafranil) is the strongest 5-HT potentiator. In the brain, increased availability of NA and 5-HT in the synaptic cleft leads to reduction of their respective turnovers in the nerve endings. The reduced turnover is reflected in the decreased concentrations of their metabolites — MHPG and 5-HIAA, respectively — in the CSF. In this context I point out that the principal metabolite of clomipramine — desmethylclomipramine — is pharmacologically active and differs from the mother substance in that it potentiates NA.

Van Praag (1977b) demonstrated a negative correlation between the therapeutic response to clomipramine (225 mg per day) and the pre-treatment CSF 5-HIAA concentration: the lower the latter concentration, the better the chance of a therapeutic effect. Träskman et al (1979) were unable to confirm this observation, but their group of patients was small, the clomipramine dosage low (150 mg) and the plasma concentration accordingly low. They did, however, establish another fact: within the group of patients with low CSF 5-HIAA values, the therapeutic response to clomipramine improved in proportion as the decrease in CSF 5-HIAA concentration during treatment was more marked. This indicates that, in the group of '5-HT-deficient' patients, 5-HT potentiation is a factor correlated to the therapeutic response. This conclusion is supported by the observation that patients with low CSF 5-HIAA values show a poor response to nortriptyline, which is a NA potentiator (Åsberg et al 1972).

In the group of patients with average to high CSF 5-HIAA values, improvement in response to clomipramine correlated with diminution of the CSF MHPG value during treatment. This seems to warrant the postulate that these patients respond to desmethylclomipramine — a clomipramine metabolite which potentiates NA. These findings support the hypothesis that the group of vital depressions comprises a more 5-HT-deficient and a predominantly NA-deficient subgroup (Goodwin et al 1978).

The selective 5-HT reuptake inhibitors now being developed have not yet been used in research into the predictive value of 5-HIAA in the CSF.

Conclusions. There are indications that CSF 5-HIAA has a predictive value for the use of 5-HTP and some tricyclic antidepressants in the treatment of depressions. None of these compounds is truly 5-HT-selective; all influence the catecholamine metabolism as well. This is why these observations do not warrant the conclusion that these compounds derive their therapeutic activity (exclusively) from their serotonergic actions. To warrant this conclusion, research of this type would have to be done with compounds which tend to 100 per cent 5-HT selectivity. Such compounds are available, but have not yet been tested in the context of this problem-definition. Perhaps such testing would be superfluous: this argumentation by no means excludes the possibility that non-MA-ergic effects of antidepressants might play a role in their therapeutic activity.

Lumbar puncture requires a clinical setting and can impose stress on the patient. Moreover, most antidepressants are of the 'broad-spectrum' type: they influence 5-HT-ergic as well as catecholaminergic processes. In view of all this, diagnostic determination of CSF 5-HIAA values is not likely soon to be used on a large scale.

3.3 CSF 5-HIAA: prognostic significance

Risk of recurrence. In the majority of vital depressive patients with diminished CSF 5-HIAA values, these abnormal findings persist after abatement of the depressive phase (van Praag 1977c). This was the first indication that we might be dealing not with a causative but with a predisposing factor, i.e. a factor that enhances the risk of a (vital) depression when the individual is exposed to psychological or somatic stress. Several subsequent observations have demonstrated the plausibility of this hypothesis. For example, the relapse rate in the '5-HT-deficient group' of vital depressions exceeded that in comparable patients without demonstrable central 5-HT disorders (van Praag & De Haan 1979). In a group of healthy test subjects, low CSF 5-HIAA values were found to correlate positively with the incidence of depression in the family (Sedvall *et al* 1980). In a group of patients with rapidly recurrent unipolar and bipolar depressions, long-term enhancement of the amount of 5-HT available in the brain, with the aid of 5-HTP, led to reduction of the relapse rate. The effect was most pronounced in patients with persistently decreased CSF 5-HIAA values (van Praag & De Haan 1980). In unipolar depression, the prophylactic potency of 5-HTP was comparable with that of lithium (van Praag & De Haan 1981).

Suicide risk. There are indications that CSF 5-HIAA values in vital depressions are related not only to the relapse rate but also to the suicidality (Banki *et al* 1981). The relation is a negative one: low 5-HIAA values correlated with high suicidality scores. Moreover, the suicide rate in the '5-HT-deficient' subgroup was found to exceed that in the 'normoserotonergic' subgroup (Åsberg *et al* 1976b; van Praag 1981); this applied in particular to violent suicides (by hanging, wrist-slashing, etc.) (Träskman *et al* 1981). Finally, a group of 119 patients who had attempted suicide were traced after a year: 10 per cent of the '5-HT-deficient' patients had meanwhile committed suicide, but no suicide had occurred in the 'normoserotonergic' group (Träskman *et al* 1981).

Conclusion. At present there are relatively strong indications that, within the group of vital depressions, diminished CSF 5-HIAA values constitute a factor which increases the risk of (a) relapse of the depression, and (b) suicide. This variable is, therefore, of prognostic significance in the tracing of high-risk cases, always assuming that these observations are confirmed by research on a larger scale.

3.4 Plasma tryptophan

The enzyme tryptophan hydroxylase, which converts tryptophan to 5-HTP, is unsaturated. Consequently this conversion increases as the amount of tryptophan available increases. The tryptophan supply is an important regulating factor in 5-HT synthesis. The amount of tryptophan transported to the brain is dependent on two variables. It is directly proportional to the plasma (free) tryptophan concentration, and indirectly proportional to the concentration of amino acids which share the mechanism of transport to the brain with tryptophan. The higher this ratio, the larger the amount of tryptophan transported to the brain, and vice versa (for review: Young & Sourkes 1977).

According to Møller et al (1980), the group of 'endogenous depressions' includes a subgroup with a reduced ratio between tryptophan and 'competing amino acids' in plasma. The absolute concentration of total and free tryptophan was normal. We may assume that a relative deficiency of tryptophan (and therefore of 5-HT) exists in the brain in these patients. The CSF 5-HIAA concentration, by the way, was not determined.

The low-ratio group showed a favourable response to oral administration of l-tryptophan; the response in the normal-ratio group was minimal.

Conclusion. The observations reported by Møller *et al* are promising both in scientific terms — the reduced tryptophan/'competing amino acid' ratio might be a cause of the reduced 5-HT turnover in the brain — and in practical terms. This ratio could perhaps be used to trace the '5-HT-deficient' subtype of vital depression with the aid of a peripheral variable. The good response of low-ratio patients to the 5-HT precursor l-tryptophan lends plausibility to this theory. Whether this variable is of prognostic significance has not been investigated.

4. Catecholamine metabolism
4.1 Urinary MHPG

MHPG is the principal NA metabolite in the CNS; in quantitative terms, vanillylmandelic acid (VMA) is of subordinate importance. In the peripheral nervous system the reverse is the case. The average contribution of the CNS to the total amount of MHPG excreted in urine is estimated to be 63 per cent (Maas *et al* 1979). This is why renal MHPG excretion is regarded as a (gross) measure of the NA metabolism in the CNS.

The first studies of renal MHPG excretion in depressions mentioned a diminished average excretion of this metabolite in a heterogeneous group of depressive patients (Maas *et al* 1968). This might indicate a reduced NA turnover in the CNS. This observation has been corroborated as well as contradicted (for review: Goodwin & Potter 1979). A possible explanation of this discrepancy might be that the group of depressions is heterogeneous in this respect. There are some indications that this explanation makes sense. For example, Goodwin & Post (1975) found that low MHPG excretors are concentrated within two groups: bipolar depressions and schizo-affective psychoses. These findings have been corroborated by others (Schildkraut *et al* 1978; Edwards *et al* 1980). MHPG excretion was decreased as compared with that in (a) a group of depressions not further differentiated, and (b) a group of recurrent non-vital depressions; and it was decreased also as compared with that in (c) the same patient in a manic phase, and (d) a normal control group (Goodwin & Post 1975; Schildkraut *et al* 1978; Post *et al* 1977). When the peripheral contribution to renal MHPG excretion was suppressed with the aid of carbidopa (a peripheral decarboxylase inhibitor), patients with bipolar depressions excreted less MHPG than normal controls (Garfinkel *et al* 1977). This supports the conclusion that reduced renal MHPG excretion is based on diminished central NA turnover.

All this does not take away the fact that there is still uncertainty about the degree of reliability of renal MHPG excretion as an index of central NA turnover. The influence of such factors as physical activity, diet and degree of tenseness on MHPG excretion has not been established with certainty. Most of the available data do indicate, however, that this influence is not very marked and probably cannot explain the above-mentioned phenomenon (for review: Hollister *et al* 1980). It should also be borne in mind that MHPG excretion shows individual day-to-day variations. Separate individual observations are, therefore, inconclusive. Finally, a recent study repudiates the contention that renally excreted MHPG is largely of central origin (Blomberg *et al* 1980).

4.2 Renal MHPG excretion: therapeutic significance

Maas *et al* (1972) found that patients showing a favourable response to imipramine or desipramine had a lower pre-treatment urinary MHPG excretion (<900µg/g creatinine) than non-responders (>1350µg/g creatinine). For the response to amitriptyline, the reverse was reported (Schildkraut *et al* 1978): the pre-treatment excretion in responders exceeded 1590 µg MHPG/g creatinine; patients with a lower excretion failed to improve. Beckman & Goodwin (1975) confirmed these findings: imipramine responders, they observed, excreted 1100 µg MHPG per 24 hours, and amitriptyline responders excreted 2170 µg. In this study the type of depression involved was not identified.

Imipramine is a stronger NA potentiator than 5-HT, while the reverse applies to amitriptyline. Desipramine potentiates NA selectively. The following construct is conceivable: low MHPG excretors respond well to imipramine and desipramine because they are NA-deficient; high MHPG excretors show a better response to amitriptyline possibly because they are 5-HT-deficient. The latter possibility is no fabrication: low CSF 5-HIAA concentrations were found in patients with a high renal MHPG excretion, and vice versa (Goodwin *et al* 1978). These data support the hypothesis that, within the group of vital depressions, there are two pathogenetically different subtypes: a predominantly NA-deficient and a predominantly 5-HT-deficient subtype (Maas 1975). The strength of this argument is limited, because imipramine and amitriptyline are not very selective in their influence on central MA.

Modai *et al* (1979) studied the amitriptyline/MHPG correlation in patients with unipolar and bipolar depressions. They, too, found that the pre-treatment MHPG excretion was higher in amitriptyline responders than in non-responders. Patients of the same type were studied by Hollister *et al* (1980), who used a far more selective antidepressant: nortriptyline. This compound is a strong NA potentiator but virtually does not potentiate 5-HT. Therapeutic result and MHPG excretion did not correlate. When a bimodal distribution was forced by comparing the six lowest MHPG excretors with the six highest excretors, a difference was in fact found: the former group showed more improvement than the latter.

4.3 Renal MHPG excretion: conclusions

It seems plausible that (a) renal MHPG excretion supplies some information about central NA metabolism; (b) the group of depressions includes patients with diminished renal MHPG excretion; (c) most of them are found within the group of bipolar and schizo-affective patients; (d) this is not an exclusive phenomenon, but is observed in other types of depression as well. The level of urinary MHPG excretion seems to have some predictive significance with regard to the therapeutic efficacy of 5-HT-potentiating and more NA-potentiating antidepressants.

These (preliminary) conclusions are based on mean values in relatively large groups of patients. No conclusion can as yet be drawn about the value of MHPG determinations in the individual patient. Since the MHPG excretion varies fairly considerably in the individual patient, there is no reason for high expectations, particularly because relatively readily standardized factors such as motor activity and nutrition seem to contribute little to this variability. Finally, the collection of 24-hour urine inconveniences both the staff and the patient and limits the practicality of the test. Whether MHPG excretion over shorter periods supplies diagnostic information has not yet been established.

No data are available on the question of whether this test provides prognostic information.

4.4 MHPG concentration in CSF

There is no agreement about the question whether the CSF MHPG concentration can be decreased in depressions (for review: Schildkraut 1978). This is probably due to careless and dissimilar depression classification.

The urinary and CSF MHPG concentrations are not correlated (Shaw et al 1973), and this is inconsistent with the theory that renal MHPG excretion is an index of NA metabolism (MHPG production) in the CNS. A possible explanation is: the baseline CSF MHPG concentration is an instantaneous measure of central NA metabolism, whereas renal MHPG excretion is a kind of integrated measure over a 24-hour period. Moreover, MHPG transport from the CNS is not susceptible to probenecid. There is no known inhibitor of this transport system. It is, therefore, impossible to study the MHPG production over a longer period via the CSF-'window'.

Conclusion. It is uncertain whether CSF MHPG values can deviate from normal in depressions. The possible significance of this variable for (a) the choice of antidepressant, and (b) the prognosis of the depression has not yet been studied.

4.5 HVA concentration in CSF

In depressions associated with inhibition of motor activity and initiative, postprobenecid HVA accumulation in CSF is diminished (van Praag & Korf 1971a; Banki 1977). This indicates a reduced DA turnover in the CNS. The phenomenon is observed in Parkinson's disease also.

Several compounds with DA-potentiating action have been demonstrated to have a therapeutic effect in depressions in that the patient was activated by them. This applies to the DA precursor L-DOPA (Goodwin et al 1970; van Praag 1974) and to piribedil, a postsynaptic DA agonist (Post et al 1978). The influence of these compounds on the patient's mood is small. Their activating effect is most pronounced in patients with deficient postprobenecid HVA accumulation. The therapeutic effect of the antidepressant nomifensine likewise shows a negative correlation with the CSF

HVA level after probenecid (van Scheyen *et al* 1977). This agent does exert an influence on the patient's mood, perhaps because it potentiates NA as well as DA.

A decreased CSF HVA concentration is syndrome-dependent: the level is normalized as the depression abates. It is, therefore, unlikely that this phenomenon could have prognostic significance, although this has not yet been studied.

Conclusion. In depressions, the phenomenon called inhibition is correlated with decreased postprobenecid HVA accumulation in CSF. It is in these patients that DA-potentiating compounds have an activating effect. Most antidepressants exert but little influence on the DA system. When a depressive patient is insufficiently activated by the traditional antidepressants, the addition of a DA potentiator can be contemplated. Potential responders could perhaps be traced by determination of the CSF HVA concentration. However, this test has not yet been used in this sense. Nor has any research been done into its possible prognostic value.

5. Discussion

It is a justifiable conclusion that disorders of central MA metabolism can occur in depressions. These disorders are concentrated in the group of vital depressions and, less evidently, in schizo-affective psychoses with pronounced depressive (melancholic) features (van Praag 1981). MA disorders are characteristic of a *proportion* of these populations. MA research consequently provides a basis for the concept of the biochemical classifiability of (vital) depressions (van Praag & Korf 1971b). In other words: apart from the traditional criteria of classification — symptomatology, aetiology and course — the criterion 'pathogenesis' should be applicable in this group.

What is the present situation of pathogenetic depression diagnosis? Two variables seem to be most promising: the 5-HIAA concentration in CSF and renal MHPG excretion. It looks as if CSF 5-HIAA values are of predictive significance, both as regards the choice of antidepressant and as regards the prognosis of the depression in terms of risk of recurrence and suicide risk. Practical problems related to lumbar puncture, however, preclude large-scale application of these tests. This is why peripherally measurable indices of central 5-HT metabolism would be important. In principle, several strategies are available to achieve this. To begin with, the *hormonal* strategy: measurement of the plasma concentration of hypophyseal hormones whose release is (partly) subject to serotonergic control. Determination of plasma prolactin as a measure of the activity in the (tubero-infundibular) DA system is the best example of this strategy.

However, the results obtained with this strategy in relation to the 5-HT system have not so far been encouraging (Westenberg *et al* 1982).

Another possibility is measurement of the *tryptophan/competing amino acids ratio* in plasma. This ratio is reduced in some vital depressive patients (Møller *et al* 1980). If these should prove to be the patients in whom the CSF 5-HIAA concentration is diminished, then the '5-HT-deficient' subgroup could be identified with the aid of a peripheral variable (see also the subsection on plasma tryptophan).

Finally, I should like to point out a very recent development: the discovery in the brain of imipramine binding sites which probably have receptor characteristics (for review: Langer & Briley 1981). A receptor is a binding site which mediates the pharmacological actions of a substance. The density of imipramine binding sites was found to parallel the 5-HT concentration. It is suspected that these sites are part of the 5-HT reuptake system in the neuron. These binding sites have been found not only in the brain but also in blood platelets. The properties of these two groups of sites are identical, and this makes it possible to study the central binding sites on the basis of peripheral findings.

A reduced density of imipramine binding sites in the blood platelets has been recently reported in depressive patients (Briley *et al* 1980). Whether this phenomenon correlates with other biochemical indicators of disturbed 5-HT metabolism remains to be established. In principle, however, the imipramine binding sites in blood platelets can be regarded as a 'window' to the central 5-HT metabolism.

Renal MHPG excretion is the second variable of suspected predictive value as regards the treatment of depressions, at least when groups are compared. The value of this test in the individual patient requires further investigation. This method, too, has practical disadvantages: the inconvenience of conscientiously collecting 24-hour urine. It would, therefore, be worthwhile to establish whether determination of plasma MHPG values might constitute an effective alternative. Preliminary findings in this respect have been encouraging (Sweeney *et al* 1980).

The hormonal 'window' seems to afford possibilities for peripheral study of the central NA metabolism. In this context I am thinking in particular of the dexamethasone suppression test. This type of research will be discussed in part II of this presentation.

6. Summary

The monoamine (MA) hypothesis postulates correlations between disorders of central MA metabolism and the pathogenesis of certain depressive symptoms. In this context, considerable research has focussed

Table 1. Preliminary conclusions about the predictive value of some variables of central MA metabolism for the treatment and the prognosis of (vital) depressions

	Deviant in depressions	Predictive value with regard to Treatment	Predictive value with regard to Prognosis
5-HT system			
CSF 5-HIAA ·	+	+	+
Tryptophan/competing amino acids ratio	+	+	?
Imipramine binding sites in blood platelets	+	?	?
NA system			
Urinary MHPG	+	+	?
CSF MHPG	±	?	?
DA system			
CSF HVA	+	+	?

+ = yes; ± = uncertain; ? = not investigated.

on the central MA metabolism in depressions in the past 20 years. The question is discussed whether abnormalities discovered in this research are of diagnostic value. In other words: do they warrant conclusions about the treatment of choice and about the prognosis of the depression? Measurements of CSF 5-HIAA and urinary MHPG are identified as the most promising 'tests'. The former provides both therapeutic and prognostic, and the latter only therapeutic information, so far as we know. Lumbar puncture and collection of 24-hour urine are hardly practicable procedures in the out-patient setting in which most depressive patients are treated. Simplification of the procedures is, therefore, a practical prerequisite. Some possible developments in this direction are discussed.

The available data support the concept of the biochemical heterogeneity of depressions. This concept implies that, in addition to the traditional criteria of classification (symptomatology, aetiology and course), the criterion 'pathogenesis' merits a place in the diagnosis of depressions.

References

Åsberg, M., Bertilsson, L., Tuck, D., Cronholm, B. & Sjöqvist, F. (1972): Indolamine metabolites in the cerebrospinal fluid of depressed patients before and during treatment with nortriptyline. *Clin. Pharmacol. Ther., 14,* 277-286.

Åsberg, M., Thorén, P., Träskman, L., Bertilsson, L. & Ringberger, V. (1976a): 'Serotonin depression': a biochemical subgroup within the affective disorders? *Science, 191,* 478-480.

Åsberg, M., Träskman, L. & Thorén, P. (1976b): 5-HIAA in the cerebrospinal fluid. A biochemical suicide predictor? *Arch. Gen. Psychiatry, 33,* 1193-1197.

Banki, C.M. (1977): Correlation between cerebrospinal fluid amine metabolites and psychomotor activity in affective disorders. *J. Neurochem., 28,* 255-257.
Banki, C.M., Molnar, G. & Vojnik, M. (1981): Cerebrospinal fluid amine metabolites, tryptophan and clinical parameters in depression. II. Actual psychopathological symptoms. *J. Affect. Disor., 3,* 91-99.
Beckman, H. & Goodwin, F.K. (1975): Antidepressant response to tricyclics and urinary MHPG in unipolar patients: Clinical response to imipramine or amitriptyline. *Arch. Gen. Psychiatry, 32,* 17-21.
Berger, P.A., Faull, K.F., Kilkowsky, J., Andersen, P.J., Kraemer, H., Davis, K.L. & Barchas, J.D. (1980): CSF monoamine metabolites in depression and schizophrenia. *Am. J. Psychiatry, 137,* 174-181.
Blomberg, P.A., Kopin, I.J., Gordon, E.K., Markey, S.P. & Ebert, M.H. (1980): Conversion of MHPG to vanillylmandelic acid. *Arch. Gen. Psychiatry, 37,* 1095-1098.
Briley, M.S., Langer, S.Z., Raisman, R., Sechter, D. & Zarifian, E. (1980): Tritiated imipramine binding sites are decreased in platelets of untreated depressed patients. *Science, 209,* 303-305.
Edwards, D.J., Spiker, D.G., Neil, J.F., Kupfer, D.J. & Rizk, M. (1980): MHPG excretion in depression. *Psychiatry Res., 2,* 295-305.
Garfinkel, P.E., Warsh, J.J., Stancer, H.C. & Godse, D.D. (1977): CNS monoamine metabolism in bipolar affective disorder. *Arch. Gen. Psychiatry, 34,* 735-739.
Goodwin, F.K., Brodie, H.K.H., Murphy, D.Z. & Bunney, W.E. (1970): L-DOPA, catecholamines and behaviour: a clinical and biochemical study in depressed patients. *Biol. Psychiatry, 2,* 341-366.
Goodwin, F.K. & Post, R.M. (1975): Studies of amine metabolites in affective disorders and schizophrenia: a comparative analysis. In Freedman, D.X. (ed.): *Biology of the Major Psychoses: A Comparative Analysis.* Raven Press, New York.
Goodwin, F.K., Cowdry, R.W. & Webster, M.H. (1978): Predictors of drug response in the affective disorders: toward an integrated approach. In Lipton, M.A., DiMascio, A., Killam, K.F. (eds.): *Psychopharmacology: A Generation of Progress.* Raven Press, New York.
Goodwin, F.K. & Potter, W.Z. (1979): Norepinephrine metabolite studies in affective illness. In Usdin, E., Kopin, I.J., Barchas, J. (eds.): *Catecholamines: Basic and Clinical Frontiers, 2.* Pergamon Press, New York.
Hollister, L.E., Davis, K.L. & Berger, P.A. (1980): Subtypes of depression based on excretion of MHPG and response to nortriptyline. *Arch. Gen. Psychiatry, 37,* 1107-1110.
Jori, A., Dolfini, E., Casati, C. & Argenta, G. (1975): Effect of ECT and imipramine treatment on the concentration of 5-hydroxyindoleacetic acid (5-HIAA) and homovanillic acid (HIVA) in the cerebrospinal fluid of depressed patients. *Psychopharmacology, 44,* 87-90.
Langer, S.Z. & Briley, M. (1981): High-affinity ^{3}H-imipramine binding: a new biological tool for studies in depression. *Trends in Neuroscience, 4,* 28-31.
Maas, J.W., Fawcett, J.A. & Dekirmenjian, H. (1968): 3-Methoxy-4-hydroxyphenylglycol (MHPG) excretion in depressive patients. *Arch. Gen. Psychiatry, 19,* 129-134.
Maas, J.W., Fawcett, J.A. & Dekirmenjian, H. (1972): Catecholamine metabolism, depressive illness, and drug response. *Arch. Gen. Psychiatry, 26,* 252-262.
Maas, J.W. (1975): Biogenic amines and depression: biochemical and pharmacological separation of two types of depression. *Arch. Gen. Psychiatry, 32,* 1357-1361.
Maas, J.W., Hattox, S.E., Green, N.M. & Landis, D.H. (1979): 3-Methoxy-4-hydroxyphenylglycol production by human brain in vivo. *Science, 205,* 1025-1027.
Modai, I., Apter, A., Golomb, M. & Wijsenbeek, H. (1979): Response to amitriptyline and urinary MHPG in bipolar depressive patients. *Neuropsychobiology, 5,* 181-184.

Møller, S.E., Kirk, L. & Honoré, P. (1980): Relationship between plasma ratio of tryptophan to competing amino acids and the response to 1-tryptophan treatment in endogenously depressed patients. *J. Affect. Disor., 2,* 47-59.

Post, R.M., Gordon, E.K., Goodwin, F.K. & Bunney, W.E. (1973): Central norepinephrine metabolism in affective illness: MHPG in the cerebrospinal fluid. *Science, 179,* 1002-1003.

Post, R.M., Stoddard, F.J., Gillin, J.C., Buchsbaum, M.S., Runkle, D.C., Black, K.E. & Bunney, W.E. jr. (1977): Alterations in motor activity, sleep and biochemistry in a cycling manic depressive patient. *Arch. Gen. Psychiatry, 34,* 470-477.

Post, R.M., Gerner, R.H., Carman, J.L., Gillin, Ch., Jimerson, D.C., Goodwin, F.K. & Bunney, W.E. (1978): Effects of a dopamine agonist piribedil in depressed patients. *Arch. Gen. Psychiatry, 35,* 609-615.

Praag, van H.M. (1969): The complementary aspects in the relation between biological and psychodynamic psychiatry. *Psychiatr. Clin., 2,* 307-318.

Praag, van H.M. (1971): The position of biological psychiatry among the psychiatric disciplines. *Compr. Psychiatry, 12,* 1-7.

Praag, van H.M. & Korf, J. (1971a): Retarded depression and the dopamine metabolism. *Psychopharmacology, 19,* 199-203.

Praag, van H.M. & Korf, J. (1971b): Endogenous depressions with and without disturbances in the 5-hydroxytryptamine metabolism: a biochemical classification? *Psychopharmacology, 19,* 148-152.

Praag, van H.M., Korf, J., Dols, L.C.W. & Shut, T. (1972): A pilot study of the predictive value of the probenecid test in application of 5-hydroxytryptophan as antidepressant. *Psychopharmacology, 25,* 14-21.

Praag, van H.M., Burg, van den, W., Bos, E.R.H. & Dols, L.C.W. (1974): 5-Hydroxytryptophan in combination with clomipramine in 'therapy-resistant' depression. *Psychopharmacology, 38,* 267-269.

Praag, van H.M. (1974): Towards a biochemical typology of depression? *Pharmacopsychiatr., 7,* 281-292.

Praag, van H.M. (1976): Het diagnostiseren van depressies. *Ned. T. Geneeskd., 120,* 2274-2281.

Praag, van H.M. (1977a): *Depression and Schizophrenia. A Contribution on their Chemical Pathologies.* Spectrum Publications, New York.

Praag, van H.M. (1977b): Evidence of serotonin-deficient depression. *Neuropsychobiology, 3,* 56-63.

Praag, van H.M. (1977c): Significance of biochemical parameters in the diagnosis, treatment and prevention of depressive disorders. *Biol. Psychiatry, 12,* 101-131.

Praag, van H.M. (1979): Central serotonin: its relation to depression vulnerability and depression prophylaxis. In Obiols, J., Ballús, C., Gonzalez Monclus, E., Pujol, J. (eds.): *Biological Psychiatry Today.* Elsevier/North-Holland Biomedical Press.

Praag, van H.M. & De Haan, S. (1979): Central serotonin metabolism and frequency of depression. *Psychiatry Res., 1,* 219-224.

Praag, van H.M. & De Haan, S. (1980): Depression vulnerability and 5-hydroxytryptophan prophylaxis. *Psychiatry Res., 3,* 75-83.

Praag, van H.M. & De Haan, S. (1981): Chemoprophylaxis of depressions. An attempt to compare lithium with 5-hydroxytryptophan. *Acta Psychiatr. Scand. Suppl.,* 191-205.

Praag, van H.M. (1981): Management of depression with serotonin precursors. *Biol. Psychiatry, 16,* 291-310.

Praag, van H.M. (1982): Depression, suicide and serotonin metabolism in the brain. In Post, R.M., Ballenger, J.C. (eds.): *The Neurobiology of Manic Depressive Illness.* Williams and Wilkins, Baltimore.

Scheyen, van, J.D., van Praag, H.M. & Korf, J. (1977): A controlled study comparing nomifensine and clomipramine in unipolar depression, using the probenecid technique. *Br. J. Clin. Pharmacol., 4,* 179S-184S.
Schildkraut, J.J. (1973): Norepinephrine metabolites as biochemical criteria for classifying depressive disorders and predicting responses to treatment: preliminary findings. *Am. J. Psychiatry, 130,* 695-699.
Schildkraut, J.J. (1978): Current status of the catecholamine hypothesis of affective disorders. In Lipton, M.A., DiMascio, A., Killam, K.F. (eds.): *Psychopharmacology: A Generation of Progress.* Raven Press, New York.
Schildkraut, J.J., Orsulak, P.J., LaBrie, R.A., Schatzberg, A.F., Gudeman, J.E., Cole, J.O. & Rohde, W.A. (1978): Toward a biochemical classification of depressive disorders. I. Differences in urinary excretion of MHPG and other catecholamine metabolites in clinically defined subtypes of depressions. *Arch. Gen. Psychiatry, 35,* 1436-1439.
Sedvall, G., Fyrö, B., Gullberg, B., Nybäck, H., Wiesel, F.A. & Wode-Helgodt, B. (1980): Relationships in healthy volunteers between concentration of monoamine metabolites in cerebrospinal fluid and family history of psychiatric morbidity. *Br. J. Psychiatry, 136,* 366-374.
Shaw, D.M., O'Keefe, R., Macsweeney, D.A., Brookshank, B.W.L., Noguera, R. & Coppen, A. (1973): 3-Methoxy-4-hydroxyphenylglycol in depression. *Psychol. Med., 3,* 333-336.
Sweeney, D.R., Leckman, J.F., Maas, J.W., Hattox, S. & Henninger, G.R. (1980): Plasma free and conjugated MHPG in psychiatric patients. *Arch. Gen. Psychiatry, 37,* 1100-1103.
Träskman, L., Åsberg, M., Bertilsson, L., Cronholm, B., Mellström, B., Neckers, L.M., Sjöqvist, F., Thorén, P. & Tybring, G. (1979): Plasma levels of chlorimipramine and its demethyl metabolite during treatment of depression. *Clin. Pharmacol. Ther., 26,* 600-610.
Träskman, L., Åsberg, M., Bertilsson, L. & Sjöstrand, L. (1981): Monoamine metabolites in cerebrospinal fluid and suicidal behaviour. *Arch. Gen. Psychiatry, 38,* 631-636.
Westenberg, H.G.M., van Praag, H.M., De Jong, J.T.V.M., Thijssen, J.H.H. & Schwarz, F. (1982): Postsynaptic serotonergic activity in depressive patients: evaluation of the neuroendocrine strategy. *Psychiatry Res., 7,* 361-371.
Young, S.N. & Sourkes, R.L. (1977): Tryptophan in the central nervous system: regulation and significance. *Adv. Neurochem., 2,* 133-191.

II. Hormonal Variables

1. The way to the anterior hypophyseal lobe

Hormone assays of sufficient sensitivity to be used on small amounts of blood have been developed in the past decade. Frequent measurements over a limited period of time have become possible, thus eliminating an important potential source of error: fluctuations in concentration, whether incidental (e.g. stress-determined) or systematic (due to intermittent hormone release), are no longer misinterpreted as abnormalities inherent in a particular syndrome. Moreover, it was established during this period that monoaminergic (MA-ergic) systems are involved in the regulation of the release of anterior hypophyseal hormones. This release was found to be directly controlled by the so-called releasing and inhibiting factors: peptide hormones produced in the hypothalamus. The production of these hormones is regulated (partly) MA-ergically. This implies that the measurement of anterior hypophyseal hormones in blood provides a kind of 'window' through which the activity of hypothalamic MA-ergic systems can be observed (for review: van Praag 1978). The most elegant example of this strategy is the determination of plasma prolactin, which supplies data on the activity of the tuberoinfundibular dopaminergic (DA-ergic) system.

These developments have made a significant contribution to the recent upswing in psycho- and neuroendocrinological research. Has this research produced tests of practical significance for the diagnosis and prognosis of depressions? To anticipate the conclusions: tests of indisputable practical value are not yet available; but there are indeed some tests that justify a high level of expectation. I shall discuss them in the following sections.

2. The dexamethasone suppression test (DST)
2.1 The CRF/ACTH/cortisol 'axis' in depressions

Some 50 per cent of all patients with endogenous depressions show cortisol hypersecretion (Sachar *et al* 1973, 1980). Cortisol production is excessive in particular during periods in which it is normally minimal: at night and in the early morning. This is not likely to be a stress phenomenon: hypersecretion occurs in apathic depressive patients as well, continues during (EEG-monitored) sleep, is not abolished by anxiolytics, and does not occur in normal individuals subject to stress of sleep deprivation (Sachar *et al* 1980).

Given intact adrenal glands, cortisol secretion virtually parallels that of ACTH. ACTH production in turn is controlled by the corticotropin-releasing factor (CRF) produced in the hypothalamus. Taking this into account, Sachar (1975) described the hypersecretion of cortisol as an expression of "disinhibition of the hypothalamic cells secreting CRF". He regarded the phenomenon as "an intrinsic part of severe depressive illness". As already pointed out, this phenomenon occurs in about 50 per cent of patients with endogenous (vital) depressions. Its specificity — the question whether it can be seen also in other categories of depressive or non-depressive patients — has not yet been adequately researched.

Observations made with the aid of the dexamethasone suppression test (DST) point in the same direction (Carroll *et al* 1976, 1981). Dexamethasone is a synthetic corticosteroid which inhibits ACTH/cortisol production by the stimulation of cortisol (feedback) receptors in the brain.

It causes a marked fall of the plasma cortisol level, and this effect persists for 24 hours or longer. This suppressive effect is less pronounced in some patients with endogenous depressions, who show an earlier 'escape' from this effect: the plasma cortisol level is normalized more quickly than it normally is (Fig. 1). Depressive patients with a disturbed DST show cortisol hypersecretion as well, but patients with cortisol hypersecretion do not necessarily show a disturbed DST (Sachar et al 1980). 'Early escape' after the DST suggests ACTH overproduction, and this in turn indicates overproduction of CRF, the compound which stimulates the hypophysis to release ACTH.

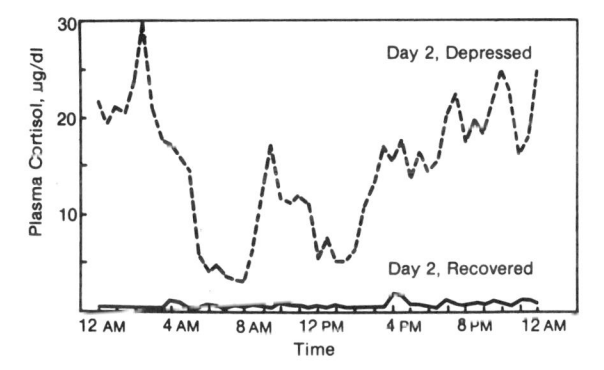

Fig. 1. Typical non-suppressor. Plasma cortisol values in a 58-year-old man suffering from bipolar depression with motor retardation, during the depression (- - -) and after recovery (—) (Carroll et al 1976).

The neuronal regulation of CRF is a complex mechanism (Lal & Martin 1980), but it is beyond doubt that noradrenergic (NA-ergic) systems exert a tonic-inhibitory influence on the secretion of this hormone. Hypofunction of hypothalamic NA-ergic systems is, therefore, a possible explanation of the disinhibition of the CRF/ACTH/cortisol system. This explanation is consistent with the MA hypothesis on the pathogenesis of endogenous (vital) depressions (see part I of this presentation). A correlation between disturbed DST and diminished renal MHPG secretion would support this hypothesis, but simultaneous studies of both variables have yet to be performed.

2.2 Changes in the DST in depressions

Several authors have reported DST disturbances in depressive patients (for review: Carroll 1980a). Unfortunately, they used a diversity of terminologies in the diagnostic classification of their patients, e.g. endogenous depression, primary depression and endogenomorphous depression. It seems likely that all were referring to the aetiologically non-specific syndrome of vital depression, but this is not certain. One group has so far reported non-confirmation of the observations made by Carroll (Holsboer et al 1980): only a small proportion of their depressive patients showed a disturbed DST; moreover, the disturbance was frequently also observed in other categories of patients. The cause of this discrepancy has remained obscure, but the most plausible explanation is that the diagnostic criteria applied in Germany differ from those in the USA.

The following subsection is confined to the findings reported by Carroll et al (1980), the only group to perform *systematic* DST studies in the past four years (an impressive piece of research work).

Table 1. Diagnostic value of the dexamethasone suppression test (DST) in vital ('endogenous') depressions (Carroll 1980a)

Investigators	Sensitivity (%)	Specificity (%)	PV+	PV—
Carroll et al (1976)	48	98	95	65
Carroll et al (1980)*	40	98	95	61
Brown et al (1979)	40	100	100	70
Schlesser et al (1979)	43	100	100	62
Mean	43	99	98	64

Sensitivity: percentage of patients with vital depression and a positive DST.
Specificity: percentage of persons not suffering from vital depression, with negative DST.
PV+: predictive value: percentage of test subjects with positive DST, suffering from vital depression.
PV—: predictive value: percentage of test subjects with negative DST, not suffering from vital depression.
*Carroll's publication in 1981 reports about 60 per cent sensitivity.

2.3 Carroll's findings with the DST

To begin with, the procedure has been standardized. At 23.30 hours the test subject is given 1mg dexamethasone by mouth. At 16.00 hours on the following day and (if possible) again at 23.00 hours, blood samples are obtained for plasma cortisol determination. The test is regarded as abnormal when the cortisol concentration in one or both samples exceeds $5\mu g/dl$. The determination at 16.00 hours identifies 78 per cent of the 'non-suppressors'; the two determinations jointly identify 98 per cent. For out-patients the afternoon determination can be accepted as sufficient on practical grounds.

A disturbed DST was found in 67 per cent of patients with endogenous depression. In Carroll's terminology: the sensitivity of the test is 67 per cent. Carroll's term endogenous depression virtually covers our term vital depression. Evidently there is a subgroup that does not show the disturbance. In other psychiatric categories (including non-endogenous depression) and in normal test subjects, a disturbed DST was observed in only 3 per cent and 4 per cent of cases, respectively. In other words: the specificity of the test is about 96 per cent. The chance that a patient with a disturbed DST is suffering from endogenous depression, that is to say the predictive value (or confidence) of the test, is very high — according to Carroll, 95 per cent: always assuming that certain somatic abnormalities have been eliminated (Table 1).

2.4 Therapeutic and prognostic value of the DST

The therapeutic value of the DST has hardly been studied so far. Interesting preliminary findings in this context were reported by Brown et al (1980, 1981), who observed that patients with a disturbed DST responded preferably to tricyclic antidepressants with a predominantly NA-potentiating effect, whereas patients with a normal DST responded preferably to 5-HT-potentiating compounds.

The former finding is consistent with the hypothesis that hyperfunction of the CRF/ACTH/cortisol system is related to NA-ergic hypofunction. The latter finding might suggest that serotonergic systems are hypofunctional in patients with an undisturbed DST. In agreement with this hypothesis is the observation that a normal DST and diminished CSF 5-HIAA values correlate (Carroll 1980b).

Brown & Shuey (1980) found in addition that non-suppressors show a better response to antidepressant medication and EST than suppressors. Since all kinds of antidepressants were used, this study warrants no conclusions about the predictive value of the DST.

Generally the dexamethasone response normalizes gradually as the depression abates. There are indications that patients who make a clinical recovery but show a persistently disturbed DST, run an increased risk of relapsing soon. This would seem to imply that restoration of the DST indicates the likelihood of a favourable prognosis, while persistence of an abnormal response suggests an unfavourable one (Goldberg 1980; Greden et al 1980; Albala & Greden 1980). However, the available data are still too scanty to warrant more or less definite conclusions.

2.5 Conclusions

An early escape after the DST seems to indicate the high probability of an endogenous (vital) depression (if certain somatic diseases have been eliminated). The phenomenon is observed in only about 60 per cent of patients with endogenous depression, and as such it supports the hypothesis of the pathogenetic heterogeneity of this group of depressive syndromes. It is to be noted, however, that so far the possibility that the phenomenon is non-specific, i.e. determined more by the degree of anxious tenseness than by the mood depression as such, has not been eliminated.

There are some indications that the DST is of predictive value with regard to therapy and prognosis, but the available data are not yet sufficient to recommend practical application of the test.

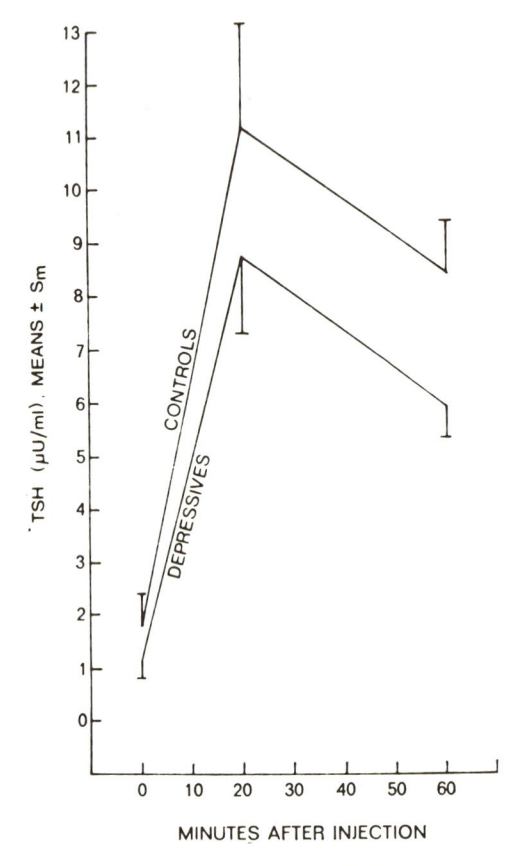

Fig. 2. TSH response to rapid intravenous injection of 500 μg TRH. The mean increase in plasma TSH in a group of vital depressive patients (n = 10) is less than that in a control group (n = 23) (van den Burg *et al* 1975).

3. TSH response to TRH

3.1 Changes in depressive patients

The thyroid hormone triiodothyronine (T3) potentiates the therapeutic effect of antidepressants, probably as a result of sensitization of β-adrenergic (NA-ergic) receptors in the brain. This prompted Prange *et al* (1972) to test thyrotropin-releasing hormone (TRH) in depressive patients.

TRH is a hypothalamic peptide which prompts the hypophysis to release thyroid-stimulating hormone (TSH), a hormone which activates the thyroid to increased hormone secretion (in addition, TRH stimulates the release of prolactin by the anterior hypophyseal lobe).

The value of TRH as an antidepressant is probably minimal (for review: van Praag & Verhoeven 1980), but an additional finding was of interest: Prange et al (1972) found that the increase in blood TSH concentration after intravenous TRH injection can be subnormal in depressions. This observation has since been repeatedly corroborated (for review: Prange 1977) (Fig. 2). When TRH is given by continuous drip instead of by injection, the difference between depressive patients and controls disappears (van den Burg et al 1975, 1976) (Fig. 3).

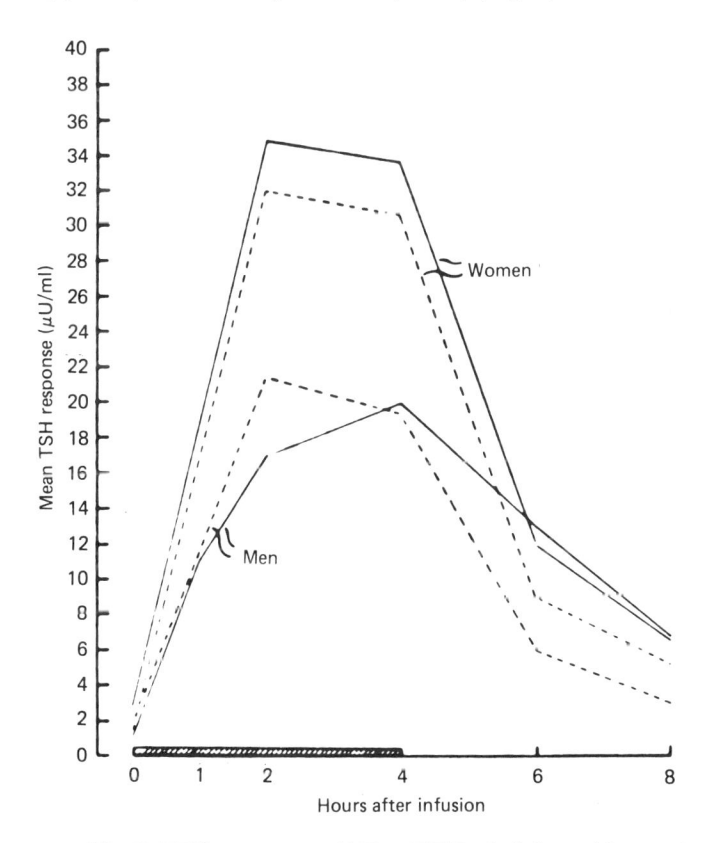

Fig. 3. TSH response to 1000 µg TRH administered by continuous drip over a 4-hour period. The TSH response in the depressive group (dashed lines) does not differ from that in the control group (continuous lines) (van den Burg et al 1976).

With regard to this test, too, the group of depressions is heterogeneous: some patients show a subnormal, others a normal response. But there is no consensus about the psychopathological identity of the TSH-deficient group. Some authors hold that the disturbed TSH response is found mainly in the unipolar group (Sachar et al 1980; Gold et al 1980), while others report it in both unipolar and bipolar patients (Linkowski et al 1981). In any case it is evident that the phenomenon is not homogeneously distributed even within a psychopathologically more or less homogenous group of depressive patients. In unipolar patients, for example, it was observed in about 50-60 per cent of cases (Extein et al 1981; Sachar et al 1980). Loosen & Prange (1980) demonstrated a negative correlation between serum cortisol level and TSH response to TRH, both in normal controls and in depressive patients. They suggested that the subnormal TSH response might result from the increased serum cortisol levels, for pharmacological doses of glucocorticosteroids are known to reduce the TSH response to TRH in normal test subjects (Re et al 1976). Others, however, found no correlation between TSH response and serum cortisol value (Kirkegaard & Carroll 1980). Moreover, no significant association was found between the incidence of a disturbed TRH test and that of a disturbed DST. Only in 30 per cent of unipolar patients with a disturbed TRH test or DST did the two disturbances occur simultaneously (Extein et al 1981). Apparently the two tests identify different subgroups.

As pointed out, TRH stimulates the release of prolactin as well as that of TSH. The prolactin response to TRH has also been reported as diminished in depressions (Mendlewicz et al 1980), but whether the TSH response is also subnormal in these patients has remained obscure.

There is still considerable uncertainty about the neuronal regulation of TRH secretion (Annunziato et al 1981), but it seems likely that NA-ergic systems promote TRH/TSH secretion. In this respect the subnormal TSH response is compatible with the MA hypothesis on depressions. The serotonergic influence is unclear. Gold et al (1977) established a negative correlation between CSF 5-HIAA values and TSH response: the lower the CSF 5-HIAA concentration, the higher the TSH response to TRH. This is not confirmed by our observation that 5-HT precursors, which significantly increase the amount of 5-HT available in the brain, exert no distinct influence on serum TSH values (Westenberg et al 1982).

3.2 Therapeutic and prognostic significance

We know of no studies which correlate the pre-treatment TSH response to therapeutic results.

Data on the possible prognostic significance of this test are scanty and not unequivocal. Sachar et al (1980) demonstrated that the disturbed TSH response persists after clinical recovery in some patients. According to

Kirkegaard & Smith (1978) and Kirkegaard & Carroll (1980), persistence of the disturbance indicates an incomplete recovery and an increased risk of quick recurrence; the disturbed TSH response should, therefore, be regarded as an indication for continued antidepressant medication. This is an interesting finding, but all in all the available data are not sufficiently conclusive to add the TRH test to the diagnostic arsenal.

3.3 Conclusions

The TSH response to TRH can be disturbed in depressive patients; the subgroup for which this is characteristic remains to be defined. There are promising indications that the test is of prognostic significance: patients with an increased risk of quick recurrence are believed to be characterized by persistence of a disturbed TSH response. The pertinent data, however, require corroboration and supplementation before practical application of the test can be recommended.

4. Growth hormone (GH) responses

4.1 Changes in depressive patients

The baseline growth hormone (GH) secretion shows a spontaneous rhythm: 6-7 bursts per 24 hours in young adults with a tendency to diminishing frequency with increasing age. Moreover, GH secretion is unstable; it is influenced by numerous incidental factors such as psychological stimuli, physical exertion, metabolic stimuli like hypoglycaemia, certain hormones and amino acids (for review: Brown *et al* 1978). In the context of hormonal influences, the stimulating effect of oestrogens merits special mention. They cause the baseline plasma GH level to vary with the phase of the menstrual cycle, and also determine a marked difference between premenopausal and postmenopausal baseline GH values. This factor has not always been taken into account in depression research. The GH response to insulin is the variable most intensively studied in this group. It has been established that this response can be subnormal in 'endogenous depressions' (Gruen *et al* 1975), but the percentage of patients in whom this occurs has not been determined. Nor has the specificity of the phenomenon been adequately studied. One publication mentions that this response can be subnormal also in prepubertal children with 'major endogenous depression' (Puig-Antich *et al* 1981).

According to Maeda *et al* (1975) TRH causes GH secretion in depressive patients but not in normal test subjects. Linkowski *et al* (1980), however, were unable to confirm this observation.

GH secretion is stimulated by DA-ergic and NA-ergic systems (Lal & Martin 1980), and consequently the plasma GH level increases in response to DA-potentiating compounds such as L-DOPA and apomorphine. There are no indications that the response to these drugs is abnormal in depressions (Gold et al 1976). Depressive patients show a subnormal response to D-amphetamine (Langer et al 1976), and amphetamine contains both DA-potentiating and NA-potentiating active components. Perhaps a deficiently functioning NA system in depressions is responsible for the difference in response. An argument in favour of this theory is that depressive patients show a deficient GH response also to desipramine — an antidepressant which potentiates NA only (Laakman 1980). All these studies concern observations made in a single institute on small numbers of patients. These findings, therefore, require corroboration and diagnostic specification.

4.2 Therapeutic and prognostic significance

There are no published studies on the possible significance of GH responses for the choice of antidepressant to be used.

Endo et al (1974) reported that the GH response to insulin returns to normal after clinical recovery. No further studies on the possible prognostic value of this test have so far been published.

4.3 Conclusions

There are indications that the GH response to certain stimuli — more specifically insulin and D-amphetamine — can be subnormal in depressions. The number of observations is still too small to warrant conclusions on (a) the specificity of the phenomenon, (b) its incidence in various categories of depression, and (c) its possible therapeutic and prognostic significance.

Table 2. Tentative conclusions on the predictive value of some hormonal variables for the treatment and prognosis of (vital) depressions

	Abnormal in depressions	Predictive value for Therapy	Prognosis
Dexamethasone suppression test (DST)	+	±	±
TRH suppression test	+	?	±
Growth hormone response to insulin	+	?	±
amphetamine	+	?	?

+ = yes; ± = uncertain; ? = not determined.

5. Discussion

This presentation does not give an exhaustive survey of hormonal disorders in (vital) depressions. I have confined myself to disorders of possible diagnostic value, i.e. of value for the choice of a particular antidepressant and for the prognosis (Table 2). The disturbances described suggest hypothalamic functional disorders. All can be brought under the denominator of disturbed MA-ergic functions, although this is by no means the only mode of explanation. Nevertheless, they support the MA hypothesis as such.

Not all depressive patients show hormonal functional disorders. These seem to be concentrated in a subgroup of the endogenous (vital) depressions, thus lending support to the concept of the pathogenetic heterogeneity of the group of vital depressions (van Praag & Korf 1971). It is not quite certain, by the way, whether the term vital depressions is appropriate for this group. Unfortunately, different authors use different systems of classification and different terminologies. Nor has it been established with certainty that these disorders are not observed outside the group of depressions. The relevant data on the DST are not unequivocal in this respect, and for the other tests this has hardly been studied at all. Research into the specificity of the phenomena discussed must, therefore, certainly not be regarded as completed.

As regards actual practice: the tests discussed are undoubtedly promising but the empirical foundation is still too weak to justify their use in practice at this time. Future research should, therefore, focus not only on specificity but also on the question of whether these hormonal disorders warrant predictions about (a) the choice of antidepressant, and (b) the prognosis of the depression.

6. Summary

The reasons behind the recent upswing in psychoendocrinology are discussed, with reference also to the relation between MA research and hormone studies. The question is raised whether hormonal research has yielded data of diagnostic value, data that warrant predictions about the choice of antidepressant and the prognosis of the depression considered.

Three function tests are discussed in this context: the DST, the TRH/TSH test, and growth hormone responses to various stimuli. These three 'tests' can all be disturbed in depressions, but probably in particular in some of the endogenous (vital) depressions. These findings, like the biochemical data, support the concept of the pathogenetic heterogeneity of the vital depressions. We do not know whether the disturbances described are all observed in the same patients or are characteristic for various subgroups. DST disturbances were found to be highly specific: characteristic of the subgroup of endogenous depressions. The specificity of the other 'tests' has not yet been adequately studied. Data on their therapeutic and prognostic significance, although promising as such, are still scanty. Any conclusion concerning their value in psychiatric practice would, therefore, be premature.

References

Albala, A.A. & Greden, J.F. (1980): Serial dexamethasone suppression tests (DST) in affective disorders. *Am. J. Psychiatry, 137,* 383.

Annunziato, L., Di Renzo, G., Quattrone, A., Schettini, G. & Preziosi, P. (1981): Brain neurotransmitters regulating TRH producing neurons. *Pharmacol. Res. Commun., 13,* 1-10.

Brown, G.M., Seggie, J.A., Chambers, J.W. & Ettigi, P.G. (1978): Psychoendocrinology and growth hormone: a review. *Psychoneuroendocrinology, 3,* 131-153.

Brown, W.A., Johnston, R. & Mayfield, D. (1979): The 24-hour dexamethasone suppression test in a clinical setting: relationship to diagnosis, symptoms and response to treatment. *Am. J. Psychiatry, 136,* 543-547.

Brown, W.A. & Shuey, I. (1980): Response to dexamethasone and subtype of depression. *Arch. Gen. Psychiatry, 37,* 747-775.

Brown, W.A., Haier, R.J. & Qualls, C.B. (1980): Dexamethasone suppression test identifies subtypes of depression which respond to different antidepressants. *Lancet I,* 928-929.

Brown, W.A. & Qualls, C.B. (1981): Pituitary-adrenal disinhibition on depression: marker of a subtype with characteristic clinical features and response to treatment. *Psychiatry Res., 4,* 115-128.

Burg, van den, W., van Praag, H.M., Bos, E.R.H., van Zanten, A.K., Piers, D.A. & Doorenbos, D.A. (1975): TRH as a possible quick-acting but short-lasting antidepressant. *Psychol. Med., 5,* 404-412.

Burg, van den, W., van Praag, H.M., Bos, E.R.H., Piers, D.A., van Zanten, A.K. & Doorenbos, D.A. (1976): TRH by slow continuous infusion: an antidepressant? *Psychol. Med., 6,* 393-397.

Carroll, B.J., Curtis, G.C. & Mendels, J. (1976): Neuroendocrine regulation in depression. I. Limbic system-adrenocortical dysfunction. II. Discrimination of depressed from non-depressed patients. *Arch. Gen. Psychiatry, 33,* 1039-1044, 1051-1058.

Carroll, B.J. (1980a): Clinical application of neuroendocrine research in depression. In Praag, van, H.M., Lader, M.H., Rafaelsen, O.J. & Sachar, E.J. (eds.): *Handbook of Biological Psychiatry,* Vol. 3. Marcel Dekker Inc., New York.

Carroll, B.J. (1980b): Desinhibition of cortisol secretion in depression. Paper read at the 12th. Congress of the Collegium Internationale Neuropsychopharmacologicum, Göteborg, 22-26 June.

Carroll, B.J., Feinberg, M., Greden, J.F., Tarika, J., Albala, A.A., Haskett, R.F., James, N.M., Kronfol, Z., Lohr, N., Steiner, M., De Vigne, J.P. & Young, E. (1980): A specific laboratory test for the diagnosis of melancholia. *Arch. Gen. Psychiatry, 38,* 15-22.

Endo, M., Endo, J., Nishikubo, M., Yamaguchi, T. & Hatotani, N. (1974): Endocrine studies in depression. In Hatotani, N. (ed.): *Psychoneuroendocrinology* 22-31. Karger, Basel.

Extein, I., Pottash, A.L.C. & Gold, M.S. (1981): Relationship of thyrotropin-releasing hormone test and dexamethasone test abnormalities in unipolar depression. *Psychiatry Res., 4,* 49-53.

Gold, P.W., Goodwin, F.K., Wehr, T., Rebar, R. & Sack, R. (1976): Growth hormone and prolactin responses to levodopa in affective illness. *Lancet II*, 1308-1309.

Gold, P.W., Goodwin, F.K., Wehr, T. & Rebar, R. (1977): Pituitary thyrotropin response to thyrotropin-releasing hormone in affective illness: relationship to spinal fluid amine metabolites. *Am. J. Psychiatry, 134*, 1028-1031.

Gold, M.S., Pottash, A.L.C., Ryan, N., Sweeney, D.R., Davies, R.K. & Martin, D.M. (1980): TRH-induced TSH response in unipolar, bipolar, and secondary depressions: possible utility in clinical assessment and differential diagnosis. *Psychoneuroendocrinology, 5*, 147-155.

Goldberg, I.K. (1980): Dexamethasone suppression test as indicator of safe withdrawal of antidepressant therapy. *Lancet I*, 376.

Goodwin, F.K., Rubovits, R., Jimerson, D. & Post, R.M. (1977): Serotonin and norepinephrine 'subgroups' in depression. *Sci. Proc. Am Psychiatr. Assoc., 130*, 108.

Greden, J.F., Albala, A.A., Haskett, R.F., James, N., Goodman, L., Steiner, M. & Carroll, B.J. (1980): Normalization of dexamethasone suppression test: a laboratory index of recovery from endogenous depression. *Biol. Psychiatry, 15*, 449-458.

Gruen, P.H., Sachar, E.J., Altman, N. & Sassin, J. (1975): Growth hormone responses to hypoglycemia in post-menopausal depressed women. *Arch. Gen. Psychiatry, 32*, 31-33.

Holsboer, F., Bender, W., Benkert, O., Klein, H.E. & Schmauss, M. (1980): Diagnostic value of dexamethasone suppression test in depression. *Lancet II*, 706.

Kirkegaard, C., Nørlem, N., Lauridsen, U.B. & Bjørem, N. (1975): Prognostic value of thyrotropin-releasing hormone stimulation test in endogenous depression. *Acta Psychiatr. Scand., 52*, 170-177.

Kirkegaard, C. & Smith, E. (1978): Continuation therapy in endogenous depression controlled by changes in the TRH stimulation test. *Psychol. Med., 8*, 501-503.

Kirkegaard, C. & Carroll, B.J. (1980): Dissociation of TSH and adrenocortical disturbances in endogenous depression. *Psychiatry Res., 3*, 253-264.

Laakman, G. (1980): Beeinflussung der Hypophysen vorderlappen Hormonsekretion durch Antidepressiva bei gesunden Probanden, neurotisch und endogene depressiven Patienten. *Nervenarzt, 51*, 725-732.

Lal, S. & Martin, J.B. (1980): Neuroanatomy and neuropharmacological regulation of neuroendocrine function. In van Praag, H.M., Lader, M.H., Rafaelsen, O.J., Sachar, E.J. (eds.): *Handbook of Biological Psychiatry, Vol. 3*. Marcel Dekker Inc., New York.

Langer, G., Heinze, G., Reim, B. & Matussek, N. (1976): Reduced growth hormone responses to amphetamine in 'endogenous' depressive patients. *Arch. Gen. Psychiatry, 33*, 1471-1477.

Linkowski, P., Brauman, H. & Mendlewicz, J. (1980): Growth hormone after TRH in women with depressive illness. *Br. J. Psychiatry, 137*, 229-232.

Linkowski, P., Brauman, H. & Mendlewicz, J. (1981): Thyrotropin response to thyrotropin-releasing hormone in unipolar and bipolar affective illness. *J. Affect. Disord., 3*, 9-16.

Loosen, P.T. & Prange, A.J. (1980): Thyrotropin-releasing hormone (TRH): a useful tool for psychoneuroendocrine investigation. *Psychoneuroendocrinology, 5*, 63-80.

Maeda, K., Kato, Y., Ohgo, S., Chihara, K., Yoshimoto, Y., Yamaguchi, N., Kuromaru, S. & Imura, H. (1975): Growth hormone and prolactin release after injection of thyrotropin-releasing hormone in patients with depression. *J. Clin. Endocrinol. Metab., 40*, 501-505.

Martin, J.B., Reichlin, S. & Brown, G.M. (1977): *Clinical Neuroendocrinology*. Davis, Philadelphia.

Mendlewicz, J., Linkowski, P. & Brauman, H. (1980): Reduced prolactin release after thyrotropin-releasing hormone in manic depression. *N. Engl. J. Med., 302*, 1091-1092.

Praag, van, H.M. & Korf, J. (1971): Endogenous depressions with and without disturbances in the 5-hydroxytryptamine metabolism: a biochemical classification. *Psychopharmacology, 19*, 148-152.

Praag, van, H.M. (1978): Neuroendocrine disorders in depressions and their significance for the monoamine hypothesis of depression. *Acta Psychiatr. Scand., 57,* 389-404.
Praag, van, H.M. & Verhoeven, W.M.A. (1980): Neuropeptides. A new dimension in biological psychiatry. In Usdin, E., Sourkes, T.C., Youdim, M.B.H. (eds.): *Enzymes and Neurotransmitters in Mental Disease.* John Wiley, New York.
Prange, A.J., Wilson, I.C., Lara, P.P., Alltop, L.B. & Breese, G.R. (1972): Effects of thyrotropin-releasing hormone in depression. *Lancet II,* 999-1002.
Prange, A.J. Jr. (1977): Patterns of pituitary responses to thyrotropin-releasing hormone in depressed patients: a review. In Fann, W.E., Karacan, I., Pokorny, A.D., Williams, R.L. (eds.): *Phenomenology and Treatment of Depression.* Spectrum Publications, New York.
Puig-Antich, J., Tabrizi, M.A., Goetz, R., Chambers, W.J., Halpern, F. & Sachar, E.J. (1981): Prepubertal endogenous major depressives hyposecrete growth hormone in response to insulin induced hypoglycaemia. *Biol. Psychiatry, 16,* 801-819.
Re, R.N., Kourides, I.A., Ridgway, E.C., Weintraub, B.D. & Maloof, F. (1976): The effect of glucocorticoid administration on human pituitary secretion of thyrotropin and prolactin. *J. Clin. Endocrinol. Metab., 43,* 338.
Sachar, E.J., Hellman, L., Roffward, H.P., Halpern, F.S., Fukushima, D.K. & Gallagher, T.F. (1973): Disrupted 24-hour patterns of cortisol secretion in psychotic depression. *Arch. Gen. Psychiatry, 28,* 19-24.
Sachar, E.J. (1975): Neuroendocrine abnormalities in depressive illness. In Sachar, E.J. (ed.): *Topics in Psychoendocrinology.* Grune and Stratton, New York.
Sachar, E.J., Asnis, G., Halbreich, U., Nathan, R.S. & Halpern, F. (1980): Recent studies in the neuroendocrinology of major depressive disorders. *Psychiatr. Clin. North Am., 3,* 313-326.
Schlesser, M.A., Winokur, G. & Sherman, B. (1979): Genetic subtypes of unipolar primary depressive illness distinguished by hypothalamic-pituitary-adrenal axis activity. *Lancet I,* 739-741.
Westenberg, H.G.M., van Praag, H.M., De Jong, J.T.V.M., Thijssen, J.H.M. & Schwarz, F. (1982): Postsynaptic serotonergic activity in depressions: can it be measured via the neuroendocrine strategy. *Psychiatry Res., 7,* 361-371.

II: EVALUATION CRITERIA

Special Problems in Evaluation of Psychotherapy

R.J. DALY

1. Introduction

In talking about measurement of the effects of psychotherapy, one has to remember that the treatment is not well understood by many colleagues. They often imagine psychotherapy as being an exotic 'soft' or 'cosmetic' treatment with unmeasured or unmeasurable outcomes, conducted only by expensively trained individuals in the secrecy of their nicely appointed offices.

Dewald (1964) has defined psychotherapy as a "psychological process between two or more individuals, in which one (the therapist) by virtue of training and position, seeks systematically to apply psychological knowledge and interventions in an attempt to understand, influence and ultimately modify the psychic experience, mental function and behaviour of the other (the patient)".

One has to decide if psychotherapy has any effects at all, good or bad, or whether psychotherapy is an effective form of treatment; if so is it an efficient form, i.e. is it cost effective?

The most extensive criticisms of the efficacy of psychotherapy are perhaps those of Hans Eysenck (1952). His pessimistic conclusions were based on 24 surveys of treatment conducted both at psychoanalytic and other clinics. They reported uncontrolled compilations of clinical statistics using ill-defined therapist judgements of patient functioning or improvement as the only diagnostic and outcome criteria. Eysenck uncritically pooled these data and compared the findings and outcome of the natural course of neurosis. One of these studies reported data collected by insurance adjusters to adjudicate disability claims, while the other reported the percentage of neurotic patients released from New York State Hospitals as recovered or improved from 1917 to 1934. He attempted to construct a base-line for psychological improvement of neurosis in the absence of treatment, i.e. a spontaneous remission rate. This remission rate was compared with recovery rates in the 24 survey studies. He concluded that spontaneous remission was as effective as treatment given during psychological therapy. Eysenck supported his view in later reviews (1960, 1965) using selected control studies.

There has been no shortage of critics to expose Eysenck's mistakes and biases (Bergin & Lambert 1978; Malan 1973). Particularly it has been pointed out that Eysenck has used essentially dissimilar populations and that spontaneous remission rates from other sources are much more variable, ranging from 18 to 67 per cent. His review of the then available literature was biased and incomplete. They also point out that the distributions of treated and control groups are often significantly different even when the means are not. In addition, data for spontaneous remission levels do not purport to show the time it takes to achieve these levels; psychotherapy may achieve the same level in less time.

Eysenck was at least the force that prompted a whole series of research efforts into psychotherapy process and outcome. Strupp (Strupp & Bergin 1969) concluded by 1969, "any set of procedures in the context of a benign human relationship, presented to, or viewed by the patients as having therapeutic value, will result in psychological or behavioural change describable as therapeutic".

Malan (1976) concluded that there were significant effect sizes in the direction of supporting the hypothesis of the efficacy of psychotherapy. He reviewed four studies which did not use psychodynamic psychotherapy. He felt the evidence for the efficacy of psychotherapy with psychosomatic conditions was fairly strong. Malan concluded "we may end this long review of reviews by stating the following:
1. That the evidence for the effectiveness of psychotherapy is now fairly strong.
2. That there is considerable evidence that dynamic psychotherapy is effective in psychosomatic conditions.
3. The evidence in favour of dynamic psychotherapy in the ordinary run of neurosis and character disorders — for which after all this form of psychotherapy was developed — is weak in the extreme."

Psychotherapy in its widest sense includes:
1. Psychoanalysis (which is not feasible as a widespread service).
2. Psychodynamic psychotherapy both brief and long-term via individual, group, family, conjoint marital therapy and miscellaneous therapies, e.g. psychodrama, cognitive therapy, etc.
3. Behavioural therapies, desensitization, flooding, modelling, social

skills training, biofeedback, relaxation training, self-management, self-monitoring, decision training.

With regard to the methodology in the evaluation of the effects of psychotherapy it is important to conduct measurements in the following areas:
1. Costs and benefits of psychotherapy.
2. Knowledge and awareness of psychotherapy
   (a) amongst colleagues,
   (b) amongst the lay population.
3. The degree of pain in the general population, the treatment of which is the task of psychotherapy.
4. The need for treatment.
5. Who is capable of providing treatment? ('Quality control')
   (a) Professional training,
   (b) Continuous assessment.
6. Outcomes in psychotherapy.

One major aspect of the changing knowledge about the efficacy of psychotherapy is that the range of available therapy has increased immensely and we have also had an increase in the options for health care delivery. VandenBos and his colleagues (VandenBos & Pino 1980) suggest that the reason for the delay in understanding the efficacy of psychotherapy has been that "previously, from the perspective of our instruments, the effects of psychotherapy constituted a weak signal obscured by high noise level". There are now many major theories of human behaviour and malfunction. Behaviourism has been applied to a wide variety of problems in many settings. New treatments such as cognitive therapy for depression (Beck 1976) have been developed to treat specific problems. Biofeedback is widely used and various behavioural treatments, particularly relaxation therapy alone or in combination with other treatments, have been used in the treatment of a wide range of acute and chronic physical health problems. Crisis intervention, brief psychotherapy, marital therapy, family therapy, and group therapy have been extensively developed. Social skills training, self-management, self-monitoring and various other treatments are now burgeoning.

Many early researchers pointed out that there was a high degree of variance between psychotherapy patients, and that results could not be obtained if patients continued to be aggregated in a manner which ignored such meaningful variation. In addition there seemed little point in regarding psychotherapy as treatment for a homogeneous condition. Obviously psychotherapists and their methods of treatment are very heterogeneous. Paul (1967) re-emphasized the need for specification in

psychotherapy research. He also suggested the need for control groups (no-treatment controls, attention placebos, etc.) and for the use of factorial designs in exploring the efficacy of psychotherapy. He pointed out that vague hypotheses such as, "Does psychotherapy work?", were virtually meaningless. Detailed questions have to be asked. 'What treatment by whom is most effective for this individual with this specific problem and under which set of circumstances?' Strupp & Hadley (1979) argued that only by considering multiple perspectives would it be possible to derive truly comprehensive evaluations or psychotherapy outcomes. Their tripartite model emphasizes three perspectives, viz. those of:
 1. The individual (patient).
 2. The mental health professional.
 3. Society (family, neighbours, insurer or government).

Regarding allegations of the positive or negative effects of psychotherapy, a recent study by Rounsaville (Rounsaville et al 1981) surveyed the frequent speculations about possible negative interactions between pharmacotherapy and psychotherapy, occurring despite growing research evidence demonstrating the greater efficacy of combined treatment. They found that six hypotheses about negative interactions between pharmacotherapy and psychotherapy when evaluated on the basis of data derived from a clinical trial of psychotherapy and tricyclic antidepressants, alone and in combination as treatment for ambulatory depression, were not supported by the data.

Another exciting area is that of cognitive therapy for depression. A one-year follow-up of depressed out-patients treated with cognitive therapy or pharmacotherapy has recently been published. This illustrates that the same rigorous methodology expected in drug trials can also be used to evaluate psychotherapy, given specific diagnostic categories and outcome measures (Kovacs et al 1981). They used a control clinical trial format with 44 non-psychotic, non-bipolar depressed out-patients who were treated with cognitive therapy or imipramine hydrochloride over a twelve-week period. Although both interventions were associated with significant reduction in levels of depression, the cognitive therapy patients showed the greater symptomatic improvement and a higher treatment completion rate. A one-year follow-up showed that despite varying clinical courses, both groups of patients remained quite well. Self-rated depressive symptomatology was significantly lower for those who one year earlier had completed cognitive therapy than for those who had been in the clinical trials pharmacotherapy group.

2. Cost-benefit and cost-effectiveness studies

No matter how much it costs, one has to look at the costs of non-provision of psychotherapy in terms of:
  (a) lengthy and repeated hospitalization
  (b) increased incidence of physical illness and disability
  (c) social costs of inadequately treated mental illness
     (i) diminished work record and productivity
     (ii) broken homes
     (iii) disturbed children
     (iv) crime
  (d) pharmacological cost
     (i) overprescribing
     (ii) addiction and dependency.

Yates & Newman (1980) suggest that there are three approaches to cost-effectiveness and cost-benefit analysis in psychotherapy research.

1. A judgemental, summative approach that compares cost and effectiveness or benefit data for one or more psychotherapy programmes.
2. A formative approach that systematically varies parameters of psychotherapy in an attempt to understand the relationship between cost and effectiveness or benefit.
3. An operations research approach that places functions describing cost-effectiveness or cost-benefit relationships into a model of the psychotherapy system and manipulates this model to maximize effectiveness or benefit or to minimize cost.

They suggest that these different approaches are compatible and can be viewed as steps in using data on costs and outcomes both to improve psychotherapy as well as to simply evaluate it.

When it comes to measuring *effectiveness* most researchers now agree that it is important to use measures from multiple interest groups including the client, the therapist and the agency. Mathematical techniques can be used to transform survey results into a single index of therapy effectiveness that includes all information from each measure selected by various interest groups (Yates 1980).

He suggests that changes in client's self-reports of 'target' behaviours, cognitions, or affects are monitored in relation to the introduction of a new process by the therapist. These are used to modify therapy procedures until they are demonstrably effective.

Mahony (1971) used an obsessional client to record two target cognitions, namely the frequency of uncontrollable self-critical obsessions together with positive thoughts about himself. By using the graphs of his client's self-reports as a feedback of the efficacy of his self-treatment, Mahony was able to optimize the effectiveness of therapy while assessing therapy outcome.

The family and friends of out-patients can supply valuable data on patients' functioning. Members of the community in which the clients may reside also have special knowledge of psychotherapy outcomes: e.g. frequency of arrest for various misbehaviours may be important measures. And, of course, measures from the therapists themselves are particularly important.

With regard to measuring benefits, there are two procedures: firstly monetary measures of therapy outcome, or secondly transforming outcome data from non-monetary measures into monetary data. Monetary measures may assess the additional money or positive benefits for a client, the patient's family and friends or agencies. Alternatively the savings and expected costs which can be attributed to therapy through experimental designs can be considered to be a monetary benefit.

Of course, there are problems in assessing effectiveness or benefits of psychotherapy. However, many researchers have observed and measured (rather than inferred or estimated as is common in other fields) the cost-effectiveness and benefits of different treatments. By the use of good experimental design, rigorous statistical tests of the relative cost-effectiveness and the cost-benefit of different therapies, therapists and other treatment parameters, are possible. With benefit or cost/effectiveness ratios, it is not possible to test if they exceed unity, when worthwhile, because the outcomes are not expressed in the same units of costs. Thus, for example, effectiveness/cost ratios are inherently inferior to benefit/cost because they lack a common unit.

When several alternative therapies or treatments produce similar effectiveness or benefit while differing in cost, obviously the decision is easy — to use the method which is the least expensive. Alternatively with treatments or therapies with the same cost one chooses that with the greatest benefit or effect. The difficulty comes where superior effectiveness is achieved only at greater cost. If then a constraint is placed on cost, so that certain methods or techniques would not be used regardless of the ensuing benefit or effectiveness, then we have a cost constraint excluding treatments which are not feasible. When we have a treatment generating outcomes that are more valuable than the resources consumed, the question then is whether it should be chosen over other treatments. When one introduces an effectiveness or benefit constraint, a minimum degree of benefit is acceptable and will exclude some economic but less effective treatment.

When one is seeking to discover the most effective or least costly sequence in the network of treatments available, it is possible to construct graphic models of cost-effectiveness relationships and one looks at the critical path in the network of all possible service sequences which shows the effectiveness attached to each path in the network.

Yates (Yates & Newman 1980) describes a network analysis model for finding the least costly route through a therapy 'maze' for heroin addiction. Hypothetical costs are in thousands of dollars between service nodes in the network. One can choose the shortest route, i.e. the least costly, through the network. With non-effectiveness data (such as recidivism rates) placed on the links in a network, effectiveness can be similarly maximized. And putting cost-effectiveness data on the links would allow cost-effectiveness to be improved. Yates suggests that similar network models can be used to depict and solve problems in sequences of therapy or skill acquisition using more sophisticated procedures.

Another form of network (called probabilistic transition models) can be analysed to decide when the cost of provision is most worth the results of treatment as measured by a probable reduction in severity of the dysfunction.

Yates describes analyses to contrast the effectiveness of treatment (measured in probable costs for society of continued or more severe alcohol abuse) to the natural probability of the client's alcohol abuse staying the same or becoming less severe. The cost of intervention at each stage then is contrasted to the probabilistic cost savings to society that the treatment would generate. Analyses showed that intervention at the second stage of abuse had the highest ratio of monetary effectiveness to treatment cost.

Yates considers the primary purpose of all psychotherapy research, including of course cost-effectiveness and cost-benefit analyses, to be the systematic and continual improvement of the cost benefit and cost-effectiveness of separate psychotherapy systems. He feels that these operations research techniques offer the most promise for helping clinics and mental health systems to continue to self-improve and self-correct their treatment procedures.

3. Cost-benefit studies

In a series of papers Follette & Cummings (1967) described psychological services and medical utilization at the Kaiser-Permanente in San Francisco over a period of two decades. In their first paper they found that the provision of psychological services was associated with the reduction of medical utilization. A group of 132 psychiatric patients were compared with high medical utilizers through clinics, out-patients, x-ray and laboratory services. Data regarding medical utilization for one year before and five years following treatment were examined. Both the patients seen for psychotherapy (ranging from one interview only to 34 interviews with a mean of 6.2 interviews) and the high medical utilizers (controls) had an average utilization significantly higher than that of the health plan average. The results of the study indicated significant declines in the medical utilization in the psychotherapy groups when compared with the control group, whose in-patient and out-patient utilization remained relatively constant throughout the six years. The most significant declines occurred in the second year after the initial interview and the 'one interview only' and 'brief psychotherapy' groups did not require additional psychotherapy to maintain the low utilization level for the five years. On the other hand after two years the 'long-term psychotherapy' group attained a level of psychiatric utilization which remained constant through the remaining three years of study.

Techniques were tried for alerting all doctors in the scheme to the possibilities of referring patients who were high utilizers for psychotherapy. This was done via a computerized psychological screening, but did not produce any referrals from the physicians so alerted. Telephone follow-up of patients suggested that there was a good effect from resolving emotional distress. It was found that one visit alone produced a 60 per cent reduction in utilization while two to eight visits produced a 75 per cent reduction.

Goldberg et al (1970) in Washington, DC, found a 30 per cent reduction in utilization of medical services following psychotherapy intervention. Jameson et al (1978) in the Blue Cross in Western Pennsylvania looked at monthly costs per patient of medical services, and by using psychotherapy intervention reduced these by $9.41 from $16.47 to $7.06.

Lesser (1979) quotes a series of psychoanalytic studies conducted in West Germany about twenty years ago by Ann-Marie Duherssen and colleagues of the Central Institute of Psychogenic Illness of the Berlin General Health Insurance Office. This was an extensive follow-up on nearly a thousand patients over five years in analytic treatment or psychoanalysis. They used careful criteria for selection for the study which included:
 1. A precise description of the illness as well as its duration.
 2. The utilization of health care especially in-hospital care.
 3. The work capacity of individuals.
 4. Self-evaluation by the patients themselves.

For the five-year study of one thousand consecutive patients, the average number of treatment hours was one hundred. Thirteen per cent of them showed at least one relapse. They reduced their medical hospitalization average from 5.3 days prior to psychotherapy to 0.78 hospital days per year after psychotherapy. (The general average for the population was 2.5 hospital days per year.) Eighty-one per cent of patients felt strongly that they had been helped.

Nowadays it may not be adequate simply to write a verbal review of many different studies of the same problem. Instead the reviewer should seek a quantitative method of dealing with his task.

Smith & Glass (1977) used what they called "meta-analysis", a technique they developed for analysing educational research. Meta-analysis is a "second level of analysis of analyses". In their study 'Meta-analysis of Psychotherapy Outcome Studies', Smith and Glass addressed themselves to the problem of pooling different studies together in order to answer such questions as, 'What kind of effect does psychotherapy produce — on anything?'. They used the idea of 'effect size' which is the mean difference between the treated and control subjects divided by the standard deviation of the control group. Thus an effect size of +1 indicates that a person at the mean of the control group would be expected to rise to the 84th percentile of the control group after treatment. The effect sizes were from very different types of outcome including self-esteem, anxiety, work or school achievement, physiological stress, etc. They found that it was easy to calculate effect sizes where means and standard deviations were reported. They were unhappy to report that often this was not the case. Thus in some studies they had to use transformations from percentage of the patients who improved, and in others had to calculate effect sizes from various inferential test statistics.

They analysed the results of nearly 475 controlled evaluations of psychotherapy and counselling and these were coded and integrated statistically. The findings provided convincing evidence of the efficacy of psychotherapy in their view. On average, the typical therapy client was better off than 80 per cent of untreated individuals. Few important differences in effectiveness could be established between many quite different types of psychotherapy. More generally, virtually no difference in effectiveness was observed between the class of all behavioural therapies (systematic desensitisation, behaviour modification) and the non-behavioural therapies (Rogerian, psychodynamic, rational, emotive, transactional analysis).

One example from their work is the effect of psychologically informed intervention on recovery from surgery. They analysed studies (ranging from brief psychotherapy or hypnosis to explicitly educational efforts) of the effects of intervention on patients facing surgery.

They combined all outcome measures from all the studies and showed that the group receiving psychologically informed intervention surpassed the non-treated group by one half a standard deviation. It is worth noting that the findings in favour of this therapy are consistently positive. Fewer than 10 per cent of the 82 indicated outcome comparisons were negative, i.e. favouring the control group. The effect size is slightly smaller than the average effect size for psychotherapy in the treatment of say alcoholism or asthma, perhaps because the interventions were briefer and simpler. They found that the effect size for the medically relevant outcomes (ES = 0.56) was greater than that for the subjective outcomes (ES = 0.42).

When one considers those studies that used duration of hospitalization after surgery as an outcome indicator, it was found that the patients who received psychologically informed intervention had hospital stays almost two days shorter than patients in the control group who did not have such intervention. They point out the cost effect of these mostly minor interventions was easy to compute from the cost of a day in the hospital.

4. Accuracy of data

Blalock & Blalock (1968) pointed out that "for scientific knowledge to be useful it must say something about the nature and importance of a particular variable in relation to one or more others, and must verify these statements by empirical findings". Thus, in research in psychotherapy we should be able to:

(1) Specify the behaviour.
(2) Avoid ambiguity about what is being measured.
(3) Ensure that measurements are valid and replicable.

Many measurements in psychotherapy studies involve self-reports. Thus, it is possible for individuals to give inaccurate information — perhaps to please the investigator or for other reasons. This problem may be tackled in different ways; e.g. in relation to smoking, Donovan (1977) went to considerable effort to rule out bias in his study of smoking and pregnancy. He found an 18 per cent discrepancy between self-reporting of smoking during pregnancy and post-partum. He also discovered that the post-partum reports revealed considerable under-reporting while pregnant. This led to the suggestion of measuring factors which were not related to self-reporting, e.g. expired carbon monoxide levels, carboxyhaemoglobin, serum/urinary/salivary thiocyanate and cotinine. Also, in Donovan's study on birth weight and intervention in smoking behaviour, the treatment group turned out to get the treatment in 31 per cent of cases only, despite an elaborate scheme of counselling. This proportion was not statistically different from controls who reported advice which they had received adventitiously. Thus the problem of knowing who does and does not get psychological treatment turns out to be surprisingly similar to that in pharmacological treatments.

Another area where one might look at the efficacy of psychological treatment is that of coronary heart disease, where the behavioural correlations and predictions have been outlined by Rosenman *et al* (1975) in their Western Collaborative Study. Roskies *et al* (1978) and Suinn & Bloom (1978) have conducted intervention studies. The Framingham Study (Dawber *et al* 1957) brought about an understanding of the relationship between diet and heart disease.

There has been a considerable debate about whether it is possible to change behaviour which predisposes to coronary heart disease. It has been estimated that the numbers required would be 100,000 subjects, free-living in the population in a double-blind trial (US Executive Committee on Diet and Heart Disease). Thus such a study may never be conducted.

There are three main issues in demonstrating changes in patterns of behaviour.
 (1) Is the behaviour susceptible to being changed?
 (2) Is it possible to achieve large enough differences in comparable groups to test the hypothesis adequately?
 (3) Can the change be demonstrated?
There are two major difficulties, viz resources and time.

5. Self-monitoring

The importance of self-awareness has been stressed in all modes of psychotherapy. A specific technique of self-monitoring has developed as an agent for self-control techniques in behavioural psychotherapy. Self-monitoring now has become an agent of change, or a mode of psychotherapy in its own right. Various aids are used to count various forms of behaviour or to measure them. These include golf-counters, parking meter timers, beads, etc. People conducting these techniques require elaborate training and reinforcement of the technique is very important. The technique basically consists in counting specified events and measurement of specified intervals.

Diaries can also be used. A typical diary would consist of columns indicating:
 (1) time
 (2) place
 (3) persons present

(4) preceding thoughts
(5) preceding actions or events
(6) subsequent thoughts
(7) subsequent actions or events
(8) comments.

Some studies have used 'time spent seated' as a measure of anxiety (higher anxiety is correlated with shorter time spent seated).

What is needed in self-monitoring approaches is:
(1) a clearly specified target behaviour
(2) a simple self-monitoring device
(3) an emphasis on the accuracy and honesty of reporting
(4) demonstration of self-monitoring strategy
(5) supervised practice in self-monitoring assignments
(6) therapist/patient agreement to allow unannounced checks on behaviour or self-monitoring accuracy
(7) the use of an independent additional outcome measures.

Thus, weight loss or weight gain are easily measured. Independent measures may also be made in relation to smoking or phobic behaviour. Self-monitoring thus provides an opportunity for measurement and an agent for treatment, all in one.

6. Conclusion

Psychotherapeutic treatments were, early on, widely criticized as being ineffective. But nowadays numerous studies are being produced measuring the efficacy of psychotherapy, and doubts have been cast, for instance, on Eysenck's handling of the data and selection of patients (Browne & Herrnstein 1975).

Carpenter (Carpenter *et al* 1981) and his colleagues have recently underlined the importance of looking at more than just methodology in assessing the outcome of treatment in psychiatry generally, but particularly in relation to schizophrenia. They say many studies are methodologically correct but not meaningful. By this they mean that the measures used have too often in the past been insufficiently comprehensive. They argue in favour of multi-dimensional measures of outcome.

The greatly increased number and range of measurements has made it feasible to evaluate psychotherapy in an objective manner. A particular problem in psychodynamic psychotherapy is that the aims are often broad-ranging; measures of outcome must necessarily reflect this, and narrow measures of symptoms may sometimes be less appropriate than in pharmacological studies. Thus an epidemiological approach may be more useful, using such objective measures as utilization of medical services or recidivism, e.g. for self-poisoning.

Cost-benefit studies now constitute a more compelling and relevant assessment of the efficacy of psychotherapy. Their global measures are often more meaningful than measures derived from the medical model.

The newer and expanding field of behavioural psychotherapy has focussed sharply on objective measurement as a monitoring device, and even as a mode of treatment (e.g. biofeedback treatment and self-monitoring treatment). Hence, less difficulty has arisen in terms of measurement.

An important point to consider is that not all types of psychotherapy are confined to the traditional field of mental illness. Of possibly greater interest nowadays is the range of psychiatric treatments for physical illness, e.g. treatment adherence in general, CHD, hypotension, smoking, obesity, etc.

It is hoped that all developments in psychiatric treatment, as with all medical treatments, will in future include a component of programme evaluation.

References

Beck, A.T. (1976): *Cognitive Therapy and the Emotional Disorders.* International University Press, New York.
Bergin, A.E. & Lambert, E. (1978): The evaluation of therapeutic outcome. In Garfield, S.L. & Bergin, A.E. (eds.): *Handbook of Psychotherapy and Behaviour Change,* 2nd ed. Wiley, New York.
Blalock, H.M. & Blalock, A.B. (1968): *Methodology in Social Research.* McGraw-Hill, New York.
Browne, R. & Herrnstein, R.J. (1975): *Psychology.* Methuen, London.
Carpenter, W.T., Heinrichs, D.W. & Hanlon, T.E. (1981): Methodologic standards for treatment outcome research in schizophrenia. *Am. J. Psychiatry, 138,* 465-471.
Dawber, T.R., Moore, F.E. & Mann, G.V. (1957): Coronary heart disease in the Framingham Study. *Am. J. Public Health, 47,* 4-23.
Dewald, P. (1964): *Psychotherapy: A Dynamic Approach.* Basic Books, New York.
Donovan, J.W. (1977): Randomized controlled trial of antismoking advice in pregnancy. *Br. J. Prev. Soc. Med., 31,* 6-12.
Eysenck, H. (1952): The effects of psychotherapy and evaluation. *J. Consult. Psychol., 16,* 319-324.
Eysenck, H. (1960): The effects of psychotherapy. In Eysenck, H. (ed.): *The Handbook of Abnormal Psychology.* Basic Books, New York.
Eysenck, H. (1965): The effects of psychotherapy. *Int. J. Psychiatry, 1,* 97-178.
Follette, W. & Cummings, N.A. (1967): Psychiatric services and medical utilization in a prepaid health plan setting. *Med. Care, 5,* 25-35.
Goldberg, I.D., Krantz, G. & Locke, B.Z. (1970): Effect of a short-term out-patients psychiatric therapy benefit on the utilization of medical services in a prepaid group practice medical programme. *Med. Care, 8,* 419-428.
Jameson, J., Shuman, L.J. & Young, W.W. (1978): The effects of out-patients psychiatric utilization on the costs of providing third party coverage. *Med. Care, 16,* 383-399.

Kovacs, M., Rush, A.J., Beck, A.T. & Hollon, S.D. (1981): Depressed out-patients treated with cognitive therapy or pharmacotherapy. *Arch. Gen. Psychiatry, 38,* 33-39.

Lesser, A.L. (1979): Psychotherapy, benefits and costs. *Rev. de Psychiatrie de l'Univ. d'Ottawa, 9,* 191-196.

Mahony, M.J. (1971): The self-management of covert behaviour. A case study. *Behav. Ther., 2,* 575-578.

Malan, D.H. (1973): The outcome problem in psychotherapy research: a historical review. *Arch. Gen. Psychiatry, 29,* 719-729.

Malan, D.H. (1976): *Toward the Validation of Dynamic Psychotherapy.* Plenum, London.

Paul, G.L. (1967): Strategy for outcome research. *J. Consult. Psychol., 31,* 109-118.

Rosenman, R.H., Brand, R.J., Jenkins, C.D., Friedman, M., Straus, R. & Wurm, N. (1975): Coronary heart disease in the Western Collaborative Study: final follow-up of 8.5 years. *JAMA, 233,* 872-877.

Roskies, E., Spevack, M., Surkis, A., Cohen, C. & Gilman, S. (1978): Changing the coronary prone (Type A) behaviour pattern in a non-clinical population. *J. Behav. Med., 1,* 201-206.

Rounsaville, B.J., Klerman, G.L. & Weissman, M.M. (1981): Do psychotherapy and pharmacotherapy for depression conflict? *Arch. Gen. Psychiatry, 38,* 24-29.

Smith, M.L. & Glass, G.V. (1977): Meta-analysis of psychotherapy outcome studies. *Am. Psychol.,* Sept., 752-759.

Strupp, H.H. & Bergin, A. (1969): Some empirical and conceptual bases for co-ordinated research in psychotherapy. *Int. J. Psychiatry, 1,* 18-90.

Strupp, H.H. & Hadley, S.W. (1979): Specific vs. non-specific factors in psychotherapy. *Arch. Gen. Psychiatry, 36,* 1125-1136.

Suinn, R.M. & Bloom, L.J. (1978): Anxiety and management training for pattern A behaviour. *J. Behav. Med., 1,* 25-38.

VandenBos, G.R. & Pino, C.D. (1980): Research on the outcome of psychotherapy. In VandenBos, G.R. (ed.): *Psychotherapy: Practice, Research, Policy.* Sage Publications, London.

Yates, B.T. (1980): *Improving Effectiveness and Reducing Costs in Mental Health.* Charles C. Thomas, Springfield, Ill.

Yates, B.T. & Newman, F.L. (1980): Findings of cost-effectiveness and cost-benefit analyses in psychotherapy. In VandenBos, G.R. (ed.): *Psychotherapy: Practice, Research, Policy.* Sage Publications, London.

Special Problems in Evaluation of Milieu Therapy

O.S. DALGARD, S. FRIIS, T. SØRENSEN and
P. VAGLUM

1. The need for evaluation of milieu therapy
In general terms, milieu therapy can be defined as a planned treatment environment where all activities and social relations are supposed to serve a common therapeutic goal. Within this broad, and rather vague definition, there are different types of milieu therapy, according to theoretical background, methods and goals, from 'the therapeutic community proper' to behaviour modification by 'token economy'.

Whereas the negative effects on patients of the traditional, custodial hospital setting have been well documented, it has been more problematic to prove the positive effects of specific types of milieu therapy. This, of course, does not necessarily imply that milieu therapy does not work, as some of the opponents seem to mean. The rather inconclusive situation shows, however, the need for more effort to be put into evaluation and for the development of evaluation methods in this field. The present economic situation, with increasing problems in getting funding for health work, makes this need even stronger.

2. Components of evaluation
Milieu therapy, not being one single therapeutic method, but rather a variety of treatment programmes consisting of different components, may be evaluated according to the same guidelines as for health programmes in general. The main components are the following, referring to WHO publications:
(a) relevance
(b) progress
(c) effectiveness
(d) efficiency
(e) impact.

(a) *Relevance* relates to the rationale for having programmes, or services and institutions, in terms of their response to essential human needs and health policies and priorities.

(b) *Progress* is concerned with the comparison of the actual with the scheduled programme delivery, the identification of reasons for achievements or shortcomings, and indications for remedies for any shortcomings. The purpose of a progress review is to facilitate the monitoring and operational control of on-going activities. In the terms of systems analysis it is a review of the use of 'inputs'.

(c) *Effectiveness* is an expression of the desired effect of a programme, service or institution in reducing a health problem or improving an unsatisfactory health situation. Thus, effectiveness measures the degree of attainment of the pre-determined objectives and targets of the programme, service or institution. The assessment of effectiveness is aimed at improving programme formulation or the functions and structure of health service and institutions through analysis of the extent of attainment of their objectives.

(d) *Efficiency* is an expression of the relationships between the results obtained from a health programme or activity and the efforts expended in terms of human, financial and other resources, health processes and technologies, and time. The assessment of efficiency is aimed at improving implementation, and adds to the review of progress by taking account of the results.

(e) *Impact* is an expression of the positive effects of a programme, service or institution on overall health development and on related social and economic development. While a programme may be effective in that it has attained its objectives, the attainment of these objectives may, in fact, make little or no contribution to overall health and related socio-economic developments.

Even if the evaluation of relevance, progress, efficiency and impact is certainly very relevant for milieu therapy programmes, the evaluation of effectiveness seems the most urgent need. In the following section we will concentrate upon this.

3. Evaluation of effectiveness

Evaluation may be more or less scientific, depending on the extent to which the methods used are designed to control for different sources of error. When evaluation is carried out on a reasonably high scientific level, one talks of 'evaluation research'. One should then be able to test out different hypotheses about the effectiveness of the programme, and explain why the programme works or fails. The strict scientific demands which have to be put to confirmatory research should, however, not prevent the stimulation of exploratory studies, where interesting hypotheses may be generated even by using rather simple methods.

In the following we will look into the problems of research design as well as possible variables and criteria in the evaluation of milieu therapy.

3.1 Design

The choice of design for the evaluation of milieu therapy programmes has to be based upon several considerations, such as the purpose of the study, the situation in which it is going to be carried out, the time and economic resources available, etc. One important decision to make is whether the study is going to be a purely descriptive, a correlational, an experimental or a quasi-experimental one.

In a *descriptive* study one is asking questions like: What type of patients are admitted to the programme? How long are they staying? How many are exposed to which parts of the therapeutic repertoire? How many are improved at discharge and at follow-up?

In a *correlational* study one will add questions such as: What is the correlation between characteristics of the patients, the length of stay and the outcome? Are there sub-groups among the patients who are having a different course of treatment?

In the *experimental* and *quasi-experimental* study the purpose will be to clarify whether the treatment programme really has a specific impact upon the course of the patient or not. This implies the use of control or comparison groups.

In all types of design, one uses three sets of variables: characteristics of the patients at admission, characteristics of the treatment and treatment milieu, and characteristics of the patients at discharge and at one or several follow-up points. In selection of variables, it is important that they are valid, theoretically linked together and able to be measured in a reliable way. In what follows, we will discuss some special problems concerning these three sets of variables in evaluation of a milieu treatment programme.

3.2 Characteristics of patients at admission

In the description of the patient population one will include data on variables which makes it comparable to other patient populations (i.e. age, sex, diagnosis, symptoms, duration of problems, socio-economic situations, etc.). In addition, it is important to include information about variables which are known to be predictive as to the course of the disease, and about variables which the treatment programme specifically tries to influence. As the patients in a milieu treatment programme are treated in a special institutional 'culture', it is also important to describe their cultural background. This is illustrated, for example, by a study of Dalgard *et al* (1977), where cultural background (rural/urban) was significantly related to expectations from treatment as well as to treatment outcome.

3.3 Treatment variables

One of the most complicated problems in the evaluation of milieu therapy is to obtain reliable and valid measures of the treatment factors. Because of the complexity of potentially therapeutic and anti-therapeutic factors, we are faced with much more intricate problems than, for example, in the evaluation of individual psychotherapy.

One problem is that the effect of milieu therapy usually is combined with the effect of specific therapeutic methods, like drug therapy, family therapy, and individual psychotherapy. Therefore, the nature of these treatment methods, and the extent to which they are used, have to be measured to allow evaluation of their effect, both separately and in interaction with the milieu therapy. As for the measuring of the milieu therapy itself, no single approach seems to have obtained general acceptance as the ideal one. We shall here briefly mention the four types of variables most commonly measured, and comment on some of their probable shortcomings.

3.3.1 Simple descriptive dimensions (e.g. ward census and staff/patient ratio)

The rationale behind measuring such dimensions as the staff/patient ratio is that it is supposed to give some sort of information about the frequency and the quality of the interaction between staff and patients. This may be so under special conditions. For instance on very poorly staffed wards an increased staff/patient ratio will probably affect the interaction in a predictable way. But for most wards it is unlikely that a single ratio can give reliable information about complex phenomena like human interaction.

3.3.2 Staff attitudes

These may be measured by rating scales, e.g. the Opinions About Mental Illness Scale (OMI) developed by Cohen & Struening (1964). It is a 51 item scale yielding five factor scores descriptively labelled: Authoritarianism, Benevolence, Mental Hygiene Ideology, Social Restrictiveness and Interpersonal Etiology.

The scale is based on the assumption that staff attitudes mediate the nature of the staff/patient interaction. Thus the OMI scores are supposed to serve as an indirect measure of this interaction. This assumption has been seriously questioned by, for example, Edelson & Paul (1977). In their experience there is no reliable connection between the OMI-scores and individual staff performance.

3.3.3 Ward atmosphere

Several rating scales have been developed for measuring the atmosphere of treatment milieus, e.g. the Perception of Ward Scales (POW) developed by Ellsworth et al (1971) and the Ward Atmosphere Scale (WAS) developed by Moos and Houts (Moos 1974a). The most applicable one seems to be the WAS. It is by far the most used of the scales, and we shall, therefore, limit our considerations to this scale. It consists of 100 items, yielding the following 10 subscales: Involvement, Support, Spontaneity, Autonomy, Practical orientation, Personal problem orientation, Anger and aggression, Order and organization, Programme clarity and Staff control.

The WAS claims to give indirect measures of the human interaction (both between the patients and between staff and patients) within a ward. Unlike the OMI, both patients and staff are asked to fill in the forms, and the scores for a given milieu are calculated separately for the two groups. The research with the WAS has mainly focussed on two areas: process evaluation of single wards and comparative investigations of the atmosphere of several wards.

Examples of process evaluation are given by Pierce et al (1972) and Verinis & Flaherty (1978). The experience of these authors is paralleled by our own (Friis 1980a): the WAS proved to be a very useful instrument in the process of changing a ward. Feedback of the milieu facilitated the restructuring of the ward, and retesting showed that the ward atmosphere had changed significantly.

In comparative investigations the WAS has proved to discriminate significantly among wards (Moos 1974c). This finding is also paralleled by our own. The atmosphere on wards with predominantly non-psychotic patients proved to be significantly different from that on wards with predominantly acute psychotic patients and that on long-term wards for chronic psychotic patients (Friis 1981).

Among non-psychosis as well as psychosis wards the atmosphere on wards with main emphasis on drug treatment was quite different from that on wards with main emphasis on interpersonal processes (Friis 1981).

A detailed discussion on the many methodological problems with the use of instruments like the WAS is given by Moos (1974b, 1974c). In this paper we shall briefly consider some of the most crucial problems.

A common objection is that the WAS only measures perceptions of the milieu, and not necessarily what is really going on. It has been stated that staff scores might be biased in the direction of what the staff considers ideal, while the patients' perception might be distorted because of their pathology. The results from extensive use of the WAS give minimal support to these objections. Even if some individuals may have quite deviant perception of a milieu, the patient and the staff groups mostly agree closely about the WAS-scores for a ward, and the mean scores for the two groups have proved to be remarkably stable in test-retest investigations, even in the presence of a nearly complete patient turn-over from test to retest. It seems important to keep in mind, however, that for the single patient his own scores, deviant or not, are probably the most valid measures of the milieu therapy he experiences. Consequently, for those few patients with deviant perception the mean scores for the ward will not be valid measures for what one might call 'the milieu therapy received'.

Another objection, given by Gunderson (1978), is that the WAS subscales either do not reflect the therapeutic actions, or that their items represent only limited aspects of what these variables can mean. These are important objections, and it is still unclear what is the connection between the ward atmosphere and the treatment outcome for different types of patients, even if our experience seems to allow some tentative suggestions (Friis 1981). Gunderson (1978) suggests the following five functional variables as the therapeutically important ones: Containment, Support, Structure, Involvement, Validation. Unfortunately he does not suggest any measurement techniques for these variables.

3.3.4 Monitoring of staff behaviour

This approach has been advocated by, for example, Edelson & Paul (1977). For such monitoring Paul *et al* (1973) have developed an assessment instrument termed the Staff-Resident Interaction Chronograph. By use of trained observers, they score the behaviour of staff members for 10 sequential one-minute periods. They have shown that the measurements have high reliability. The validity may, however, still be questioned. It is, for instance, unclear to what degree this monitoring really does measure the important therapeutic activities, and the patient perception of staff behaviour does not seem to be taken into consideration. The procedure necessitates greater resources (of time, people and money) and does not so easily lend itself to comparative investigations as the rating scales. This procedure seems best suited for intensive study of relatively few wards.

A common objection to all the mentioned measures of milieu therapy is that they neglect description of the organizational level of institutions and that they ignore the fact that the treatment milieu is an open system in continuous interaction with the surrounding society. Obviously both the organizational structure and the interaction with the society are of prime importance for the nature and the effects of a treatment milieu. The available data do not indicate, however, that these factors have any profound effect on, for example, the milieu perception. It seems more reasonable to believe that differences in organizational structure and in the milieu interaction with the society will influence the staff behaviour and the atmosphere of the milieu. Consequently the effect of such differences may indirectly be measured by monitoring of staff behaviour or by use of the WAS.

3.4 Criteria of outcome

Criteria of outcome in milieu therapy do not differ in principle from the criteria used in the evaluation of psychiatric treatment in general. They are mainly based on change in the patient's condition and psychological functioning before and after treatment.

As in the evaluation of other psychiatric treatment methods, a change in symptoms is usually considered an important part of outcome-criteria in milieu therapy. For this purpose a number of symptom rating scales have been developed, as described by Cronholm & Daly in this volume.

As milieu therapy, however, does not focus exclusively on symptom reduction, but rather aims towards improvement of interpersonal behaviour and learning of social skills, outcome-criteria based on symptoms alone are not sufficient.

To what extent symptom removal is contributing to a change in these social dimensions, is to a great extent an empirical question. It is quite possible that the different dimensions of personal improvement follow different courses of development, and as mentioned earlier, it is, therefore, important that the outcome-criteria chosen are in accordance with the theoretical background and specific aims of the programme under consideration.

Also in the field of social relations and functioning there have been developed valid and reliable instruments, the so-called Social Adjustment Scales. The content of these are usually occupational, community, marital, parental and economic. As pointed out by Weissman (1975) there is a strong need for standardization of methods between studies, and it seems good advice to include intact a standard and widely used scale, and to supplement later with innovations.

Whatever outcome-criteria are used, it is of great importance at what time the evaluation takes place. There may be good reasons for evaluating the patient's condition on his discharge from the programme. Experience from different studies, however, indicates that this does not tell much about how the patient will manage in the community.

The crucial evaluation should, therefore, take place after the patient is back in his own surroundings. On the other hand it will be unsatisfactory to make this evaluation too long after the discharge. At this later time it can be difficult to decide what is causing the observed change in the patient's condition and way of life, the treatment or other uncontrolled factors in milieu.

Ellsworth (1975) strongly underlines the need for evaluating the patient's condition and social functioning in the community. Although patients themselves are in the best position to describe their feelings of felt distress and troublesome symptoms, their reports on social dimensions are not particularly reliable or valid. Ellsworth, therefore, recommends rating by other significant variables in the patient's social network as giving the most valid information on socially significant behaviour. The relationship to the important members in the social network is in itself decisive as to the future. On these grounds Ellsworth has worked out a Personal Adjustment and Role-Skill scale (PARS III) containing dimensions such as: interpersonal involvement, confusion, anxiety, agitation-depression, alcohol/drug improvement, household management, employment and outside social.

A recent development in the field of outcome-criteria is the quality of life approach. This seems to be a promising future criterion for the evaluation of psychiatric treatment programmes, particularly for the more chronic psychiatric population.

There is no full agreement on definition and indicators of outcome. The most satisfactory criterion in the long term seems to be the patient's subjective experience on a multitude of dimensions which are supposed to be central for the person's experience of happiness, such as: involvement, living up to one's potentialities, freedom and control over one's own life, self-confidence and self-respect. During recent years American surveys (Andrews & Withey 1976, Campbell *et al* 1976) have made important progress in the methodology in this field.

Even if there is disagreement on definition and indicators of quality of life, the concept is of great interest. If properly used, quality of life could reduce the other outcome-criteria to preliminary goals on the way to the ultimate goal: a better quality of life for the patient. The definition of quality of life will, however, depend on priorities of values, on the part of

Evaluation of milieu therapy

professionals, the patients, and society in general. It is important to make these priorities explicit.

3.5 Control groups

If the progress of a patient is satisfactory, and especially if the progress is following a logical sequence over time which is in accordance with the theoretical model of the programme, this, of course, supports the assumption that the treatment really affects the course. The ultimate verification of this, however, requires a study which includes the use of control or comparison groups.

In experimental studies, one usually assigns subjects to different treatment and no-treatment groups in a random fashion, and gathers complete data on all subjects. Ideally the researcher varies the treatment variable, keeping all other variables constant. This design is difficult to apply in milieu therapy research. Often it will be impossible to admit patients at random and to keep all variables except the treatment variables constant. When two different treatment programmes are to be compared, there may also be problems in keeping the treatment variables constant over time in both programmes.

As to the no-treatment group, which is usually an important part of treatment research, it is almost impossible to accomplish such a group in milieu therapy research. Patients who are in need of institutional care will not continue to be untreated even if they are initially refused admission. In a study of young drug abusers applying for a stay in a therapeutic community ward in Oslo, 95 per cent of those who were not admitted got another type of institutional treatment during the following three years (Vaglum & Fossheim 1980).

When randomization of patients is impossible, it is still important to do evaluation studies including comparison groups. One may then use one of the several quasi-experimental designs which have been developed and evaluated. (See Campbell 1974.) When a new milieu treatment programme is introduced or an old programme is used for new patient groups, the design called 'interrupted time series' may be very useful, as shown in a study of the results in different phases in a therapeutic community programme for young drug abusers, conducted by one of the authors (Vaglum & Fossheim 1980). In such a design, it is very important that the new programme is introduced abruptly, and that the system of measurement is kept constant through the different time periods.

As the patients are not randomized to the different groups, the results of quasi-experimental studies must be carefully evaluated in relation to the different possible threats to the internal validity. Campbell (1969) mentions nine such sources of error, including selection biases, differential loss of respondents from the comparison groups, alternation of the system of measurement, and regression artefacts due to the pseudoshifts in scoring which may occur when repeated measures are taken on initially extreme groups.

To control for selection biases, it is especially important to assess the different patient groups with regard to variables of known prognostic value. To avoid the regression artefact, for instance when using 'interrupted time series', the introduction of the new policy should not immediately follow a wide fluctuation in the prior series. The effect of a quickly introduced corrective measure in response to an acute problem, is very hard to distinguish from the ordinary reversion to trend found in any unstable series. There are, however, statistical methods which can be used to make corrections for such regression effects by estimating residual change scores (Nunnally 1975).

4. Psycho-social problems in evaluation of milieu therapy

As underlined by Group for the Advancement of Psychiatry (1959) there are in addition to serious formal problems, special psychological problems connected with psychiatric research: The personality of the investigator may well influence his observations; the responses of the subject may be shaped to a significant but undetermined extent by the impact of the investigation; the emotionally charged significance of the characteristic data of psychiatry may well bring prejudice to the research activities. To control these sources of error the importance of consultation, supervision and multiple observers and data analysts is stressed.

In the evaluation of milieu therapy, these and other psycho-social problems make research particularly difficult. These problems include:

    Getting a numerous and professionally heterogeneous staff to keep loyally to a specific treatment model.

    Resistance in the staff against measurement and classification of psychological phenomena, like symptom rating scales and diagnosis, a resistance which seems particularly strong among psychiatrists who conceive psychopathology in an interpersonal frame of reference.

Problems like this, of course, make the giving of information to staff about the general idea of the study, and other motivational work, a very important part of the research preparations. At the same time one should be cautious not to unveil the specific hypotheses to be tested in the study.

The most difficult problem, however, is the anxiety and resistance among administration and staff related to evaluation of their programme. It seems to be a characteristic of public officials to win confidence by advocating programmes and reforms as though they were certain to be successful. If public officials or administrators have committed themselves in advance to the efficacy of their programme, they are not in a good position to risk learning of failure. Under these circumstances, lack of concrete evidence increases their feeling of security. Addressing this problem, Campbell (1969) has made the following pertinent recommendation:

"Administrators should stop advocating in advance that a particular approach will solve the problem, and focus instead on identifying the seriousness of the problem and the importance of finding adequate solutions. Within this framework, the administrator, agency head, or legislator would propose that different approaches to the problem be tried and evaluated, and that the most effective be adopted."

Resistance from clinical staff appears to stem primarily from the fear that their efforts may not be measurably effective. As pointed out by Ellsworth (1973) and others, clinicians are not likely to co-operate in a process that might demonstrate their ineffectiveness. If this is so for the single clinician, the resistance against critical evaluation is likely to be even stronger in the complex social system of a therapeutic milieu, where the system as such may be threatened by disintegration if the dominating belief and values are made the subject of a critical investigation.

As stressed by Ellsworth (1975) and others, one way of reducing the personal threat to staff is by stressing that it is the programme or treatment concept that is being evaluated, not the personal competence of staff members themselves. When it comes to the institution as such, we would add that co-operation about evaluation is most likely, and probably only possible, if the institution is granted future existence, though in an altered form, if the evaluation turns out to be negative.

After all, co-operation between researchers and administrators as well as clinicians depends most heavily on the extent to which the evaluation itself is based on professional skills and sound clinical knowledge.

References

Andrews, F.M. & Withey, S.B. (1976): *Social Indicators of Well-Being: Americans' Perceptions of Life Quality.* Plenum, New York.

Campbell, A., Converse, P.E. & Rodgers, W.L. (1976): *The Quality of American Life.* Russel Sage Foundation, New York.

Campbell, D.T. (1969): Reforms as experiments. *Am. Psychologist, 24,* 409-429.

Campbell, D.T. (1974): Quasi-experimental designs. In Riecken, H. & Boruch, R. (eds.): *Social Experimentation. A Method for Planning and Evaluating Social Intervention.* Academic Press, London.

Cohen, J. & Struening, E.L. (1964): Opinions about mental illness: hospital social atmosphere profiles and their relevance to effectiveness. *J. Consult. Psychol., 28:4,* 291-298.

Dalgard, O.S., Berg-Larsen, R. & Popstad, O. (1977): Evaluering av et psykiatrisk behandlingsopplegg. *Nord psykiat. tidsskr., 31,* 73-89.

Edelson, R.I. & Paul, G.L. (1977): Staff 'attitude' and 'atmosphere' scores as a function of ward size and patient chronicity. *J. Consult. Clin. Psychol., 45:5,* 874-884.

Ellsworth, R. et al (1971): Milieu characteristics of successful psychiatric treatment programmes. *Am. J. Orthopsychiatry, 41:3,* 427-441.

Ellsworth, R.B. (1975): Consumer feedback in measuring the effectiveness of mental health programmes. In Struening, E.L. & Guttentag, M. (eds.): *Handbook of Evaluation Research.* Sage, London.

Friis, S. (1980a): The ideal ward — ideal for whom? *Scand. J. Psychiatry, 34,* 120-128.

Friis, S. (1980b): From enthusiasm to resignation in a therapeutic community. *J. Oslo City Hosp., 31,* 51-54.

Friis, S. (1981): What kind of ward atmosphere is therapeutic for psychotic and for non-psychotic patients? *J. Norweg. Med. Assoc., 101,* 848-852. (English translation available from the author.)

Group for the Advancement of Psychiatry (1959): *Some Observations on Controls on Psychiatric Research.* Publications Office, 104 East 25th Street, New York.

Gunderson, J.G. (1978): Defining the therapeutic process in psychiatric milieu. *Psychiatry, 41,* 327-335.

Moos, R.H. (1974a): *Ward Atmosphere Scale Manual.* Consulting Psychologists Press Inc., Palo Alto, California.

Moos, R.H. (1974b): *The Social Climate Scales. An Overview.* Consulting Psychologists Press Inc., Palo Alto, California.

Moos, R.H. (1974c): *Evaluating Treatment Environments. A Social Ecological Approach.* John Wiley & Sons, New York.

Nunnally, J.C. (1975): The study of change in evaluation research: principles concerning measurement, experimental design, and analysis. In Struening, E.L. & Guttentag, M. (eds.): *Handbook of Evaluation Research.* Sage, London.

Paul, G.L. et al (1973): Objective performance outcomes associated with two approaches to training mental health technicians in milieu and social-learning programmes. *J. Abnorm. Psychol., 82:3,* 523-532.

Pierce et al (1972): Changing ward atmosphere through staff discussion of the perceived ward environment. *Arch. Gen. Psychiatry, 26,* 35-41.

Vaglum, P. & Fossheim, I. (1980): Differential treatment of young drug abusers. A quasi-experimental study of a therapeutic community in a psychiatric hospital. *J. Drug. Issues, 10,* 505-515.

Verinis, J.S. & Flaherty, J.A. (1978): Using the Ward Atmosphere Scale to help change the treatment environment. *Hosp. Community Psychiatry, 29,* 238-240.

Weissman, M.M. (1975): The assessment of social adjustment. *Arch. Gen. Psychiatry, 32,* 357-365.

III: RATING METHODS IN EVALUATION OF TREATMENT

The AMP Rating Methods

B. WOGGON

1. Development of the AMP system

In 1965 the Association for Methodology and Documentation in Psychiatry (AMP) was founded by several German-speaking psychiatrists from Germany, Switzerland and Austria (Angst *et al* 1969). It was the aim of these psychiatrists to develop together a system for the documentation of psychopathological and somatic symptoms which are characteristic for the description of psychiatric patients. In 1971 the first edition of the AMP manual was published (Scharfetter 1971), followed by the second edition in 1972 (Scharfetter 1972). This manual contained a detailed description of every item, especially of the psychopathological symptoms. In 1979 the third, revised edition of the manual was published and the name of the system was changed to AMDP (AMDP 1979). One of the reasons for this change was to prevent further confusion with cyclic AMP. Equally important was the wish to emphasize that the new version of the system has been the result of many years of methodological work and many intense discussions.

Today the new edition of the AMDP system has been used in several hospitals for the routine documentation of psychiatric patients, especially in Berlin and Munich. Methodological examination of the new version — for example, of the inter-rater reliability or the construction of subscales — is not finished. For the moment it is, therefore, impossible to give a detailed synopsis of the AMDP system. In this situation I will concentrate on the following subjects: 1. Training of raters; 2. Instructions for raters; 3. Development of AMP short forms, especially two second-order scales, which will most probably survive the change from AMP to AMDP; 4. Comparison between AMDP system and other well-known rating scales.

During the last AMDP meeting in 1980 it was reported that the system has been translated into 11 languages (Baumann & Faehndrich 1981). One of these translations has given me a lot of help in preparing this paper: 'The North American Adaptation of the AMDP System' by William Guy and Thomas Ban (in preparation).

2. Description of the AMDP assessment documents

AMDP consists of five integrated parts, each printed on a single sheet of paper: 1. Anamnesis — Demographic data; 2. Anamnesis — Life events; 3. Anamnesis — Historical data; 4. Psychopathological symptoms; 5. Somatic signs. This paper concentrates on parts 4 and 5, the rating of psychopathological and somatic symptoms.

The 100 psychopathological symptoms and 40 somatic signs are clearly arranged into groups, a useful help for the rater, especially the beginner (Tables 1 and 2).

Table 1. Groups of psychopathological symptoms

1.	Disorders of consciousness (4)*
2.	Disturbances of orientation (4)
3.	Disturbances of attention and memory (6)
4.	Formal disorders of thought (12)
5.	Phobias and compulsions (6)
6.	Delusions (14)
7.	Disorders of perception (6)
8.	Disorders of the ego (6)
9.	Disorders of affect (21)
10.	Disorders of drive and psychomotility (9)
11.	Circadian rhythms (3)
12.	Other disturbances (9)

*Number of symptoms.

Table 2. Groups of somatic signs

1.	Sleep disturbances (5)*
2.	Appetite disturbances (4)
3.	Gastrointestinal disturbances (7)
4.	Cardiac-respiratory disturbances (4)
5.	Other autonomic disturbances (5)
6.	General disturbances (6)
7.	Neurological disturbances (9)

*Number of symptoms.

3. Training

Before making the first AMP rating it is essential to be familiar with the definitions of the symptoms. Therefore the first step for the beginner is to read and re-read the manual. Afterwards the training should start with supervised interviews. In our hospital we do not use video-taped interviews but live interviews. The trainings take place in a group setting, one patient being interviewed by one of us, the others listening. At the end of the interview each of us is allowed to ask additional questions. This first part of our weekly inter-rater training lasts on average one hour. During the second hour each rater completes independently the psychopathological form. Afterwards the interviewer presents his findings symptom by symptom, disagreements with other raters being subject to discussion. This discussion is followed by a short summing up, a syndrome diagnosis and if possible a nosological diagnosis. For a new rater, at least 10 supervised interviews and ratings are necessary before being able to use the AMDP system independently. Therefore, the described inter-rater trainings are supplemented by interviews supervised by an experienced rater. In my group every new rater needs on average two months before being able to use the AMDP system.

4. Instructions for raters

At the beginning it can be helpful to have the AMDP forms at hand while interviewing. Personally I do not like the situation where the interviewer looks at the symptom-list while trying to interview a psychiatric patient on very intimate topics. The experienced raters who are listening can ask supplementary questions on symptoms which have been forgotten by the beginner. Even experienced raters can forget symptoms during an interview, but the rating can be completed by asking additional questions afterwards.

A trained rater needs on average 45 minutes to make a complete AMDP interview (Woggon *et al* 1978). Often only 30 minutes are necessary; with other patients more time is needed. In my opinion it is very important for the rater to give himself enough time to develop a good contact with the patient, which is especially needed for the judgement of affective symptoms.

Every evaluation of psychopathological and somatic symptoms is based on a cross-section of a specific time period, for example, 24 hours. The rating of longer periods is difficult because it is not so easy for the patient to remember the intensity of symptoms experienced yesterday or during the last week.

For AMDP ratings a combination of subjective and objective information is needed. This confluence of the patient's own impressions and external observations creates problems, especially because of differences between subjective and objective information (Woggon 1979c).

For many symptoms it is difficult to judge whether they are related to a psychiatric illness or to the personality of the patient. Because of this difficulty the assessment of AMDP symptoms should be descriptive. This problem is part of the general discussion on defining deviations from the norm. In my opinion it is impossible to give general guidelines concerning this problem.

As shown in Fig. 1 the rating of each symptom can be represented by four judgemental steps.

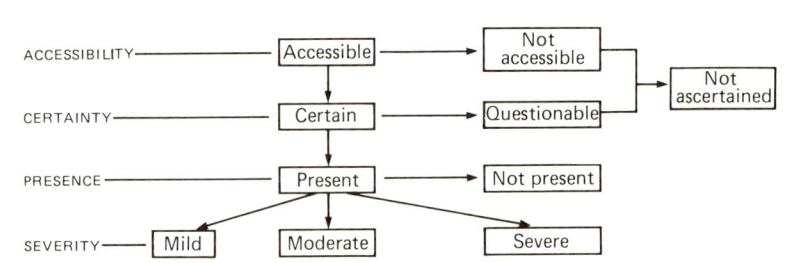

Fig. 1. Decision tree (from Guy & Ban, in preparation).

```
ACCESSIBILITY ──────── Accessible ──────► Not accessible ──┐
                                                            ├──► Not
CERTAINTY ──────────── Certain ────────► Questionable ─────┘    ascertained
                          │
PRESENCE ─────────────► Present ───────► Not present
                       ↙  ↓  ↘
SEVERITY ────── Mild  Moderate  Severe
```

A symptom is accessible and thus rateable when the necessary information is available. A mute patient cannot provide the necessary information for rating formal disorders of thought. In such cases the symptom should be rated as not ascertained.

Certainty refers to the reliability of the information. If the rater is uncertain about the presence or absence of a symptom he should rate the symptom as not ascertained.

After having resolved the question of certainty, the rater should decide whether a symptom is present or absent. If a symptom is present the degree of severity should be estimated as mild, moderate or severe. Since both intensity and duration of a symptom affect the judgement, it is sometimes very difficult to come to an agreement on the degree of severity. With fluctuating symptoms, the highest intensity should be rated.

5. Development of two second-order scales

It is the concept of the AMDP system to obtain for every patient as detailed a picture as possible. Therefore, we prefer to use the complete rating forms instead of short forms.

The examination of inter-rater reliability has shown that syndromes or subscales are much more reliable than single symptoms (Baumann & Woggon 1979; Woggon et al 1978). Using the AMDP system in research projects makes it necessary to have reliable syndromes for the performance of statistical data analyses.

Using factor analyses several slightly different primary scales have been published, giving the possibility for a differentiated representation of psychopathology. In Zurich we have developed primary scales (Baumann & Angst 1975) and second-order scales (Woggon & Dittrich 1979). In contrast to the multifactorial solution the bifactorial structure of the AMP system was shown to have a very good stability. The bifactorial structure could be reproduced in different patient samples, with reduced item pool and during 20 days of psychopharmacological treatment (Angst et al 1979; Woggon et al (1980).

Originally the first factor or second-order scale of the AMP system (Manic-Depressive Syndrome) consisted of 27 items. The factor is bipolar, combining 20 depressive symptoms and 7 manic symptoms. The second factor (Schizophrenic Syndrome) originally consisted of 25 items. Both factors showed a high correlation with normal distribution ($\tau = 0.99$ and 0.97) Therefore, a logarithmic transformation was not necessary, in contrast to the primary scales (Baumann & Angst 1975). To obtain a similar scale for the second-order and primary scales, a T-transformation ($\mu = 50$; $\sigma = 10$) was performed. For the Manic-Depressive Syndrome T is 40 if no symptoms are present; T is less than 40 if only manic symptoms are present (range T = 20-80). In the Schizophrenic Syndrome T is 31 if no symptoms are present (range T = 31-80).

Three aspects of reliability were examined:

1. Internal consistency: The internal consistency was calculated using the formula of Kuder-Richardson (K-R 20), adapted to Crombachs Alpha (Novick 1967). For the Manic-Depressive Syndrome the internal consistency is $\tau_{tt} = 0.91$ and for the Schizophrenic Syndrome $\tau_{tt} = 0.89$.

2. Inter rater reliability: The inter-rater reliability was determined using the product-moment-correlation and the κ-coefficient (Tinsley & Weiss 1975). The inter-rater reliability of the Manic-Depressive Syndrome is $\tau = 0.87$ and $\kappa = 0.77$. For the Schizophrenic Syndrome the inter-rater reliability is $\tau = 0.76$ and $\kappa = 0.73$.

3. Retest reliability (24 hours): For the Manic-Depressive Syndrome the retest reliability is $\tau = 0.89$ and $\kappa = 0.93$. The Schizophrenic Syndrome has a retest reliability of $\tau = 0.90$ and $\kappa = 0.86$ (for detailed description see Woggon & Dittrich 1979).

Two aspects of the validity were examined:

1. Differentiation between patients with schizophrenia and affective

psychoses was highly significant (Woggon & Dittrich 1979).

2. Comparison with three well-known rating scales: The Manic-Depressive Syndrome showed close correlations to the Hamilton Depression Scale (Hamilton 1960, 1967), to the factor 'Anxious depression' of the Brief Psychiatric Rating Scale (Mombour et al 1975; Overall & Gorham 1962) and to the factors 'Excitement' and 'Retardation and apathy' of the In-patient Multidimensional Psychiatric Scale (Lorr et al 1963a, b; 1966). The Schizophrenic Syndrome showed high correlations to the factor 'Thinking disturbance' of the BPRS and three factors of the IMPS: 'Paranoid projection', 'Perceptual distortion' and 'Motor disturbances' (Woggon 1979b).

The above-mentioned results concerning reliability and validity of the two second-order scales have been obtained using the AMP system and not the AMDP system. Fortunately the changes from AMP system to AMDP

Table 3. Mania-Depression Scale (Woggon & Dittrich)
Goteberg Version 21 June 1980*

1. Acquisition (11)**
2. Inhibition (15)
3. Retardation (16)
4. Restriction (18)
5. Delusions of guilt (42)
6. Apathy (60)
7. Depression (63)
8. Hopelessness (64)
9. Anxiety (65)
10. Feelings of inadequacy (71)
11. Guilt (73)
12. Lack of drive (80)
13. Inhibition of drive (81)
14. Social withdrawal (92)
15. Suicidal tendencies (95)
16. Difficulty in falling asleep (101)
17. Interrupted sleep (102)
18. Shortened sleep (103)
19. Decreased appetite (106)
20. Flight of ideas (22)
21. Euphoria (66)
22. Exaggerated self-confidence (72)
23. Increased drive (82)
24. Logorrhoea (88)
25. Excessive social contact (93)
26. Lack of feeling ill (97)

DEPRESSION +   MANIA —
(items 1-19)   (20-26)

*Adapted from the 2nd to the 3rd German edition and translated into English by the AMDP International Secretariat. In Guy & Ban (in prep.).
**Item number in the AMDP System.

Table 4. Schizophrenia Syndrome Scale (Woggon & Dittrich)
Goteberg Version 21 June 1980*

1. Apperception (9)**
2. Paralogia (23)
3. Thought blocking (24)
4. Incoherence (25)
5. Neologisms (26)
6. Suspiciousness (27)
7. Delusional mood (33)
8. Delusional perceptions (34)
9. Delusional irruption (35)
10. Delusional ideas (36)
11. Delusional dynamics (38)
12. Delusions of reference (39)
13. Delusion of persecution (40)
14. Verbal hallucinations (48)
15. Visual hallucinations (50)
16. Bodily hallucinations (51)
17. Olfactory/gustatory hallucinations (52)
18. Depersonalization (54)
19. Thought broadcasting (55)
20. Thought withdrawal (56)
21. Thought insertion (57)
22. Other feelings of influence (58)
23. Irritability (68)
24. Ambivalence (75)
25. Parathymia (76)
26. Emotional rigidity (79)

*Adapted from the 2nd to the 3rd German edition and translated into English by the AMDP International Secretariat. In Guy & Ban (in prep.).
**Item number in the AMDP System.

system make little difference to the symptoms included in the two scales. They have been adapted from AMP to AMDP and translated into English by the AMDP International Secretariat (Guy & Ban, in preparation). The new names are Mania-Depression Scale and Schizophrenia Syndrome Scale. Tables 3 and 4 show the symptoms of both scales. The Mania Depression Scale shows only one difference from the original Manic-Depressive Syndrome: one depressive symptom, 'feeling ill', is lacking. The new Mania-Depression Scale consists of 26 symptoms. The score is calculated by adding the grades of severity of the 19 depressive symptoms and subtracting the grades of severity of the 7 manic symptoms. More differences exist between the new Schizophrenia Syndrome Scale and the original Schizophrenic Syndrome. Four combined symptoms have been divided into two symptoms; these symptoms are incoherence/neologisms, delusional irruption/ideas, visual/olfactory hallucinations, thought broadcasting/withdrawal. Two very similar symptoms have been combined into one symptom: objective and subjective aspects of thought blocking were combined to thought blocking. Two symptoms are lacking in the new scale: autism and negativism. The new scale consists of 26 symptoms compared to 25 symptoms in the original syndrome. The score is calculated by adding the grades of severity of all symptoms.

The described changes seem to be not very important. Nevertheless it is planned to repeat all investigations concerning subscales on a new sample of patients documented by means of the new AMDP system in Berlin and Munich. These new scales are now available. Furthermore we hope that there will be no principal differences between old and new scales because otherwise it will be difficult to compare results of previous and new research projects.

6. Comparison between the AMDP system and other well-known rating scales

The aim of this comparison between the AMDP system and other well-known rating scales is to show differences from the rater's point of view. This means that my comparison will not be a statistical or methodological one, but a summary of opinions of raters working in my group.

Since 1969 we have used the AMP system for the assessment of psychopathological symptoms in most of our research projects, including psychopharmacological trials. The AMP system has so far been mostly used in German-speaking countries. Therefore, we wanted to use rating scales from English-speaking countries in addition to the AMP system. We thought this to be important for the comparison between our own results and the findings of others. In trials of antidepressants, in addition to the AMP system, we use the Hamilton Depression Rating Scale and in trials with antipsychotic drugs we use the Brief Psychiatric Rating Scale. Furthermore we have some experience with the In-patient Multidimensional Psychiatric Scale which we have used mainly for the psychopathological description of patients in studies where comparisons between psychopathological symptomatology and psychometric tests were examined. Since 1977 we have been occupied with the development of a German version of the Comprehensive Psychopathological Rating Scale, which could soon be finished.

We use a 24-item version of the Hamilton Depression Scale (National Institute of Mental Health), which includes the original 17-item version (Hamilton 1960), the 24-item version (CIPS 1977), plus the following 3 symptoms: helplessness, hopelessness and worthlessness (Baumann 1976). For the statistical evaluation we use two one-dimensional scores: the sum of items 1-17 and of items 1-24. The scores are calculated by adding the grades of severity of the items. In contrast to the proposal of Hamilton we work with only one rater. From the rater's point of view the Hamilton Scale is very easy to handle; raters like it. Unfortunately it is not suitable for the assessment of schizophrenic symptoms.

Therefore, in trials with antipsychotic drugs, we use a German translation of the 18-item version of the Brief Psychiatric Rating Scale (Mombour *et al* 1975; Overall & Gorham 1962). For data analyses we use the 4-factor solution (Overall 1974). Working with the BPRS is not as easy as using the Hamilton Depression Scale, especially because the grades of severity (1-7) are not described. This is the same difficulty as with the AMDP system. On the other hand in the BPRS we do not rate symptoms but symptom groups, which is easier for beginners. For well trained raters, familiar with the AMDP system, the definitions of the symptoms seem to be not sufficiently differentiated.

We have less experience with the In-patient Multidimensional Psychiatric Scale (Lorr *et al* 1963a; 1963b; 1966). We use the German translation of Flegel, Maeder and Missel (Mombour *et al* 1973). The IMPS assesses only symptoms which can be observed during the interview or which the patient himself describes during the interview. Information about the patient from nurses cannot be included. From the clinical point of view this is a disadvantage, but from the methodological point of view it is an advantage, especially concerning inter-rater reliability. The grades of severity are not described. Although Mombour (1972) gave a very positive judgement in his overview on rating scales, the IMPS was not very successful in the German-speaking part of Europe, especially in the field of psychopharmacological trials. Personally I do not understand this phenomenon; perhaps competition played a role. Many of the German-speaking psychiatrists have been engaged in the development of the AMDP system during recent years. We found the IMPS easier to handle than the AMDP system, especially for beginners in the field of psychopathology.

In 1978 we performed our first comparison between the AMP system and the Comprehensive Psychopathological Rating Scale, using a preliminary German translation (Woggon 1979a). During this study we realized that some items had been badly translated. In the meantime a better translation has been worked out (Kuny *et al* 1983) and a second comparison between the AMP system and CPRS has been performed in 170 psychiatric in-patients, mainly suffering from endogenous psychoses (Kuny 1982; Maurer 1982). The two raters had a very good impression of the CPRS. The accurate descriptions of the symptoms are most helpful. The CPRS is easily communicable and needs less time than the AMDP system. The approach towards a differentiation between reported and observed symptoms is positive, but is not always possible. The description of the four grades of severity is very helpful, but in some items the steps are different for content and quality of the symptoms and not as expected for intensity. During the second comparison study the use of half-steps was found very helpful, and made the decision process much easier. The 65 items of the CPRS represent the most important psychopathological symptoms but the AMDP system gives an even more differentiated and comprehensive picture of psychopathology. Unfortunately this is only an advantage in the hands of well-trained raters with a detailed knowledge of psychopathology. The CPRS seems to be more suitable for the assessment of depressive symptomatology than the AMDP system, while for schizophrenic symptoms the AMDP system seems more suitable and differentiated. As expected the inter-rater reliability of CPRS symptoms is much better than the inter-rater reliability of AMP symptoms (Kuny 1982).

7. Summary

Since 1979 a new edition of the AMP system has been available, called the AMDP system. AMDP should be used only by well-trained raters. Instructions for raters are given. Two second-order scales of the AMP system are described which will probably survive the change from AMP to AMDP. Based on experience with several different rating scales, a comparison is made from the rater's point of view between AMDP system, Hamilton Depression Scale, Brief Psychiatric Rating Scale (BPRS), Inpatient Multidimensional Psychiatric Scale (IMPS) and Comprehensive Psychopathological Rating Scale (CPRS).

References

AMDP/Arbeitsgemeinschaft für Methodik und Dokumentation in der Psychiatrie (ed.) (1979): *Das AMDP-System. Manual zur Dokumentation Psychiatrischer Befunde*. 3rd ed. Springer-Verlag, Berlin.

Angst, J., Battegay, R., Bente, D., Berner, P., Broeren, W., Cornu, F., Dick, P., Engelmeier, M.-P., Heimann, H., Heinrich, K., Helmchen, H., Hippius, H., Poeldinger, W., Schmidlin, P., Schmitt, W. & Weis, P. (1969): Das Dokumentations-System der Arbeitsgemeinschaft für Methodik und Dokumentation in der Psychiatrie. *Arzneimittel-Forsch, 19*, 339-405.

Angst, J., Dittrich, A., & Woggon, B. (1979): Reproduzierbarkeit der Faktorenstruktur des AMP-Systems. *Int. Pharmakopsychiatry, 14*, 319-324.

Baumann, U. & Angst, J. (1975): Methodological development of the AMP system. In Boissier, J.R., Hippius, H., Pichot, P. (eds.): *Neuropsychopharmacology. Proc. IX Congr. of the CINP, Paris 1974*, 72-78. Excerpta Medica, Amsterdam.

Baumann, U. (1976): Methodische Untersuchungen zur Hamilton-Depressions-Skala. *Arch. Psychiatr. Nervenkr. 222*, 359-375.

Baumann, U. & Woggon, B. (1979): Inter-rater-Reliabilität bei Diagnosen, AMP-Syndromen und AMP-Symptomen. *Arch. Psychiatr. Nervenkr. 227*, 3-15.

Baumann, U. & Faehndrich, E. (1981): Recent development concerning the AMDP system. AMDP Congress 1980. *Pharmacopsychiatr. 14,* 74-76.

CIPS (Collegium Internationale Psychiatriae Scalarum) (1977): *Internationale Skalen für Psychiatrie.*

Guy, W. & Ban, Th.: North American adaptation of the AMDP system. *Manual for the Documentation of Psychiatric Assessment* (in preparation).

Hamilton, M. (1960): A rating scale for depression. *J. Neurol. Neurosurg. Psychiatry, 23,* 56-62.

Hamilton, M. (1967): Development of a rating scale for primary depressive illness. *Br. J. Soc. Clin. Psychol. 6,* 278-296.

Kuny, S. (1982): Inter-rater-Reliabilität der deutschsprachigen CPRS. Med. Diss., Zürich.

Kuny, S., Maurer, M., Luckner, N. von & Woggon, B. (1983): Deutschsprachige Version der CPRS. *Int. Pharmacopsychiatry,* in press.

Lorr, M., Klett, C.J. & McNair, D.M. (1963a): *Syndromes of Psychosis.* Pergamon Press, Oxford.

Lorr, M., Klett, C.J., McNair, D.M. & Lasky, J.J. (1963b): *In-patient Multidimensional Psychiatric Scale (IMPS).* Consulting Psychologists Press, Palo Alto, California.

Lorr, M., McNair, D.M., Klett, C.J. & Lasky, J.J. (1966): *In-patient Multidimensional Psychiatric Scale (IMPS) revised.* Consulting Psychologists Press, Palo Alto, California.

Maurer, M. (1982): Konstruktion deutschsprachiger CPRS-Skalen. Med. Diss., Zürich.

Mombour, W. (1972): Verfahren zur Standardisierung des psychopathologischen Befundes, parts 1 and 2. *Psychiatr. Clin. 5,* 73-120; 137-157.

Mombour, W., Gammel, G., Zerssen, D. von & Heyse, M. (1973): Die Objektivierung psychiatrischer Syndrome durch multifaktorielle Analyse des psychopathologischen Befundes. *Nervenarzt 44,* 352-358.

Mombour, W., Kockott, G. & Fliege, K. (1975): Die Brief Psychiatric Rating Scale (BPRS) von Overall und Gorham bei akuten paranoid-halluzinatorischen Psychosen. Untersuchungen zu einer deutschen Uebersetzung der BPRS. *Pharmakopsychiatr. 8,* 279-288.

Novick, M.R. (1967): Coefficient alpha and the reliability of composite measurement. *Psychometrika 32,* 1-13.

Overall, J.E. (1974): The Brief Psychiatric Rating Scale in psychopharmacology research. In Pichot, P. (ed.): *Psychological Measurements in Psychopharmacology.* Karger, Basel, pp.67-78.

Overall, J.E. & Gorham, D.R. (1962): The Brief Psychiatric Rating Scale. *Psychol. Rep. 10,* 799-812.

Scharfetter, Ch. (1971): *Das AMP-System. Manual zur Dokumentation psychiatrischer Befunde. 1.* Springer, Berlin.

Scharfetter, Ch. (1972): *Das AMP-System. Manual zur Dokumentation psychiatrischer Befunde. 2.* Springer, Berlin.

Tinsley, H.E.A. & Weiss, D.J. (1975): Inter-rater-reliability and agreement of subjective judgements. *J. Counselling Psychol. 22,* 358-376.

Woggon, B. (1979a): Comparison between Comprehensive Psychopathological Rating Scale (CPRS) and Association for Methodology and Documentation in Psychiatry (AMP) System. *Prog. Neuro-Psychopharmacol. 3,* 423-427.

Woggon, B. (1979b): Untersuchung zur Validität der übergeordneten AMP-Skalen durch Vergleiche mit der Hamilton-Depressions-Skala, BPRS und IMPS. *Int. Pharmacopsychiatry, 14,* 338-349.

Woggon, B. (1979c): Einstufung von AMP-Syndromen bezüglich Fremd- und Selbstbeurteilung. *Int. Pharmacopsychiatry, 14,* 158-169.

Woggon, B., Baumann, U. & Angst, J. (1978): Inter-rater-Reliabilität von AMP-Symptomen. *Arch. Psychiatr. Nervenkr. 225,* 73-85.

Woggon, B. & Dittrich, A. (1979): Konstruktion übergeordneter AMP-Skalen: 'manisch-depressives' und 'schizophrenes' Syndrom. *Int. Pharmacopsychiatry 14,* 325-337.

Woggon, B., Dittrich, A., Luckner, N. von & Keller, W. (1980): Untersuchung zur Stabilität der faktoriellen Struktur des AMP-Systems im Behandlungsverlauf. *Int. Pharmacopsychiatry, 15,* 360-364.

The Comprehensive Psychopathological Rating Scale (CPRS)

B. CRONHOLM

The Swedish Medical Research Council supports improvement of research methodology *inter al.* by setting up *ad hoc* 'planning groups'. In 1971 such a group comprising 15 psychiatrists, psychologists and clinical pharmacologists was formed and given the task of studying problems concerning the evaluation of change in psychiatric symptomatology with treatment. Jan-Otto Ottosson, M.D. and professor of psychiatry at the University of Gothenburg, was the chairman and leader of the group. The main interest was soon centred on the use of rating scales. Inquiries to psychiatric departments and drug companies in Scandinavia revealed that a great number of different scales were used, but also that none of them could be recommended for common use. For that reason the group decided that a new rating scale should be developed and a working team was formed. It consisted of three psychiatrists (M. Åsberg, C. Perris and G. Sedvall) and one psychologist (D. Schalling). Later on, the English psychiatrist S.A. Montgomery was added to the group. An English version of the 'Comprehensive Psychopathological Rating Scale (CPRS)' was published in 1978 by Åsberg *et al.* See also Åsberg & Schalling (1979).

General problems of rating are discussed in the introductory paper (Cronholm & Daly). It may be added that rating essentially is a systematization of what we are doing in all clinical evaluation, even if it implies quantifying and measuring what may seem too subjective, too subtle and too elusive for any measurement to be possible. It is easily forgotten that any clinical statement about the severity of a disorder and about improvement or deterioration is essentially some sort of quantification.

From the very beginning it was agreed that the new scale should be developed with the explicit purpose of being useful for measuring change in severity of a mental disorder during treatment. It should be of use for comparison between an active drug and placebo, or between two or more different drugs. This means that the items included should be sensitive to change in the disorder studied. On the other hand it was not necessary that they had any diagnostic specificity — the scale was not to be used as a diagnostic instrument. As a matter of fact, very few symptoms in themselves are really specific to any particular psychiatric disorder. Many symptoms are quite unspecific and appear as an integral part in most psychiatric syndromes. This holds true, for example, for inner tension, lassitude and sadness.

It was a leading idea that the scale should be able to serve as a pool of items, from which subscales could be used in studies of different psychiatric syndromes or disorders. For that reason the scale should be comprehensive and cover a broad range of psychiatric symptomatology. The use of subscales for studies of different psychiatric syndromes is necessary. Inclusion of items that do not belong to the syndrome studied will be of no positive value and the rating of them highly influenced by random factors. Their inclusion would only lower the reliability of the instrument. Subscales may be developed on the basis of *a priori* assumptions, but more rational procedures, based on empirical studies seem to be preferable (Montgomery & Åsberg 1979; Cronholm & Daly, this volume).

The final scale comprises 65 items. All of them are listed in Table 1. The items were selected on the basis of clinical experience and after perusal of the literature, but of course also with respect to the special purpose of the scale. The aim of sensitivity to change of course meant that items indicating more or less constant personality traits had to be avoided. Signs or symptoms that are not linearly related to severity of a disorder, for example morning insomnia or diurnal variation, were also excluded. As underlined in the introductory paper (Cronholm & Daly), 'atoms' of behaviour have to be avoided but also too comprehensive, global statements. All items included are thus somewhere in between these two extremes. However, to keep the number of items within reasonable limits, closely related signs or symptoms have had to be condensed into one item. Thus, ideas of guilt or sin and an unrealistic pessimism as regards success or the future in general were condensed into the item 'Pessimistic thoughts'. The item 'Disrupted thoughts' includes such different aspects of thought disorder as thought blocking, insertion, withdrawal or broadcasting. Under the heading 'Lack of appropriate affect' both blunted and incongruous affects were included. The designers of the scale avoided items that require extensive knowledge and a unitary opinion among raters about some specific theories or frames of reference. For that reason such psychoanalytical

Table 1. CPRS Item List

Reported variables	Observed variables
1. Sadness	41. Apparent sadness
2. Elation	42. Elated mood
3. Inner tension	43. Hostility
4. Hostile feelings	44. Labile emotional responses
5. Inability to feel	45. Lack of appropriate emotion
6. Pessimistic thoughts	46. Autonomic disturbances
7. Suicidal thoughts	47. Sleepiness
8. Hypochondriasis	48. Distractability
9. Worrying over trifles	49. Withdrawal
10. Compulsive thoughts	50. Perplexity
11. Phobias	51. Blank spells
12. Rituals	52. Disorientation
13. Indecision	53. Pressure of speech
14. Lassitude	54. Reduced speech
15. Fatiguability	55. Specific speech defect
16. Concentration difficulties	56. Flight of ideas
17. Failing memory	57. Incoherent speech
18. Reduced appetite	58. Perseveration
19. Reduced sleep	59. Overactivity
20. Increased sleep	60. Slowness of movement
21. Reduced sexual interest	61. Agitation
22. Increased sexual interest	62. Involuntary movements
23. Autonomic disturbances	63. Muscular tension
24. Aches and pains	64. Mannerisms and postures
25. Muscular tension	65. Hallucinatory behaviour
26. Loss of sensation or movement	66. Global rating of illness
27. Derealization	67. Assumed reliability of the rating
28. Depersonalization	
29. Feeling controlled	
30. Disrupted thoughts	
31. Ideas of persecution	
32. Ideas of grandeur	
33. Delusional mood	
34. Ecstatic experiences	
35. Morbid jealousy	
36. Other delusions	
37. Commenting voices	
38. Other auditory hallucinations	
39. Visual hallucinations	
40. Other hallucinations	

constructs as defence mechanisms, coping strategies, latent anxiety and latent hostility, etc., were not included. The designers also avoided several terms that are commonly used by psychiatrists to describe the mental state of patients but also are closely attached to diagnostic categories. This holds true for, for example, anxiety, depression, thought disorder, and paranoia. Some of these terms are quite ambiguous: 'depression' may mean either an isolated symptom that is common in many psychiatric disorders, or a diagnostic category. During construction of the scale it was found that the raters often had difficulties in giving up their diagnostic prejudices. For example, they hesitated to call a schizophrenic patient depressed even if they agreed that there was no doubt that he was sad, because they considered the disorders 'depression' and 'schizophrenia' as being mutually exclusive. The problem was solved by substituting the term 'Sadness' for 'Depression'.

It is very well known that there may be a more or less conspicuous discrepancy between what a person tells us and our own observations during an interview. Denial or dissimulation of symptoms is not uncommon. An obviously sad patient may tell us that he feels all right. Hallucinations may be denied at the same interview that the patient talks to his 'voices'. For this reason the designers of the scale decided to separate 40 reported symptoms and 25 observed signs. The proportion may be advantageous from the point of view of reliability as the inter-rater reliability of reported symptoms is as a rule higher than that of observed ones.

The constructors of the CPRS devoted much effort to making the description of the items and their scale steps as unambiguous and clear as possible. The description of the items should preferably give all information needed by the rater and also help him to formulate adequate questions. Many deficiencies in the text were found and corrected during the evaluation of preliminary versions that were tried on a great number of patients.

It was the ambition of the constructors to use, as far as possible, a quite simple and non-technical language. Technical terms are to a high degree dependent on implicit assumptions, varying among different psychiatrists due to their training within different frames of reference. To the individual psychiatrist his own frame of reference mostly is accepted as self-evident, and he may be unaware that other psychiatrists may find other frames just as self-evident. Such differences among psychiatrists, of course, tend to lower inter-rater reliability. The risk of such mutual misunderstandings will be much less when a non-technical language is used.

Another advantage of using a non-technical language is that it makes possible training of raters without formal psychiatric education — for example, nurses or private practitioners — to use the scale. High inter-rater reliabilities were shown for raters from different disciplines when rating depressed patients with the CPRS (Montgomery *et al* 1978a).

Scaling severity of psychiatric symptoms has to be more or less arbitrary. However, it is desirable to make the procedure as explicit as possible and not to use such vague terms as 'mild', 'moderate' or 'severe' without further qualifications. In the CPRS, severity is graded according to intensity and frequency of the symptoms. In order to reach some consistency between definitions of scale steps for different items, the following general rule was used in their construction:

- 3 should be a description of an extreme degree of the symptom, e.g. unrelenting dread or anguish in 'Inner tension';
- 2 a description of subjective experiences or behaviour that would always or almost always be considered clearly pathological in the circumstances, e.g. continuous feelings of inner tension overlaid with intermittent panic;
- 1 a description that could apply to a pathological deviation from the individual's own norm, but might also represent the habitual state of some people, e.g. occasional feelings of edginess and ill-defined discomfort;
- 0 absence of the particular symptom.

The rater is instructed to rate in accordance with the scale text, even if this means that a patient whom he feels to be in his habitual state has to be given a positive score. A patient who has recovered after an illness thus does not always receive zero scores on all items.

However, for some variables individual variation is so wide that application of the rule above would limit the use of the scale for assessing change. This holds true for, for example, sexual interest and sleep. The habitual level of functioning for one individual may be an important, illness-related malfunctioning in another. For that reason, an intra-individual standard has to be used. The patient is explicitly asked to compare his present state to his own habitual functioning, which is then taken to be the norm.

Even if only the scale steps 0-3 have definitions, the use of half-steps is strongly recommended. It makes possible a more varied grading in seven steps instead of only four.

The rating with CPRS should be based on a flexible, clinical interview. The subject is encouraged to describe in his own words, and in detail, the symptoms that are relevant to him. The interviewer then completes the information obtained by means of questions about areas that have not been fully covered. On the basis of the information given by the subject and his own observations during the interview, the rater scores the relevant items.

In a hierarchy of scales, rating scales cannot claim to be more than ordinal scales. This means that from a puristic point of view very few, if any, arithmetic operations are permissible. However, in many situations a sum of scores on relevant items is used as an estimate of the severity of a more or less hypothetical, underlying disease process. In spite of theoretical objections this procedure works well especially in depressive states, where severity of individual symptoms is linearly related to global estimates of severity (Bech *et al* 1975; Montgomery & Åsberg, 1979). However, a schizophrenic patient with florid symptoms is not necessarily worse off, or more severely 'ill', than one who denies any subjective symptoms. During improvement the total score may *rise* due to better insight and better contact with the rater, thus giving a paradoxical estimate of deterioration. Of course, such problems make difficulties when CPRS — or some other rating scale — is used in evaluation of treatment.

The changes in severity of illness during treatment are most commonly estimated in one of three ways. The difference between pre-treatment and treatment or post-treatment scores has the most evident face value. The method means that the scores are handled as belonging to an interval scale. Another estimate is per cent change in score. This means handling the scores as belonging to a ratio scale. The most reliable and theoretically most sound way of estimating change is — somewhat paradoxically — to use final scores only without considering the initial ones. An empirical study of patients with depressive illness has shown that the choice between these estimates is of little consequence since they are highly correlated, 0.84-0.96 (Träskman *et al* 1979).

As already mentioned, even such simple arithmetical operations as addition and subtraction are theoretically not permissible with scores obtained from a rating scale, since an assumption of equal intervals is not justified.

To work out quotients or percentages is still worse as it presumes not only equidistances but also an absolute zero. However, more or less severe attacks of bad conscience will easily be overcome by considering the practical value of such procedures. To a large extent this holds true also for more complicated mathematical and statistical calculations such as means, *t*-tests, correlations and even analysis of variance. However, in some situations it is wise to apply instead non-parametric statistics.

The first versions of the CPRS were in Swedish but already during its development it was also translated into English. Naively, we may tend to think that translation just means substituting a foreign word for the well-known one in our own language. As soon as we really try, we will find that translation is not at all simple. We cannot be confident that a word in one language has an exact synonym in another; this is rather the exception than the rule. For that reason, translation always means interpretation and re-writing to attain as closely as possible the same meaning of one or more sentences in two different languages. This is very important when definitions of variables in a rating scale are translated from one language to another. As a matter of fact, development of the English parallel text unveiled linguistic weaknesses in the early, Swedish versions. The translation procedure thus contributed to improvement of both versions. Whether the translation has been successful and the two versions thus really parallel has to be controlled by means of testing inter-rater reliability between pairs of raters using versions in different languages. The depression subscales of the CPRS in Swedish and English have shown fully acceptable parallelism (Montgomery et al 1978b).

References

Åsberg, M., Montgomery, S., Perris, C., Schalling, D. & Sedvall, G. (1978): A Comprehensive Psychopathological Rating Scale (CPRS). *Acta Psychiatr. Scand., Suppl. 271*, 5-27.

Åsberg, M. & Schalling, D. (1979): Construction of a new psychiatric rating instrument, the Comprehensive Psychopathological Rating Scale (CPRS): *Prog. Neuro-Psychopharmacol. 3*, 405-412.

Bech, P., Gram, L.F., Dein, E., Jacobsen, O., Vitger, J. & Bolwig, T.G. (1975): Quantitative rating of depressive states. *Acta Psychiatr. Scand., 51*, 161-170.

Montgomery, S., Åsberg, M., Jörnestedt, L., Thorén, P., Träskman, L., McAuley, R., Montgomery, D. & Shaw, P. (1978a): Reliability of the CPRS between the disciplines of psychiatry, general practice, nursing and psychology in depressed patients. *Acta Psychiatr. Scand., Suppl. 271*, 29-32.

Montgomery, S., Åsberg, M., Träskman, L. & Montgomery, D. (1978b): Cross cultural studies of the use of CPRS in English and Swedish depressed patients. *Acta Psychiatr. Scand., Suppl. 271*, 33-37.

Montgomery, S. & Åsberg, M. (1979): A new depression scale designed to be sensitive to change. *Br. J. Psychiatry, 134*, 384-389.

Träskman, L., Åsberg, M., Bertilsson, L., Cronholm, B., Mellström, B. & Thorén, P. (1979): Plasma levels of chlorimipramine and its demethyl metabolite during treatment of depression. Antidepressant effect in biochemical subgroups. *Clin. Pharmacol. Ther. 26*, 600-610.

The Use of Rating Scales for Affective Disorders

P. BECH

1. Introduction

The growing tendency to construct new rating scale systems seems not to be based on intensive analyses of their predecessors. This seems especially to be the case in the field of affective disorders (e.g. Snaith 1981). Thereby the effort to obtain international standards for recording clinical data, for example, in the evaluating of psychiatric treatment, has been delayed. This overview is an attempt to reconsider the use of the prevailing rating scales for affective disorders. In this connection it is important to realize that rating scales are more than operational definitions of clinical data at the level of observation. Rating scales contain, moreover, specific criteria by which the various items of the scale can be combined to syndromes or diagnoses.

In this overview most emphasis will be laid on the rules for combination of items. There are two different elements of such combinations, namely (1) quantitative elements, when measuring the severity of affective states, and (2) qualitative elements when measuring the diagnosis of affective illnesses.

2. Quantitative rating scales for affective states

2.1 General considerations

A symptom rating scale is an instrument for measuring the severity of affective states. Therefore, such scales must contain the most characteristic and observable symptoms for measuring states like depression, anxiety or mania.

Traditionally, the rule for combination of the individual symptoms within quantitative scales is the summed scale score or the total score. However, the resistance shown by clinicians toward the use of rating scales exactly reflects their scepticism about the value of summing different symptoms to a total score. This scepticism is, moreover, shared by statisticians, because the scores obtained by rating scales are categorized values, not truly numerical values. In the statistical inference, therefore, statistical models for categorized data should be used, and only when evidence has been obtained by such analyses can the individual item score be combined to a single total score. The quantitative rating scale which has been the object for most analyses is the Hamilton Depression Scale (Hamilton 1960), and our analysis of this scale will focus on the evidence for using a total score as the rating for depressive states.

2.2 The Hamilton Depression Scale (HDS)

Four different methods for testing the use of total scores of the HDS have been introduced, namely (1) global clinical assessment, (2) item-total score relationship, (3) factor analysis, and (4) the Rasch model.

2.2.1 The global clinical assessment

Statistical methods for testing the relationship between each item of the HDS and the global clinical assessment have been discussed elsewhere (Bech et al 1975a). Our results showed that only 6 of the 17 HDS items validly followed the global assessment (the items were: depressed mood, guilt, work and interests, retardation, psychic anxiety, and general somatic symptoms — in the following called the melancholic items).

2.2.2 Item-total score relations

One of the simplest ways to evaluate whether a rating scale is a uni-dimensional measurement of depressive state is item-total score correlations. Items that correlate most highly with the corresponding total score of the remaining items are the most relevant items. This method is, however, limited, because it depends on the specific characteristics of the patient material on which it has been developed. Thus, correlation analyses are likely to form rather than to test hypotheses. Evaluation of the HDS by such item-total score correlations showed, however, that the six melancholia items were among the items with significant correlation coefficients (Bech & Rafaelsen 1980).

2.2.3 Factor analysis

Factor analysis has been used as a tool for determining internal structures in a rating scale. When a number of items show high inter-correlation among themselves, a general factor will emerge, and such a factor has often been considered as an argument for summing items to total scores. However, comparisons of factors in different studies are difficult and complex. Concerning the HDS the various factor analytic studies have produced divergent results (e.g. Bech & Rafaelsen 1980), but interesting findings of factor structure across weekly ratings have emerged (Rosenberg et al 1981).

2.2.4 The Rasch model

The most appropriate statistical method to test for summing items when measuring the severity of affective states is logistic models, for example, the Rasch model (Rasch 1980). It is a powerful characteristic of the Rasch model that it directly controls whether the summed scale score is a sufficient measure of depressive state. However, the technique of estimation by Rasch models is a complicated procedure, and there exists no 'rapid' Rasch computer program for persons without a statistical background. Using the Rasch analysis we have confirmed that the sum of the 6-item HDS subscale is a uni-dimensional measure of severity of depression, in contrast to the 17-item HDS (Bech et al 1981).

2.3 The Bech-Rafaelsen Melancholia Scale (MES)

However, to cover the spectrum of manic-melancholic states we decided to develop an 11-item melancholia scale in which the HDS-item of retardation was subdivided into motor, verbal, emotional, and intellectual components. All these forms of melancholic retardation have been included in the Cronholm-Ottosson Depression Scale (Cronholm & Ottosson 1960). Our melancholia scale should, therefore, be conceived as an attempt to co-ordinate these prevailing observer scales in the field of depression (Table 1).

It is often held that there is a lower limit for the number of items on a rating scale owing to the problem of inter-observer reliability. However, the MES has been found to have a reliability equal to the HDS (Bech & Rafaelsen 1980; Rafaelsen et al 1981). Item-total score correlation of the MES has also been found adequate (Bech & Rafaelsen 1980; Rafaelsen et al 1981). Studies to test the scale for objectivity using logistic models are continuing. It is, however, important to realize that so far our inquiries are limited to the sample of hospitalized patients. Our preliminary investigations of patients in general practice have shown that the definition of each melancholia item on a five-point scale is difficult to use. Therefore, we have redefined the items on a two-point scale (0 = absent and 1 = present), and this GP-version of our melancholia scale has shown to be a reliable instrument in the GP-setting. The MES is included in the sample of scales found useful for psychopharmacological research (van Riezen 1983).

Table 1. Quantitative melancholia and mania scales

MELANCHOLIA		MANIA
	(1) Mood level	
	(2) Self-esteem	
Decreased	(3) Motor activity	*Increased*
	(4) Verbal activity	
	(5) Intellectual activity	
	(6) Emotional contact	
(7) Anxiety		(7) Hostility
(8) Tiredness and pains		(8) Noisy behaviour
(9) Suicidal impulses		(9) Increased sexual interest
	(10) Sleep disturbances	
	(11) Working capacity	

2.4 The Bech-Rafaelsen Mania Scale (MAS)

In the field of manic states no observer scale analogue to the HDS has as yet been established. One of the first mania scales, the Beigel Mania State Scale (Beigel *et al* 1971), is a rating scale to be administered by the nursing staff. In our validation study of the Beigel scale we found that only a sub-group of the 26 items followed a global clinical assessment of mania (Bech *et al* 1975b). On this background we developed our mania scale to be administered by psychiatrists (Bech *et al* 1978). When constructing the MAS we had consulted a short Swedish mania scale (Petterson *et al* 1973). Adequate inter-observer reliability of the MAS has been obtained, and item-total score correlations are of statistical significance (Bech *et al* 1979). The scale (Table 1) has now been translated into French (Jouvent *et al* 1980) and German (Gastpar 1980). Studies to test the scale for objectivity using logistic models are continuing. The MAS is included in the sample of scales found useful for psychopharmacological research (van Riezen 1983).

2.5 The Hamilton Anxiety Scale (HAS)

The association between states of anxiety and depression has often made it difficult to evaluate the relative efficacy of cyclic antidepressants, monoamineoxidase inhibitors, beta-adrenergic blockers, and benzodiazepines in the treatment of depressive disorders. In controlled drug trials in depressive disorders it has, therefore, been customary to use quantitative rating scales both for depression and anxiety. In such studies the HAS has been used to measure anxiety. However, this scale was originally constructed for quantifying anxiety in patients with a diagnosis of anxiety neurosis. We have evaluated the inter-observer reliability and item-total score correlations of the HAS in patients with depressive disorders (Rafaelsen *et al* 1981). The results showed that the inter-observer reliability was adequate. However, the item-total score correlations indicated that the HAS was no uni-dimensional scale for anxiety. The subgroup of intercorrelated items showed a factor which was very similar to the factor of psychic anxiety found by Hamilton (1969). Thus, the use of the HAS in patients with depressive disorders calls for further validation studies.

2.6 Error of Type II in clinical trials

The probability of Type I error in clinical trials is the risk which one takes if one accepts that two treatments differ, when in fact they do not. The Type I error is called the significance level α; thus, a 5 per cent significance level for a clinical trial means that the maximum acceptable probability of a Type I error has been set at 5 per cent. However, in clinical trials decisions regarding the rejection of the null hypothesis at the level of α are commonly made without reference to Type II, or β, error. As stated by MacRae (1976) the Type II error is when two treatments do actually differ, but the trial fails to demonstrate this difference. For specified α and sample size the value of β will decrease with increase in the difference between the outcome measure of the two treatments. For any specified sample size, therefore, it is important to have a sensitive and relevant outcome measure. The Type II error operates in clinical trials when a multi-dimensional rating scale has been used as the outcome measure by its total score, and can consequently be reduced by using an adequate, one-dimensional scale.

3. Qualitative rating scales for affective disorders
3.1 General considerations

In diagnostic or qualitative rating scales the absence of items plays the same role as the presence of items. This is in contrast to quantitative scales in which it is only the presence of items that counts. Thus, the relationship between items and diagnosis is a combination of negative and positive item values.

There are two main rules or models of item-combinations leading to psychiatric diagnoses: (1) the logical decision-tree model, and (2) statistical models.

3.1.1 The logical decision-tree model

This model for combination of clinical data is usually based on the hierarchy structure of psychiatric diagnoses (e.g. Jaspers 1959; Kendell

1975). At the top of the hierarchy are the organic psychoses. Next in the order are the schizophrenic psychoses. Thus schizophrenia has logical priority over affective disorders. However, the significance of the hierarchical element within the area of affective disorders is very complex, apart from the fact that mania has the third position in the order of psychiatric disorders. The problem is that the logical decision-tree based on the hierarchical model requires pathognomonic symptoms, and within the spectrum of affective disorders such symptoms are often lacking. Thus, the reliability of the classification of affective disorders by the logical decision-tree model is low compared with schizophrenia (e.g. Helzer *et al* 1978 — concerning the Feighner criteria, and Williams & Spitzer 1981 — concerning DSM III).

3.1.2 Statistical models (the WHO Depression Scale and the Newcastle indices)

Among the various statistical models that have been used to derive item-combinations of diagnostic importance within the affective disorders, it is the multivariate analysis that has been the most successful (e.g. Kendell 1975). The Newcastle scales for the diagnosis of depression (endogenous versus reactive) are based on multivariate analysis (e.g. Carney *et al* 1965; Roth *et al* 1974; Gurney 1971; Bech *et al* 1980). However, when using the Newcastle Scales the logical decision-tree model has been used in that organic psychoses and schizophrenia have been excluded beforehand. The positive and negative weighting scores found by the multivariate analysis makes it possible to use the summated item scores as the rating for the patient. Thereby, relatively complex criteria, involving numerous alternative combinations of items, can be expressed quite simply, and the weighted sum of the score on each of the 10 items places the patient-ratings on a 'dimension' from endogenous to reactive depression.

The original Newcastle items are defined on two-point scales, but preliminary results from our group showed that by using three-point scales from the WHO Depression Scale (Sartorius *et al* 1980) the inter-observer reliability will improve. Moreover, the first Newcastle index (N-I, Carney *et al* 1965) has a higher inter-observer reliability than the second Newcastle index (N-II, Gurney 1971). On the other hand, when using the relationship between plasma levels of imipramine or clomipramine and outcome as an index of external validity, we found that both Newcastle Scales were valid (Bech *et al* 1980). However, our results are limited to hospitalized patients. As stated by Spitzer & Williams (1980) the logical decision-tree has an obvious advantage over statistical models in that it does not require a data base and does not depend on the specific characteristics of the patient sample on which it has been developed — unlike multivariate analysis.

4. The combined use of qualitative and quantitative rating scales in endogenous depression

4.1 Hospitalized patients

In clinical research it is of great importance to work with homogeneous groups of patients. In research on depressed in-patients we will recommend both a quantitative rating scale (to ensure that every patient is severely depressed, e.g. a score on the MES of 15 or more) and a qualitative rating scale (to ensure that every patient has an endogenous depression, e.g. a score on the N-I of 6 or more). Eventually, a modified version of the WHO Depression Scale can contain both these quantitative and qualitative aspects in evaluating hospitalized patients with affective disorders.

4.2 Patients in general practice

Psychiatric disorders are often missed in general practice because doctors are trained to look for symptoms of the major psychiatric illnesses, which, however, are uncommon in the setting of general practice. On the other hand, Goldberg (e.g. Goldberg & Huxley 1980) and Gastpar (e.g. Gastpar *et al* 1980) have found that training in interview techniques can improve the ability of doctors to detect minor psychiatric symptoms. Especially in the field of affective disorders a carefully taken interview is needed because many patients interpret their complaints somatically rather than psychologically.

In their study on the diagnosis of depression in general practice Gastpar *et al* have used a WHO-screen scale, which is included in our GP-melancholia scale. We have developed diagnostic criteria for endogenous somatization depression (Bech & Jørgensen 1981), for which we have used a combination of quantitative and qualitative rating scales (Table 2). According to criteria A in Table 2 only patients with somatic complaints but without demonstrable organic findings are included in this GP-study. By pilot studies the general practitioners are trained to perform a detailed psychiatric interview to look for a depressive syndrome (criteria B). The quantitative scale for criteria B is our GP-melancholia scale, and we have defined the depressive syndrome by the presence of at least five of the eleven items. However, the GP-melancholia scale remains to be evaluated by use of the logistic Rasch model.

Table 2. Diagnostic criteria for endogenous somatization depressions

A: Somatic complaints without demonstrable organic findings
B: A depressive syndrome
C: Not associated with organic mental disorder or schizophrenia
D: No severe psychosocial stressors
E: No neurotic personality traits

According to criteria C in Table 2 we have used the logical decision-tree model when excluding patients with organic mental disorders and schizophrenia. Moreover, by criteria D in Table 2, depressive reactions are excluded because these conditions have a ready explanation as understandable responses to adversity (e.g. Bebbington *et al* 1981). Finally, neurotic personality traits are excluded in accordance with criteria E in Table 2. This criterion is important because a standardized interview can induce symptoms in neurotic patients. For example, the Eysenck concept of neuroticism covers the 'yes'-response (Eysenck & Eysenck 1969). However, one of the limitations of observer rating scales is that neurotic personality traits are difficult to define operationally. However, Vanggaard (1979) has made careful analysis of the neurotic secondary gain, which he conceives as a personality trait that is inconsistent with the diagnosis of endogenous depression. Thereby this concept can play a double role, as it both invalidates the quantitative rating of depression and excludes endogenous depression. However, our GP-study is still continuing.

A modification of the WHO Depression Scale, especially at the level of personality traits, might indicate that this scale can contain both a GP-version and a version for hospitalized patients.

5. Conclusion and summary

The prevailing rating scales for affective disorders have been reviewed. The scales were subdivided into quantitative and qualitative (diagnostic) scales.

It was shown that different rules for item-combinations exist within the two groups of rating scales (Table 3).

The quantitative scales have to be improved for minimizing the errors of Type II, which have to be taken into account in controlled clinical trials. Scales for melancholia, anxiety and mania were discussed, and it was shown that the number of item-categories is important for the setting in which the scales are intended to be used (hospital versus general practice).

Concerning the qualitative scales it was shown that the Newcastle indices can be extracted from the WHO Depression Scale. Moreover, whereas the Newcastle index of endogenous depression is limited to hospitalized patients, the WHO scale seems to have value in general practice also.

As stated by Snaith (1981) the time has now arrived for a moratorium to be declared upon the publication of new scales and for researchers to spend their energy in taking a careful look at existing scales to see how they may be improved and to compare their properties. Among the scales for affective disorders, the WHO depression* scale and the AMDP-system (Association for Methodology and Documentation in Psychiatry) should be reconsidered and modified with a view to building bridges between the various scales now available.

Table 3. Models for combination of clinical data

Classes of clinical data		Models	Scales
A	B		
+ +	0	Rasch	Quantitative
+	—	Hierarchy structure	Qualitative
+	—	Multivariate analysis	Qualitative

+ +, present in severe degree; +, present; 0, not present; —, present but weighted negatively.
A, depressive symptoms; B, psychosocial stressors.

References

AMDP (ed.) (1979): *Das AMDP-system.* 3rd ed. Springer, Berlin.
Bebbington, P.E., Tennant, C. & Hurry, J. (1981): *Adversity and the Nature of Psychiatric Disorder in the Community,* vol. 3, pp.345-366.
Bech, P., Gram, L.F., Dein, E., Jacobsen, O., Vitger, J. & Bolwig, T.G. (1975a): Quantitative rating of depressive states. *Acta Psychiatr. Scand. 51,* 161-170.
Bech, P., Bolwig, T.G., Dein, E., Jacobsen, O. & Gram, L.F. (1975b): Quantitative rating of manic states. *Acta Psychiatr. Scand. 52,* 1-6.
Bech, P., Rafaelsen, O.J., Kramp, P. & Bolwig, T.G. (1978): The mania rating scale: scale construction and inter-observer agreement. *Neuropharmacology, 17,* 430-431.
Bech, P., Bolwig, T.G., Kramp, P. & Rafaelsen, O.J. (1979): The Bech-Rafaelsen Mania Scale and the Hamilton Depression Scale. *Acta Psychiatr. Scand. 59,* 420-430.
Bech, P. & Rafaelsen, O.J. (1980): The use of rating scales exemplified by a comparison of the Hamilton and the Bech-Rafaelsen Melancholia Scale. *Acta Psychiatr. Scand., Suppl. 285,* 128-131.
Bech, P., Gram, L.F., Reisby, N. & Rafaelsen, O.J. (1980): The WHO Depression Scale: relationship to the Newcastle Scales. *Acta Psychiatr. Scand. 62,* 140-153.
Bech, P. & Jørgensen, B. (1981): Endogenous somatization depressions in general practice. Paper presented at the Prevention and Treatment of Depression meeting, Amsterdam, May 1981.
Bech, P., Allerup, P., Gram, L.F., Reisby, N., Rosenberg, R., Jacobsen, O. & Nagy, A. (1981): The Hamilton Depression Scale. *Acta Psychiatr. Scand. 63,* 290-299.
Beigel, A., Murphy, D.L. & Bunney, W.E. (1971): The manic-state rating scale. *Arch. Gen. Psychiatry, 25,* 256-262.

Carney, M.W.P., Roth, M. & Garside, R.F. (1965): The diagnosis of depressive syndromes and prediction of ECT response. *Br. J. Psychiatry, 111,* 659-674.

Cronholm, B. & Ottosson, J.-O. (1960): Experimental studies of the therapeutic action of electroconvulsive therapy in endogenous depression. The role of the electrical stimulation and of the seizure studied by variation of stimulus and modification by lidocaine of seizure discharge. In Ottosson, J.-O. (ed.): Experimental studies of the mode of action of electroconvulsive treatment. *Acta Psychiatr. Neurol. Scand., Suppl. 145,* 69-97.

Eysenck, H.J. & Eysenck, S.B.G. (1969): *Personality Structure and Measurement.* Routledge & Kegan Paul, London, pp.116-117.

Gastpar, G. (1980): Personal communication.

Gastpar, M., Gilsdorf, V. & Gastpar, G. (1980): Diagnosis of depression in general practice. Paper presented at the WHO International Symposium on Diagnosis and Treatment of Depression. Washington, DC.

Goldberg, D. & Huxley, P. (1980): *Mental Illness in the Community.* Tavistock, London.

Gurney, C. (1971): *Diagnostic Scales for Affective Disorders.* Proceedings of the Fifth World Conference of Psychiatry. Mexico City, p.330.

Hamilton, M. (1960): A rating scale for depression. *J. Neurol. Neurosurg. Psychiatry, 23,* 56-62.

Hamilton, M. (1969): Diagnosis and rating of anxiety. *Br. J. Psychiatry, Special Publication No. 3,* 76-79.

Helzer, J.E., Clayton, P.J., Pambakian, R. & Woodruff, R.A. (1978): Concurrent diagnostic validity of a structured psychiatric interview. *Arch. Gen. Psychiatry, 35,* 849-853.

Jaspers, K. (1959): *General Psychopathology.* Manchester University Press, Manchester, pp.611-612.

Jouvent, R., Lecoubier, Y., Puech, A.J., Simon, P. & Widlöcher, D. (1980): Antimanic effect of clonidine. *Am. J. Psychiatry, 137,* 1275-1276.

Kendell, R.E. (1975): *The Role of Diagnosis in Psychiatry.* Blackwell, London.

MacRae, K.D. (1976): Statistical aspects of trial design. In Good, C.S. (ed.): *The Principle and Practice of Clinical Trials.* Churchill Livingstone, Edinburgh, pp.87-92.

Petterson, U., Fyrö, B. & Sedvall, G. (1973): A new scale for the longitudinal rating of manic states. *Acta Psychiatr. Scand. 49,* 248-256.

Rafaelsen, O.J., Gjerris, A., Bolwig, T.G., Kramp, P., Bojholm, S., Andersen, J. & Bech, P. (1981): Hamilton Anxiety Scale: Evaluation of homogeneity and inter-observer reliability in patients with depressive disorders. Paper presented at WPA Symposium on Psychopathology of Anxiety and its Management. Cairo.

Rasch, G. (1980): *Probabilistic Models for some Intelligence and Attainment Tests.* University of Chicago Press, Chicago.

Riezen, H. van (1983): *Scales Useful for Clinical Psychopharmacological Research.* Reviews in Pure and Applied Pharmacological Sciences (in press).

Rosenberg, R., Bech, P. & Allerup, P. (1981): The Hamilton Depression Scale: Factor analysis of some data fitting a Rasch model. Paper presented at the Third World Congress of Biological Psychiatry, Stockholm, July 1981.

Roth, M., Garside, R. & Gurney, C. (1974): Classification of depressive disorders. In Angst, J. (ed.): *Classification and Prediction of Outcome of Depression.* Schattauer, Stuttgart, pp.3-26.

Sartorius, N., Jablensky, A., Gulbinat, W. & Ernberg, G. (1980): Application of WHO scales for the assessment of depressive states in different cultures. *Acta Psychiatr. Scand., Suppl. 285,* 204-211.

Snaith, R.P. (1981): Rating scales. *Br. J. Psychiatry, 138,* 512-514.

Spitzer, R.L. & Williams, J.B.W. (1980): Classification of mental disorders and DSM III. In Kaplan, H., Freedman, A. & Sadock, B. (eds.): *Comprehensive Textbook of Psychiatry.* Williams & Wilkins, New York, pp.1035-1072.

Vanggaard, T. (1979): *Borderlands of Sanity*. Munksgaard, Copenhagen.
Williams, J.B.W. & Spitzer, R.L. (1981): The reliability of the diagnostic criteria of DSM III. In Wing, J.K., Bebbington, P. & Robins, L.E. (eds.): *What Is A Case?* Grant McIntyre. London, pp.107-114.

Self-Rating Scales in the Evaluation of Psychiatric Treatment

D. von ZERSSEN

1. Introduction

The primary goal of psychiatric treatment is to cure or, at least, to improve mental disorders at the lowest possible risk for the patient. The reduction of symptoms usually serves as a measure of success in reaching this goal. Therefore, the quantification of psychiatric symptoms is a basic requirement for the evaluation of the efficacy of therapeutic efforts. The introduction of modern psychopharmacological treatment and also that of behaviour therapy in psychiatry has stimulated the development of a psychopathometric approach (von Zerssen 1980; von Zerssen & Möller 1980) which is surveyed comprehensively by Cronholm & Daly in this volume. The authors rightly point out that, with respect to rating procedures, "self-rating may be complementary to expert rating", because "different aspects may be observed and the sources of error" are different (von Zerssen & Cording 1978). In the following paper these statements will be commented on in more detail.

2. General considerations

As compared with expert rating (Mombour 1972; Pichot & Olivier-Martin 1974), self-rating is simpler because it does not require highly skilled specialists (well-trained psychiatrists or clinical psychologists) as raters; the patients themselves rather perform the task of indicating the presence or absence of disturbances and, in some rating scales, also that of marking their degree (frequency/intensity). The disturbances in question are usually specified in a questionnaire whether for one global rating (e.g. that of 'inner tension') or for the rating of several (up to more than 100) items. They may also be presented in a graphical form as in the Visual Analogue Scale (Luria 1975).

Scale values are derived from the patient's check marks on the questionnaire, using a 'key' which can be programmed for electronic data processing. The scoring procedure is thus executed only by the patient, by technical personnel, and, if available, by a computer. The scale values may be based on a global rating or, as sum-scores, on a number of scores obtained from individual items. In unidimensional scales, the items of a questionnaire all belong to one construct (e.g. 'anxiety'), in two- or multi-dimensional scales, they are distributed among two or more constructs (e.g. 'anxiety', 'hostility' and the like). Generally, the constructs are either conceived as clinical syndromes or represent dimensions of factorial analyses of questionnaire items. This is also analogous to the conception of clinical rating scales.

Besides the different kinds of raters (either experts or the patients themselves) there is another basic difference between expert rating and self-rating, which lies in the content of the scales: Whereas clinical rating refers to signs *and* symptoms, self-rating by its very nature is restricted to symptoms (complaints) alone, since it is hardly possible to observe one's own behaviour from outside and to judge the inadequacy of one's own thinking and performance, particularly in a state of severe mental abnormality. Therefore, it is not very meaningful to ask a patient whether he believes in events that really do not take place but rather whether he is persecuted by so-and-so (if, from the point of view of the constructor of the scale, this seems extremely unlikely or even impossible).

Another limitation of self-ratings is that they cannot be usefully applied to patients who are unco-operative or of a very low intelligence (verbal IQ below 80) or otherwise impaired in their judgement or performance and are thus unwilling or unable to meet the demands of the test instruction. Consequently, self-ratings are not recommended for the assessment of psychopathology in oligophrenic, demented or severely psychotic patients. The domain of their application is rather the investigation of psychopathic, neurotic, psychosomatic or only mildly to moderately psychotic patients or patients with special mental problems (such as sexual deviations or insufficiencies, eating disturbances, etc.).

Due to the subjective nature of any kind of rating, there are several biases inherent in patients' self-ratings (Prusoff *et al* 1972a). Besides the lack of insight regarding the abnormality of the inner experience and the external behaviour of psychotic patients, which has just been pointed out, a more or less conscious tendency to simulate sickness or good health has to be considered (de Soto & Küthe 1959). To a certain extent, this tendency can be controlled by a scale composed of complaints which are too common to be totally denied and, at the same time, too adverse to be fully accepted by the majority of people (von Zerssen 1976a/c: scale for the assessment of 'denial of illness'). Other aspects of 'response style', such as saying 'yes' or 'no', are not so relatively specific for clinical self-ratings and are, therefore, extensively dealt with in the psychological literature on self-rating, particularly with respect to personality traits (Berg 1967).

Owing to their lower sensitivity to change, personality inventories (like the MPI: Eysenck 1959) are not as important for therapeutic studies as symptom-scales. They may be of use as predictors of response to therapeutic measures but of less use as indicators of a patient's response to treatment, with the exception of personality changes under long-lasting psychotherapy in severe neuroses and in personality disorders (Smith *et al* 1980).

Another type of rating for the evaluation of psychiatric treatment is concerned with side-effects, particularly those of physical or chemical agents (ECT, drugs). However, for this purpose self-rating is relatively seldom used, although it should be possible to identify a large number of complaints induced by such agents. At present, therapeutic effects and side-effects are not distinguished in self-ratings, but to a certain extent this is true also in expert ratings (Busfield *et al* 1962). They can be separated only by the direction of change under therapy: A decrease in the values of symptom-scales during the course of treatment points to a therapeutic effect, an increase in the values is indicative of side-effects (at least, if an interruption of the therapeutic procedure is followed by a decrease in the scale values).

The quality of a scale can be estimated according to several criteria (Lienert 1969) of which objectivity, reliability and validity are generally acknowledged. These three criteria can all be expressed in quantitative terms, usually as correlation coefficients.

Objectivity, i.e. the degree of independence of scale values of the investigator, is almost perfect in self-ratings, which can be regarded as one important advantage of these ratings as compared with expert ratings.

Reliability refers to the degree of agreement between a subject's values, as compared with other subjects' values, on the same scale at different times (stability) or on parts of the same scale at the same time (consistency). All scales based on additive item-scores should possess high internal consistency and, in the case of personality scales, also high temporal stability, whereas symptom-scales should be highly sensitive to change. For this reason, the test-retest reliability (stability) of symptom-scales may be rather low, at least in patients with marked changes in their clinical condition (as, hopefully, in most therapeutic trials). Fortunately enough, there is usually no trend in the scores of repeatedly administered rating-scales, as is the case with most performance tests which are influenced by learning (see Fig. 1) and which are, therefore, only of limited value in therapeutic trials, at least if the temporal course of the disorder under treatment has to be analysed in detail.

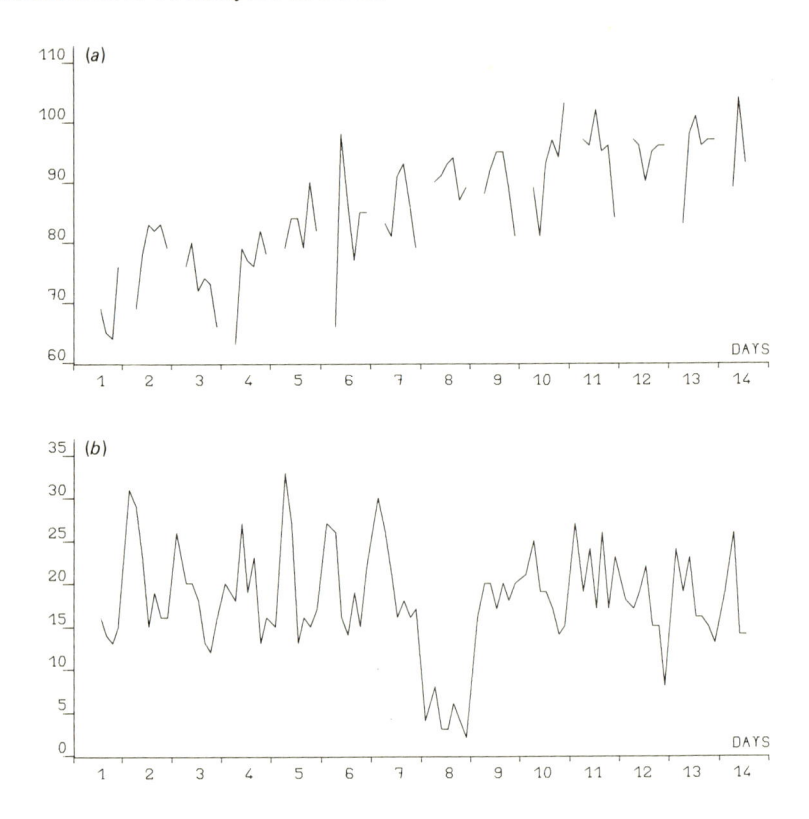

Fig. 1. Course-patterns of repeated measurements by a performance-test (calculating) and a self-rating mood-scale in a male patient with endogenous depression. (*a*) Pauli test (modified: number of calculations in 2 min). (*b*) Value of the mood-scale Bf-S/Bf-S' (von Zerssen 1976d; see Table 1). Measurements were taken every 3 hours from 7 a.m. to 10 p.m. and, with the mood-scale, also once at night (2.30 a.m.) during a drug-free period in the hospital. During this time the patient was mildly to moderately depressed, particularly in the morning, and hypomanic on day 8. This is reflected adequately by the mood-scale but not by the performance test.

Validity designates the degree of agreement between the scale values and the variable to be measured (a trait variable as in personality scales or a state variable as in symptom-scales). For the validation of scales constructed to evaluate response to treatment, the sensitivity of scale values (and of all underlying item-scores) to the changes in the patient's clinical condition should be elucidated. Unfortunately, this task has been rather neglected in the construction and in the final validation of the majority of clinical self-rating scales.

Besides high objectivity, reliability and validity there are some other criteria that qualify a scale as a valuable tool for research and clinical practice. These are:

1. The existence of *normative values* from the general population and *comparative values* from clinical samples.
2. *Comparability* with equal (parallel) or similar scales.
3. *Economy* with respect to test material, manpower (experts for rating, etc.) and time consumed by the entire assessment procedure (application and evaluation). Except for a few very voluminous tests, for example, the Minnesota Multiphasic Personality Inventory (MMPI) with more than 550 items (Hathaway & McKinley 1951), this criterion is fulfilled to a marked extent by most self-rating scales used for evaluating psychiatric therapy. This is particularly true of global assessment scales. From the point of view of cost-benefit analyses of instruments used for evaluating psychiatric treatment, the economic aspect is a very important one.
4. *Usefulness* referring to the need for the scale in question: for example, a lack of similar scales of at least equal quality with respect to the other criteria. This test, unlike the others just mentioned, is failed by many of the scales in clinical use, either because they are outmoded or because there were already better ones at hand when the new scales were constructed.

3. Examples of scales

3.1 Survey

Table 1 lists some of the self-rating scales most often employed in European countries for the evaluation of psychiatric treatment. All of them are available in various languages (e.g. the KSb-S in German, English, Swedish, French, Italian and Spanish). One widely used personality inventory (Eysenck's MPI) is included in the list because this test or a similar one (e.g. the Eysenck Personality Inventory, EPI: Eysenck & Eysenck 1971) has sometimes served as a predictor of response to treatment, particularly in psychopharmacological experiments with healthy volunteers (Janke *et al* 1979) or even as a criterion of change in personality structure during long-term psychotherapy. Owing to the instruction which does not restrict the rating to the 'usual self' (Kendell & DiScipio 1968) or to the premorbid characteristics of the patient (von Zerssen 1979, 1982; von Zerssen *et al* 1970), the scale values are markedly influenced by actual mental disorders such as depressive episodes (Coppen

& Metcalfe 1965). This has to be taken into account when the test is administered to patients during their illness. It may then be advisable to change the instruction accordingly (asking for the 'usual self' at the time *before* the onset of the patient's disorder) or to use scales primarily constructed to evaluate *pre*morbid personality traits (von Zerssen 1982).

In the USA several other self-rating scales, symptom-scales as well as personality inventories (or a mixture of both as the MMPI), are or were in use for the evaluation of psychiatric treatment, among others the Clyde Mood Scale (Clyde 1963), the Multiple Affect Adjective Check List (Zuckerman & Lubin 1965), the Hopkins Symptom Checklist (Derogatis *et al* 1973), and its revised version, the Self-Report Symptom Inventory, 90 items — Revised (SCL-90-R: Derogatis 1977).

Special mention should be made of self-rating global improvement scales which proved particularly useful in the self-evaluation of patients under antidepressants (McNair 1974) and of the Subject's Treatment Emergent Symptom Scale (STESS 1976) constructed primarily for the evaluation of side-effects of psychopharmacological treatment in children but also applicable in adults. The scale is, however, not basically different from other scales which are composed mainly of somatic complaints (e.g. the Beschwerden-Liste B-L/B-L'; see Table 1 and von Zerssen 1981) and is less well validated than most of them (Baumann & Stieglitz 1980).

The Early Clinical Drug Evaluation Unit (ECDEU) System (Guy 1976), developed at the National Institute of Mental Health (NIMH), constitutes a collection of a number of Anglo-Saxon scales for expert ratings, nurses' ratings and self-ratings recommended for psychopharmacological investigations. This system served as a model for a collection of scales from Anglo-Saxon or German speaking countries by the Collegium Internationale Psychiatriae Scalarum (CIPS 1981). Some of the CIPS-scales of German origin (e.g. the KSb-S, see Table 1) are also at hand in English and other translations. This may facilitate international comparisons of various treatments on the basis of scale values.

3.2 *Scales from a psychiatric information system*

At the Max-Planck-Institut für Psychiatrie (MPI-P) in Munich, a Psychiatric Information System (PSYCHIS München) was developed (Barthelmes & von Zerssen 1978) for, among other purposes, the evaluation of in-patient care. For this aim, the patient's mental status is documented at admission and discharge by means of expert ratings according to the In-patient Multidimensional Psychiatric Scale (IMPS: Lorr & Klett 1967) and by means of self-ratings, using a series of clinical self-rating scales (Klinische Selbstbeurteilungs-Skalen, KSb-S: von

Table 1. Clinical self-rating scales most commonly used in various European countries

Scales (References)	Abbreviation	Content	Number of items	Comments
Clinical Self-Rating Scales (von Zerssen 1976) from the Psychiatric Information System (PSYCHIS, Munich; Barthelmes & von Zerssen 1978)	KSb-S			Parallel forms (S' or L') to all scales with standard values from a representative sample of the West German population (for subjects with an IQ $\geq$ 80)
List of Somatic Complaints (von Zerssen 1976b; Stieglitz et al 1980)	B-L/B-L' B-L^0*	Physical and general complaints (B/B')	24/24/17	The items from B-L^0 are not scored but merely serve to provide further information about the individual complaints
Paranoid-Depression Scale (von Zerssen 1976c)	PD-S/PD-S'	Paranoid (P/P') and depressive (D/D') tendencies	43/43	Control scales: denial of illness (Kv-S), motivation (M) and discrepancy (Dk) between responses to parallel forms
Depression Scale (von Zerssen 1976c)	D-S/D-S'	As above (D/D')	16/16	Subscale from PD-S/PD-S' (without control scales)
Mood Scale (von Zerssen 1976d)	Bf-S/Bf-S'**	Actual state of well-being	28/28	Particularly sensitive to change
Depression Inventory (Beck et al 1961)	D-I	As in D-S/D-S'	21	No standard values, no manual
Fear Survey Schedule (Wolpe & Lang 1964)	FSS-III	Phobias	72	Rather an inventory of items than a scale
Maudsley Personality Inventory (Eysenck 1959)	MPI	Trait variables: extraversion and neuroticism	48	Conceived as a personality inventory, not as a symptom-scale
Self-Rating Anxiety Scale (Zung 1971)	SAS	Anxiety	20	No standard values, no manual
Self-Rating Depression Scale (Zung 1965)	SDS	As in D-S/D-S'	20	No standard values, no manual
Visual Analogue Scale (Zealley & Aitken 1969; Luria 1975)	VAS	As in Bf-S/Bf-S'	—	No standard values, no manual, but particularly sensitive to change

*B-L, Beschwerden-Liste. **Bf-S, Befindlichkeits-Skala.

Zerssen 1976a-d; see Table 1). One of these, a mood scale called 'Befindlichkeits-Skala' (Bf-S and its parallel version Bf-S'), is also administered every other day during in-patient treatment. In addition, a short verbal intelligence test, the subscale 'Information' of the Wechsler Scale (Wechsler 1958), and a series of personality inventories for retrospective evaluation of premorbid personality (separate scales for self-rating and for relatives' rating) are applied at admission (von Zerssen 1982). Together with basic biosocial and medical data (including final psychiatric diagnoses, type and success of treatment according to clinical impression, etc.), the item-scores and scale values derived from them are stored in a data bank which also contains a subset of analogous data from two samples ($n_1 = 1952$ and $n_2 = 1537$) of the general population (n_1: von Zerssen 1976a; n_2: Dilling *et al* 1983; n_1 and n_2: von Zerssen & Weyerer 1982).

The KSb-S fulfil all the aforementioned criteria, a fact which distinguishes them from almost all other self-rating scales in use for the evaluation of psychiatric treatment (von Zerssen 1976a-d, 1979). Therefore, we will restrict the exemplification of scales used for this purpose mainly to these instruments (all of which exist in two parallel forms, see Table 1). They cover those aspects of the 'subjective status' (Jaspers 1963) of mental patients that have been repeatedly elicited as relatively independent of each other in factor-analytic studies of symptom-scales (von Zerssen 1976a), namely somatic complaints (B-L/B-L'), psychically experienced distress of an anxious-depressive type (D-S/D-S'), and psychotic features of a paranoid type (P-S/P-S'). Moreover, the actual reduction of a patient's general feeling of well-being is ascertained every other day, using an adjective checklist, the mood scale called 'Befindlichkeits-Skala (Bf-S/Bf-S'). This particular scale is also employed for repeated measurements (up to every three hours daily for two and more weeks) in special research projects (see also Linden & Krautzig 1981; Schwarz & Strian 1972), for example, on chronobiological aspects of endogenous depression (Dirlich *et al* 1981; von Zerssen & Cording 1978; von Zerssen *et al* 1983).

The factorial structure based on the intercorrelations among the KSb-S, together with two short verbal intelligence tests (or one of these and social strata), is presented in Table 2 for a representative sample of the general population (FRG; n = 1666; age range 20-64 years) and in Table 3 for a group of psychiatric in-patients investigated at admission (MPI-P; n = 127; similar distribution of sex and age as in the general population sample). It can be easily recognized that in both samples the parallel forms of each subscale and, in the general population sample, the two verbal intelligence tests reach almost the same specifically high loadings on one factor per subscale, with the exception of the D-scales which do not enter a separate factor; their loadings are rather distributed over factors constituted by other scales, mainly those concerning actual reduction of well-being (Bf-Bf′) and somatic complaints (B/B′). There is, however, no apparent relationship of any of the self-rating scales to verbal intelligence and/or social strata.

Table 2. Factorial structure of the KSb-S and two verbal intelligence tests from data of a general population survey (n = 1666)

	I	II	III	IV	V	h^2
Bf	**0.91**	0.16	—0.14	0.05	—0.03	0.88
Bf′	**0.92**	0.17	—0.12	0.04	—0.02	0.89
B	0.21	**0.92**	—0.15	0.15	0.00	0.94
B′	0.23	**0.89**	—0.21	0.12	—0.01	0.90
P	0.09	0.10	—0.09	**0.87**	0.01	0.78
P′	0.07	0.14	—0.16	**0.85**	—0.03	0.77
D	**0.53**	**0.44**	—0.30	**0.40**	—0.15	0.75
D′	**0.57**	**0.42**	—0.27	**0.41**	—0.07	0.75
Kv	—0.18	—0.18	**0.90**	—0.14	—0.02	0.89
Kv′	—0.17	—0.19	**0.90**	—0.17	—0.01	0.90
INF	0.03	—0.09	—0.06	0.05	**0.84**	0.72
MWT	—0.04	0.06	0.05	—0.08	**0.84**	0.72
% total variance	20.46	17.85	15.91	15.77	11.90	81.89

From von Zerssen (1976a). Result of principal component analysis with orthogonal rotation according to the scree test (Cattell 1966).
INF, subtest of the Wechsler Scale (Wechsler 1958).
MWT, Mehrfach-Wortwahl-Test (Merz *et al* 1975).
For abbreviations of the KSb-S subscales see Table 1.

Table 3. Factorial structure of the KSb S, a verbal intelligence test and social strata from data of psychiatric in-patients (various diagnoses) at admission (n = 127)

	I	II	III	IV	V	VI	h^2
Bf	**0.88**	0.21	—0.10	0.04	0.05	0.03	0.83
Bf′	**0.84**	0.21	—0.22	—0.01	—0.03	0.10	0.81
B	0.31	**0.87**	—0.21	0.13	0.02	—0.04	0.92
B′	0.28	**0.85**	—0.32	0.03	—0.08	—0.03	0.91
P	—0.04	0.26	—0.05	**0.88**	—0.04	0.12	0.86
P′	0.19	—0.05	—0.17	**0.90**	0.02	—0.04	0.88
D	**0.56**	**0.61**	—0.26	0.22	—0.12	0.00	0.82
D′	**0.69**	**0.46**	—0.28	0.25	—0.08	—0.02	0.84
Kv	—0.19	—0.30	**0.86**	—0.12	0.07	0.01	0.89
Kv′	—0.25	—0.23	**0.86**	—0.14	—0.11	0.06	0.89
INF	—0.10	—0.06	—0.03	—0.02	**0.97**	0.18	0.99
SOC. STRATA	0.09	—0.04	0.05	0.06	0.18	**0.97**	0.99
% total variance	21.61	19.64	15.43	14.53	8.53	8.40	88.14

From von Zerssen (1976a). Result of principal component analysis with orthogonal rotation according to the scree test (Cattell 1966).
INF, subtest of the Wechsler Scale (Wechsler 1958).
For abbreviations of the KSb-S subscales see Table 1.

In a factor-analytic comparison of the items from the B-, the D-, and the P-scales of the KSb-S (without the parallel versions, the control scales and the Bf-scales) with the items of three self-rating scales from the literature — the Self-rating Depression Scale (SDS: Zung 1965), the Self-rating Anxiety Scale (SAS: Zung 1971) and a 20-item version of Eysenck's Psychoticism-Scale (Eysenck & Eysenck 1972; see Baumann & Dittrich 1975) — the subscales of the KSb-S, including the D-scale, proved to be much more homogeneous than the other scales (Wittmann 1978; von Zerssen 1979). This was true of the data from psychiatric in-patients (n = 185), healthy controls (n = 129) and, consequently, all subjects together (n = 314). Moreover, the KSb-S discriminated much more effectively than the SAS and the Psychoticism Scale between subgroups of the clinical (n = 94) and control samples (n = 91) which were equalized in their composition according to sex, age, and verbal intelligence. Only the SDS was almost as effective in this respect as the D-scale, which had the highest discriminatory power (see Table 4). Similar results were obtained in comparisons of clinical subgroups (paranoid psychotics, non-paranoid schizophrenics, depressives, neurotics with the exception of neurotic depressives) and in intra-individual comparisons of the same patients' state at admission and discharge from the hospital. The results referred to indicate so far that marked differences may exist in the construct validity and the clinical usefulness of some of the scales listed in Table 1.

Table 4. Ranking of scales according to the rate of misclassifications and to the phi-coefficient from a comparison of psychiatric in-patients (n = 94) and healthy controls (n = 91)

	% minimum misclassifications	Phi
D	19.5	0.61
SDS	24.9	0.50
B	32.4	0.35
P	32.9	0.33
Psychoticism	35.1	0.30
SAS	39.5	0.21

For abbreviations of scales see Table 1.

4. Examples of application

In a French-Canadian drug trial of two antidepressants in 37 depressed patients (Bobon *et al* 1981), self-ratings on the basis of Zung's SDS and the mood scale Bf-S/Bf-S' (Heimann *et al* 1975) were employed in addition to expert rating according to the Hamilton Rating Scale for Depression (Hamilton 1960). As shown in Fig. 2, changes of the patients' clinical condition as rated by clinicians are reflected concordantly by Bf-

S/Bf-S' values but not by the values of the SDS (see also Arfwidsson *et al* 1974). This supports the assumption of a particularly high sensitivity of Bf-S/Bf-S' to changes in a patient's emotional state (as, for example, related to depression). This assumption is also confirmed by the application of Bf-S/Bf-S' in other investigations of drug response, as illustrated in the following examples.

Fig. 2. Observer-ratings (HAMD scores: right ordinate) and self-ratings (Bf-S, Bf-S', SDS scores: left ordinate) for 18 patients on amitriptyline and 19 patients on trazodone, double-blind conditions (from Bobon *et al* 1981).

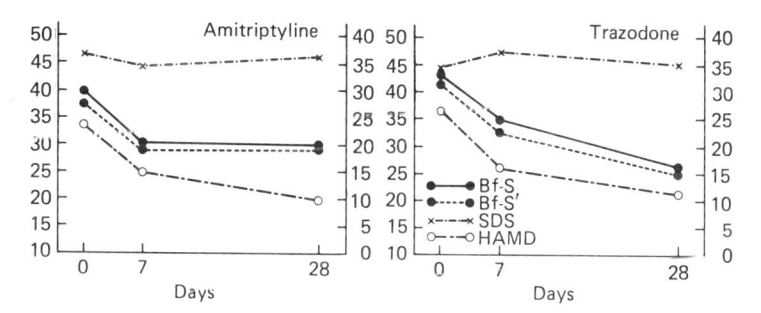

The standardized administration of scales to all in-patients treated at the Psychiatric Department of the MPI-P, in connection with the standardization of therapeutic routines, provides the basis for a retrospective-prospective evaluation of treatment response according to scale values. In the years from 1974 to 1976, for instance, patients with the diagnosis of endogenous depression (according to the ICD-8 Glossary: WHO 1974) were treated primarily with one of the new tetracyclic antidepressants maprotiline (1974/75) and mianserin (1975/76), respectively, whereas before and after that time the classical tricyclic antidepressant amitriptyline was the drug of first choice. In case of serious side-effects or of insufficient therapeutic effects after at least two weeks, another antidepressant could be substituted for the first drug. Data of 76 patients treated first with either amitriptyline or one of the new drugs (19 patients in each drug group: amitriptyline 1970-74 — maprotiline 1974/75 — mianserin 1975/76 — amitriptyline 1976-78) were available for a comparison of clinical efficacy (von Zerssen & Cording-Tömmel 1981).

The four drug groups were very similar in their composition according to sex, age, social data, severity and subtypes of depression, etc. Criteria of drug response were: replacement of the first antidepressant by another and decrease in scale values of Bf-S/Bf-S' after one, two, and three weeks of medication (and other indices of change in scale values under treatment with the first drug (Cording-Tömmel 1982)). Statistical comparisons were performed using non-parametric tests.

In these comparisons, mianserin proved to be replaced by another drug significantly more often than maprotiline and amitriptyline. This could be shown not to depend on a bias of the physicians who were in charge of the patients but rather on the comparatively low clinical efficacy of the drug, using Bf-S/Bf-S' values at the time of change in medication as a measure of response to treatment. Moreover, the differences between Bf-S/Bf-S' values after one, two, and three weeks of medication and the last values before medication (see Fig. 3a-c) were significantly smaller in patients treated with mianserin than in those treated with one of the other drugs. (After four weeks of medication, the number of patients still under mianserin was too small for a statistical comparison!)

Fig. 3. Improvement according to Bf-S/Bf-S' with the first antidepressant after one week (n = 76), two weeks (n = 76) and three weeks (n = 56) during in-patient treatment of patients with endogenous depression. Am.I, amitriptyline 1970-74; Ma., maprotiline 1974/75; Mi., mianserin 1975/76; Am.II, amitriptyline 1976-78; n.s., not significant (from von Zerssen & Cording-Tömmel 1981).

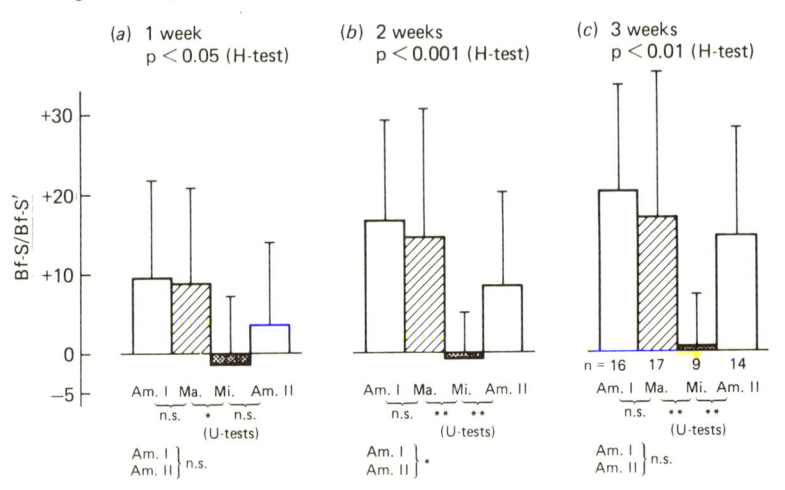

In accord with the literature, there was a trend to a reduced drug response over the years (most likely due to an increasing selection of drug-nonresponders for in-patient treatment), but this could not explain the findings regarding the low therapeutic efficacy of mianserin. When patients with Bf-S/Bf-S' values below a cut-off point indicating the borderline between moderate and severe distress before medication, i.e.

patients with only mild to moderate disturbances, were excluded from the analysis, the results for the 17 patients remaining in each group were thoroughly in accord with the findings of the first analysis (Cording-Tömmel 1982).

The conclusions drawn from this comparison of drug efficacy according to scale values of a self-rating instrument could be criticized in view of the many positive reports on mianserin's antidepressive properties in the literature (Montgomery 1980). Meanwhile, however, results of a well-controlled drug trial (Kragh-Sörensen 1981) seem to substantiate the findings and conclusions of the retrospective-prospective study dealt with here, thus underlining the validity of the methodological approach in which repeated self-ratings play a crucial role in evaluating therapeutic efficacy.

In a similar way, one problem regarding the side-effects of the neuroleptic treatment of schizophrenia could be successfully attacked. In a comparison of scale values of the IMPS and the KSb-S of schizophrenic patients assessed at admission and discharge, a marked decrease not only in psychotic features but also in depressive symptomatology was found (Möller et al 1981). This finding contradicts the notion of 'pharmacogenic depression' as a frequent side-effect of neuroleptic medication, at least during the first weeks or months of treatment. However, patients with this type of side-effect might have been discharged only after the cessation of a pharmacologically induced depression. Therefore, the values of the mood scale Bf-S/Bf-S′ were analysed over the whole course of neuroleptic treatment of schizophrenic in-patients of the MPI-P's Psychiatric Department.

A 'depressive episode' during treatment was defined operationally as an increase of at least three subsequent scale values of Bf-S/Bf-S′ above a cut-off point indicating the borderline between a mild and a moderate degree of subjective distress. With respect to repeated self-ratings according to Bf-S/Bf-S′ during hospitalization, only records of patients with a well-documented course of in-patient treatment of at least three weeks' duration (n = 237 out of a total of 280 cases) were analysed by means of a computer program (Möller & von Zerssen 1981). The results show that 'depressive episodes' as defined above occurred predominantly in patients who had entered the hospital in a depressed state (according to the Bf-S/Bf-S′ values at admission) and that in only 14 per cent of all 237 patients were 'depressive episodes' not preceded by a depressed state at admission. As it is not even certain that in these 14 per cent the episodic depression was indeed induced by the patients' neuroleptic medication, it can be inferred from the results that the frequency of 'pharmacogenic

Table 5. Course patterns of actual mood according to BF-S/BF-S' in schizophrenic in-patients (n = 72)

Course pattern of depression	Description	Reference pattern	Frequency
I. 'Decreasing depression'	Depressive mood scores on admission, decreasing scores during hospital stay		16 (22%)
II. 'Constant depression'	Depressive mood scores during (approximately) the whole hospital stay		17 (24%)
III. 'Recidive depression'	Depressive mood scores on admission, after decreasing to normal scores development of one or more depressive periods IIIa: normal scores on discharge IIIb: depressive scores on discharge		6 (8%) IIIa: 4 IIIb: 2
IV. 'Newly developed depression'	Normal mood scores on admission, development of one or more depressive periods during hospital stay IVa: normal scores on discharge IVb: depressive scores on discharge		12 (17%) IVa: 7 IVb: 5
V. 'No depression'	No depressive mood scores during (approximately) the whole hospital stay		19 (26%)
VI. 'Others'	Not classifiable		2 (3%)

From Möller & von Zerssen (1982).

depression' due to neuroleptics in the acute treatment of schizophrenia has been over-estimated by most authors who did not employ a psychopathometric approach to the problem.

The same conclusion can be drawn from a visual classification of the course of scale values of Bf-S/Bf-S' during in-patient treatment in a cohort of 72 patients with schizophrenic or similar paranoid psychoses, followed up five to seven years after their hospitalization at the MPI-P (Möller & von Zerssen 1982; see Table 5). Only 17 per cent of the patients in this sub-sample developed a 'depression' during in-patient treatment without having been depressed on admission. The method of visual classification seems to be a promising approach to the analysis of longitudinal data based on large series of measurements as obtained by the repeated administration of self-rating scales even in the absence of expert ratings. In as far as expert ratings were performed in this or similar studies on depression arising from acute neuroleptic treatment of schizophrenics (e.g. Knights & Hirsch 1981), the results are in accord with those reported here (Möller & von Zerssen 1982). This can be regarded as a validation of the results achieved by means of self-ratings.

Whereas therapeutic effects can be expected only if there is a disorder to be cured or, at least, a symptom to be abolished, side-effects of treatment can also be observed in the absence of any symptomatology. This is often the case in psychopharmacological experiments with healthy volunteers. Here self-rating scales constructed to measure a change in the clinical condition of patients may be used for the measurement of side-effects, i.e. the induction of symptoms by the drugs under investigation. This is exemplified by a figure illustrating the influence of a new pharmacological agent (an antaminicum with antidepressive properties) on the previously well-balanced subjective state of a healthy subject investigated at the pharmacological laboratory of a drug company (Fig. 4)*. It is quite obvious that, as compared with low scale values of Bf-S/Bf-S' throughout the day before the drug trial, there is a marked reduction in subjective well-being (as reflected by increasing scale values), which parallels the blood level of the drug. Very similar patterns of changes in the blood levels and the self-ratings were observed in the two other subjects undergoing this drug trial. The results confirm the validity of the scale values of Bf-S/Bf-S' as a measure of reduction in subjective well-being (in this case mainly due to the sedative properties of an antaminicum) and point to the importance of discriminating symptoms of a disorder from side-effects of medication (and, of course, other influences) in therapeutic trials with patients.

*The author is indebted to Dr. med. H. Sieroslawski, Medical Department of Dr K. Thomae GmbH, Biberach/FRG, for providing the figure and an exposé on the drug WA 335 (Danitracen), 1976.

Fig. 4. Changes in Bf-values and in the blood level of an antaminicum (WA 335) during a drug trial in a healthy male volunteer.

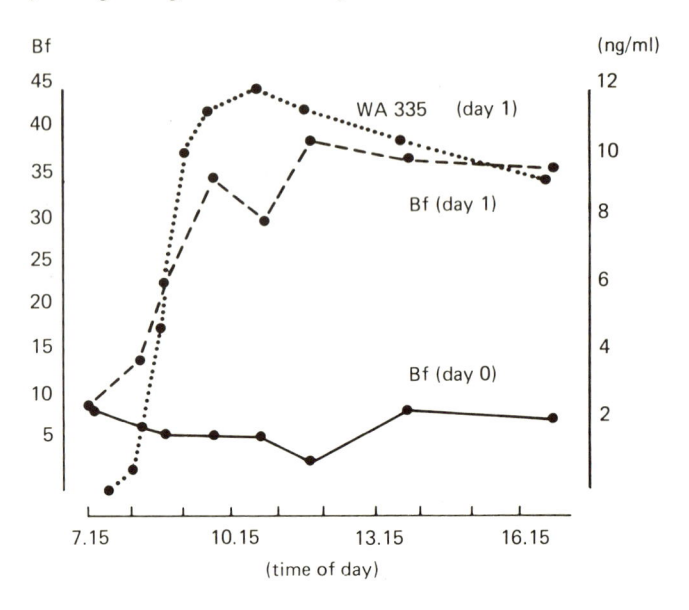

Finally, an example of the predictive value of personality inventories in therapeutic trials is chosen from a research project on the differential efficacy of cognitive and behavioural therapy in patients with severe neurotic depression. The project conducted at the Psychiatric Department of the MPI-P is still in progress (de Jong *et al* 1981). The intermediate analysis of data from 40 subjects shows that the outcome criterion (total score of the Beck Depression Inventory at discharge, chosen for comparison with results of similar investigations in the USA) correlates significantly and in opposite directions with extraversion (negatively) and neuroticism (positively) as measured by a modified version (von Zerssen 1979, 1982) of the ENNR (Brengelmann & Brengelmann 1960) and, moreover, with subscales of the Premorbid Personality Inventories mentioned above (scales for a neurotic personality structure and oral dependence, both of which are closely related to neuroticism). This result may reflect merely a generally poor prognosis in neurotic depression of intraverted and basically neurotic personalities and may not be specific for the response to special modes of treatment since similar results were obtained in a six-month follow-up of former in-patients with this type of depression, who had received other kinds of therapy (Kerr *et al* 1970). Nevertheless, it seems necessary to be aware of a possible influence of personality traits on prognosis and response to treatment in any therapeutic trial and, therefore, to include the assessment of personality by means of self-rating scales more often than is usual in such investigations.

5. Conclusions

The statement of Cronholm & Daly (see above) that "self-rating may be complementary to expert rating" could be substantiated in this article. Moreover, evidence was provided for the validity of self-rating of changes in the well-being of psychiatric patients and healthy volunteers and for the usefulness of repeated self-ratings during therapy even if, for economic reasons, no simultaneous ratings could be performed by experts. New methodological approaches to the evaluation of psychiatric treatment are made possible on this basis: for example, the retrospective-prospective evaluation of standardized clinical treatment routines or the visual classification of graphical plots of scale values in an attempt to evaluate different types of changes in symptomatology under treatment. The duration of such research projects may extend to several years without impairing the validity of ratings in spite of a considerable change in research personnel because the ratings are executed by the patients and the administration of the scales and the subsequent scoring procedures can be routinely performed by technical personnel without special training in clinical psychiatry and rating procedures.

The main task of the investigator in the evaluation of psychiatric treatment by means of self-rating scales is to design the study (Möller & Benkert 1980), to select appropriate scales, to control the performance of the investigation and, finally, to interpret the results meaningfully (no self-rating scale, for example, can be regarded as a direct measure of clinical depression but may be used as an indicator of the presence of depression and the degree of subjective distress induced by it).

The following recommendations regarding the use of self-rating scales should be considered in preparing a research project on the response to psychiatric treatment:

1. Utilize scales already available (Cautela & Upper 1976; CIPS 1981; Guy 1976; Pichot & Olivier-Martin 1974; Tasto 1977) and add new ones, specifically constructed for the intended project, only if they are complementary to the other scales or if duplication is being used for validation purposes.
2. Consult a specialist in the clinical application of self-rating scales if you are not familiar with it yourself. This is also recommended with respect to the interpretation of the results. But even if you are a specialist in this field, do consult the test-manuals in preparing the study and, later on, in interpreting the findings.

3. Pay attention to the instruction and motivation of patients and staff members for an adequate use of self-rating.
4. Introduce a measure of verbal intelligence for the selection of patients, particularly if the sample size is expected to be small, and exclude cases with an estimated verbal IQ below 80 (according to the standards of the Wechsler Scale).
5. Do not rely exclusively on self-ratings, but combine them with other measures, above all expert ratings and, if possible, systematic observation, performance tests, etc. (Baumann & Seidenstücker 1977; Cronholm & Daly, this volume; Prusoff et al 1972b; Raskin et al 1969; von Zerssen & Möller 1980).
6. Make use of series of repeated measurements with short and simple scales to fill the gap between pre- and post-treatment values and include visual analyses in the evaluation of the data.

It is the author's impression that clinicians, at least in Europe, have tended to underestimate the value of self-rating procedures as research tools, whereas clinical psychologists have tended to overestimate them. A more extensive exchange of opinions and experiences may provide a more balanced view on both sides and thereby lead to an appropriate use of self-rating scales in the evaluation of psychiatric treatment.

References

Arfwidsson, L., d'Elia, G., Laurell, B., Ottosson, J.-O., Perris, C. & Persson, G. (1974): Can self-rating replace doctor's rating in evaluating anti-depressive treatment? *Acta Psychiatr. Scand. 50,* 16-22.

Barthelmes, H. & Zerssen, D. von (1978): Das Münchener Psychiatrische Informationssystem (PSYCHIS München). In Reichertz, P.L. & Schwarz, B. (eds.): *Informationssysteme in der medizinischen Versorgung. Ökologie der Systeme.* Schattauer, Stuttgart, 138-145.

Baumann, U. & Dittrich, A. (1975): Konstruktion einer deutschsprachigen Psychotizismus-Skala. *Z. Exp. Angew. Psychol. 22,* 421-443.

Baumann, U. & Seidenstücker, G. (1977): Zur Taxonomie und Bewertung psychologischer Untersuchungsverfahren bei Psychopharmakaprüfungen. *Pharmakopsychiatr. 10,* 165-175.

Baumann, U. & Stieglitz, R.-D. (1980): Ein Vergleich von vier Beschwerdenlisten. *Arch. Psychiatr. Nervenkr. 229,* 145-163.

Beck, A.T., Ward, C.H., Mendelson, M., Mock, J. & Erbaugh, J. (1961): An inventory for measuring depression. *Arch. Gen. Psychiatr. 4,* 561-571.

Berg, I.A. (1967): *Response Set in Personality Assessment.* Aldine Publishing Company, Chicago.

Bobon, D.P., Lapierre, Y.D. & Lottin, T. (1981): Validity and sensitivity of the French version of the Zerssen Bf-S/Bf-S' self-rating mood scale during treatment with trazodone and amitriptyline. *Prog. Neuropsychopharmacology, 5,* 519-522.

Brengelmann, J.C. & Brengelmann, L. (1960): Deutsche Validierung von Fragebogen der Extraversion, neurotischen Tendenz und Rigidität. *Z. Exp. Angew. Psychol. 7,* 291-331.

Busfield, B.L. Jr., Schneller, P. & Capra, D. (1962): Depressive symptom or side-effect? A comparative study of symptoms during pre-treatment and treatment periods of patients on three antidepressant medications. *J. Nerv. Ment. Dis. 134,* 339-345.

Cattell, R.B. (1966): The scree test for the number of factors. *Multivar. Behav. Res. 1,* 245-276.

Cautela, J.R. & Upper, D. (1976): The behavioural inventory battery: the use of self-report measures in behavioural analysis and therapy. In Hersen, M. & Bellack, A.S. (eds.): *Behavioural Assessment: A Practical Handbook.* Pergamon Press, Oxford, 77-109.

CIPS (1981): Collegium Internationale Psychiatrae Scalarum (eds.): *Internationale Skalen für Psychiatrie.* Beltz, Weinheim.

Clyde, D.J. (1963): *Manual for the Clyde Mood Scale.* Biometr. Lab., University of Miami, Coral Gables, Florida.

Coppen, A. & Metcalfe, M. (1965): Effect of a depressive illness on MPI scores. *Br. J. Psychiatry, 111,* 236-239.

Cording-Tömmel, C. (1982): *Zur Wirksamkeit von Mianserin und Maprotilin im Vergleich zu Amitriptyln bei schwerer endogener Depression.* Diss. Med. Universität, München.

de Jong, R., Henrich, G. & Ferstl, R. (1981): A behavioural treatment programme for neurotic depression. *Behav. Anal. Modif. 4,* 275-287.

Derogatis, L.R., Lipman, R.S., Rickels, K., Uhlenhuth, E.H. & Covi, L. (1973): The Hopkins Symptom Checklist (HSCL): a measure of primary symptom dimensions. In Pichot, P. (ed.): *Psychological Measurement: Problems in Psychopharmacotherapy.* Karger, Basel.

Derogatis, C.R. (1977): SCL-90. *Administration. Scoring and Procedures.* Manual I for the revised version and other instruments of the psychopathology rating scale series. Johns Hopkins University School of Medicine, Baltimore.

De Soto, C.B. & Küthe, J.L. (1959): The set to claim undesirable symptoms in personality inventories. *J. Consult. Psychol. 23,* 496-500.

Dilling, H., Weyerer, S. & Castell, R. (1983): *Psychische Erkrankungen in der Bevölkerung.* Enke, Stuttgart (in press).

Dirlich, G., Kammerloher, A., Schulz, H., Lund, R., Doerr, P. & Zerssen, D. von (1981): Temporal co-ordination of rest-activity cycle, body temperature, urinary free cortisol, and mood in a patient with 48-hour unipolar-depressive cycles in clinical and time-cue-free environments. *Biol. Psychiatry, 16,* 163-179.

Eysenck, H.J. (1959): *Manual of the Maudsley Personality Inventory.* University of London Press, London.

Eysenck, H.J. & Eysenck, S.B.G. (1971): *Manual of the Eysenck Personality Inventory* (1st ed. 1964), 4th ed. University of London.

Eysenck, S.B.G. & Eysenck, H.J. (1972): The questionnaire measurement of psychoticism *Psychol. Med. 2,* 50-55.

Guy, W. (1976): *ECDEU Assessment Manual for Psychopharmacology.* Rev. ed, Rockville, Maryland.

Hamilton, M. (1960): A rating scale for depression. *J. Neurol. Neurosurg. Psychiatry, 23,* 56-62.

Hathaway, S.R. & McKinley, J.D. (1951): *Minnesota Multiphasic Personality Inventory: Manual.* Psychological Corporation, New York.

Heimann, H., Bobon-Schrod, H., Schmocker, A.M. & Bobon, D.P. (1975): Auto-evaluation de l'humeur par une liste d'adjectifs, la 'Befindlichkeits-Skala' (BS) de Zerssen. *Encephale 1,* 165-183.

Janke, W., Debus, G. & Longo, N. (1979): Differential psychopharmacology of tranquilizing and sedating drugs. *Mod. Probl. Pharmacopsychiatry, 14,* 13-98.

Jaspers, K. (1963): *General Psychopathology,* 7th ed. University of Chicago Press, Chicago.

Kendell, R.E. & DiScipio, W.J. (1968): Eysenck personality inventory scores of patients with depressive illness. *Br. J. Psychiatry, 114,* 767-770.
Kerr, T.A., Schapira, K., Roth, M. & Garside, R.F. (1970): The relationship between the Maudsley Personality Inventory and the course of affective disorders. *Br. J. Psychiatry, 116,* 11-19.
Knights, A. & Hirsch, S.R. (1981): 'Revealed' depression and drug treatment for schizophrenia. *Arch. Gen. Psychiatry, 38,* 806-811.
Kragh-Sörensen, P. (1981): Antidepressant treatment in elderly patients. Lecture held at WPA/APA regional meeting, Oct.30-Nov.3. Manuscript. New York City, N.Y.
Lienert, G.A. (1969): *Testaufbau und Testanalyse,* 3rd ed. Beltz, Weinheim.
Linden, M. & Krautzig, E. (1981): Befindlichkeitsmessung in kurzzeitigen Abständen: ein experimenteller Beitrag zur Validierung der Befindlichkeitsskala (Bf-S) nach von Zerssen. *Pharmakopsychiatr 14,* 40-41.
Lorr, M. & Klett, C.J. (1967): *Manual for the In-patient Psychiatric Scale* (revised). Consulting Psychologists Press, Palo Alto, California.
Luria, R.E. (1975): The validity and reliability of the Visual Analogue Mood Scale. *J. Psychiatr. Res. 12,* 51-57.
McNair, D.M. (1974): Self-evaluations of antidepressants. *Psychopharmacology, 37,* 281-302.
Merz, J., Lehrl, S., Galster, V. & Erzigkeit, H. (1975): Der MWT-B — ein Intelligenzkurztest. *Psychiatr. Neurol. Med. Psychol.* Leipz. *27,* 423-428.
Möller, H.-J. & Benkert, O. (1980): Methoden und Probleme der Beurteilung der Effektivität psycho-pharmakologischer und psychologischer Therapieverfahren. In Biefang, S. (ed.): *Evaluationsforschung in der Psychiatrie: Fragestellungen und Methoden.* Enke, Stuttgart, 54-128.
Möller, H.-J. & Zerssen, D. von (1981): Depressive Symptomatik bei Aufnahme und Entlassung stationär behandelter schizophrener Patienten. *Nervenarzt, 52,* 525-530.
Möller, H.-J., Zerssen, D. von, Werner-Eilert, K. & Wueschrer-Stockheim, M. (1981): Psychopathometrische Verlaufsuntersuchungen an Patienten mit Schizophrenien und verwandten Psychosen. *Arch. Psychiatr. Nervenkr. 230,* 275-292.
Möller, H.-J. & Zerssen D. von (1982): Depressive states occurring during the neuroleptic treatment of schizophrenia. *Schizophr. Bull., 8,* 109-117.
Mombour, W. (1972): Verfahren zur Standardisierung des psychopathologischen Befundes. *Psychiatr. Clin.* (Basel) *5,* 73-120, 137-157.
Montgomery, S.A. (1980): Maprotiline, nomifensine, mianserin, zimelidine: a review of antidepressant efficacy in in-patients. *Neuropharmacology, 19,* 1185-1190.
Pichot, P. & Olivier-Martin, R. (eds.) (1974): *Psychological Measurement in Psychopharmacology. Mod. Probl. Pharmacopsychiatry, 7.* Karger, Basel.
Prusoff, B.A., Klerman, G.L. & Paykel, E.S. (1972a): Concordance between clinical assessments and patients' self-report in depression. *Arch. Gen. Psychiatry, 26,* 546-552.
Prusoff, B.A., Klerman, G.L. & Paykel, E.S. (1972b): Pitfalls in the self-report assessment of depression. *Can. Psychiatr. Assoc. J. 17,* 101-107.
Raskin, A., Schulterbrandt, J., Reatig, N. & McKeon, J.J. (1969): Replication of factors of psychopathology in interview, ward behaviour and self-report ratings of hospitalized depressives. *J. Nerv. Ment. Dis. 148,* 87-98.
Schwarz, D. & Strian, F. (1972): Psychometrische Untersuchungen zur Befindlichkeit psychiatrischer und intern-medizinischer Patienten. *Arch. Psychiatr. Nervenkr. 2,* 70-81.
Smith, M.L., Glass, G.V. & Miller, T.I. (1980): *The Benefits of Psychotherapy.* Johns Hopkins Press, Baltimore.
STESS (1976): Subject's Treatment Emergent Symptom Scale. In Guy, W. (ed.) *ECDEU Assessment Manual for Psychopharmacology.* Rev. ed. Rockville, Maryland, 347-350.

Stieglitz, R.-D., Baumann, U., Tobien, H.H. & Zerssen, D. von (1980): Zur Stichprobenunabhängigkeit und Zeitinvarianz von Testkennwerten bei einer Beschwerden-Liste. *Z. Exp. Angew. Psychol. 27,* 631-654.
Tasto, D.L. (1977): Self-report schedules and inventories. In Ciminero, A.R., Calhoun, K.S., & Adams, H.E. (eds.): *Handbook of Behavioural Assessment.* Wiley, New York, 153-193.
Wechsler, D. (1958): *The Measurement and Appraisal of Adult Intelligence,* 4th ed. Williams and Wilkins, Baltimore.
WHO (1974): *Glossary of Mental Disorders and Guide to their Classification for Use in Conjunction with the International Classification of Diseases,* 8th rev. World Health Organization, Geneva.
Wittmann, B. (1978): Untersuchung über die faktorielle und klinischdiagnostische Differenzierbarkeit der Syndrome Angst und Depression in der klinischen Selbstbeurteilung sowie über die Beziehung zwischen den Fragebogendimensionen 'Paranoide Tendenzen' und 'Psychotizismus'. Diss. med. Universität München.
Wolpe, J. & Lang, P.J. (1964): A fear survey schedule for use in behaviour therapy. *Behav. Res. Ther. 2,* 27-30.
Zealley, A.K. & Aitken, R.C.B. (1969): Measurement of mood. *Proc. R. Soc. Med. 62,* 993-996.
Zerssen, D. von, Köller, D.-M. & Rey, E.-R. (1970): Die prämorbide Persönlichkeit von endogen Depressiven. Eine Kreuzvalidierung früherer Untersuchungsergebnisse. *Confin. Psychiatr.* (Basel) *13,* 156-179.
Zerssen, D. von unter Mitarbeit von D.-M. Köller (1976): Klinische Selbstbeurteilungs-Skalen (KSb-S) aus dem Münchener Psychiatrischen Informations-System (PSYCHIS München), Manuale. (a) Allgemeiner Teil; (b) Die Beschwerden-Liste; (c) Paranoid-Depressivitäts-Skala. Depressivitäts-Skala; (d) Die Befindlichkeits-Skala. Beltz, Weinheim.
Zerssen, D. von & Cording, C. (1978): The measurement of change in endogenous affective disorders. *Arch. Psychiatr. Nervenkr. 226,* 95-112.
Zerssen, D. von (1979): Klinisch-psychiatrische Selbstbeurteilungs-Fragebogen. In Baumann, U., Berbalk, H. & Seidenstuecker, G. (eds.): *Klinische Psychologie. Trends in Forschung und Praxis 2.* Huber, Bern, 130-159.
Zerssen, D. von (1980): Psychopathomethrische Verfahren und ihre Anwendung in der Psychiatrie. In Peters, U.H. (ed.): *Die Psychologie des 20. Jahrhunderts.* Kindler, Zürich, 149-169.
Zerssen, D. von & Möller, H.-J. (1980): Psychopathometrische Verfahren in der psychiatrischen Therapieforschung. In Biefang, S. (ed.): *Evaluationsforschung in der Psychiatrie.* Enke, Stuttgart, 129-166.
Zerssen, D. von (1981): Körperliche und Allgemeinbeschwerden als Ausdruck seelischer Gestörtheit. *Therapiewoche, 31,* 865-876.
Zerssen, D. von & Cording-Tömmel, C. (1981): Is Mianserin a potent anti-depressant? Paper read at the 3rd World Congress on Biological Psychiatry, Stockholm.
Zerssen, D. von (1982): Personality and affective disorders. In Paykel, E.S. (ed.): *Handbook of Affective Disorders.* Churchill Livingstone, Edinburgh.
Zerssen, D. von, Dirlich, G. & Fischler, M. (1983): The influence of an abnormal time routine and therapeutic measures on 48-hour cycles of affective disorders. Chronobiological considerations. In Wehr, T.A. & Goodwin, F.K. (eds.): *Circadian Rhythms in Psychiatry.* Boxwood Press, Los Angeles, California.
Zerssen, D. von & Weyerer, S. (1982): Sex differences in rates of mental disorders. *Int. J. Ment. Health, 11,* 9-45.
Zuckerman, M. & Lubin, B. (1965): *Manual for the Multiple Affect Adjective Check List.* Educational and Industrial Testing Service, San Diego, California.
Zung, W.W.K. (1965): A self-rating depression scale. *Arch. Gen. Psychiatr. 12,* 63-70.

Zung, W.W.K. (1971): A rating instrument for anxiety disorders. *Psychosomatics, 12,* 371-379.

Methods for Measuring Social Adjustment

H. KATSCHNIG

1. Introduction

The advent of community psychiatry in the last two decades has stimulated interest in measuring the outcome of psychiatric treatment not only in terms of absence of psychopathological symptoms but also in terms of the quality of life of the individual. Although a certain correlation between type and intensity of psychopathology on the one hand and social maladjustment on the other hand does not seem improbable, it has now been firmly established that they may also be independent of each other (Weissman *et al* 1974).

It seems inappropriate nowadays to look at the outcome of psychiatric illness merely in terms of symptoms and not also in terms of social functioning of the individual. How well do schizophrenic patients fare after the symptoms of the acute episode have receded and after they have been discharged from hospital? Do they work? Do they live in a family? Do they have friends? Can they care for themselves? Are their social relationships satisfying? These and similar questions are increasingly asked in follow-up studies and in many research centres efforts have been made to arrive at a standardized way of assessing what is usually called the social adjustment of a psychiatric patient.

2. Terminological and theoretical issues

On the most global level social adjustment can be defined as the equilibrium between an individual and his environment. More precisely it can be regarded as the functioning of an individual in specific social roles. Theoretically a discrepancy in this person-environment fit may result from a disability on the side of the individual or from disturbances in the social environment. Practically this equilibrium has to be regarded as a continuous dynamic process of an individual trying to cope with environmental demands either by adjusting to the environment, by actively changing the environment or his relation to it, or even by leaving his old environment and looking for a new one. Subjective psychological processes like denial may lead to a certain degree of social adjustment which could be judged by an outside observer as undesirable and even as a disguised form of social maladjustment.

It should be evident from these considerations that social adjustment is a complex process rather than a state and that there may be a number of pitfalls when efforts are made to measure it. The situation is further complicated by the multiplicity of terms used in this field, a selection of which is presented in Table 1.

Table 1. Terms used in the literature for social adjustment or aspects of it

Positive
Social adjustment
Social role adjustment
Social skills
Social competence
Social effectiveness
Social attainment
Social integration

Neutral
Social performance
Role performance
Social behaviour
Social functioning
Adaptive functioning
Environmental adaptation

Negative
Social handicap
Social maladjustment
Social impairment
Social disability
Social disablement
Social dysfunction
Social ineffectiveness
Social inadequacy

The term chosen by a specific author is likely to indicate his theoretical position. A number of terms put the emphasis on the social skills of the individual, while others clearly underline the relationship between the individual and his environment, both types of terms reflecting different theoretical positions of the author.

Social maladjustment in psychiatric patients may either be conceived of as being a direct result of incapacitating symptoms — like thought disorders in schizophrenia which impair an individual's communication abilities — or as behaviour problems resulting from experiences during illness — like inability to care for oneself after a prolonged stay in a mental hospital. Wing (1976) has called the symptom-related impairment 'primary handicap' and has chosen the term 'secondary handicap' for impairments related to social learning or the unlearning of certain types of behaviour in the role of the mental patient. The therapeutic consequences may be quite different in these two cases; pharmacological treatment in the first instance, social skills training in the second.

A fundamentally different approach to achieving an equilibrium — though on a reduced level of functioning — consists in reducing environmental demands through providing alternative milieus in sheltered living and working arrangements. A schizophrenic patient who may have too little responsibility on the ward of a mental hospital and is overburdened in the community may be well adjusted and lead a satisfying life with the resources of a therapeutic community with fellow patients. Instead of providing an alternative environment it may be also well worth trying to change the environment of the patient (e.g. his family through family therapy).

It is evident that fundamentally divergent value decisions about the desirability of a certain structure of society and equally fundamentally divergent assumptions about the nature of human beings and of personal relationships cannot be left out when questions of social adjustment are discussed. Is it healthy to adapt to the stressful environment of our industrialized societies and are we justified in sending a patient back to work at any price? Can we decide for a schizophrenic patient that it would be better for him to return to his family and call the failure to do so 'maladjustment'? Although there may be considerable agreement that being married constitutes a higher degree of social adjustment than being single, a substantial minority in western societies would argue against this opinion. So the difficult question has to be considered whether, in the context of psychiatric research and therapy, social adjustment should be regarded as relevant only if a patient does not achieve or loses a certain degree of social adjustment or social integration which he in fact wants to achieve or retain. These and similar principal questions have to be borne in mind throughout this paper although they will not be discussed any further. The lack of agreed social norms clearly besets this field.

Table 2. Definition of rating for outcome (from Tsuang *et al* 1979)

Status	Good = 3	Rating Fair = 2	Poor = 1
Marital	Married or widowed	Divorced or separated	Single, never married
Residential	Own home or relatives' residence	Nursing or county home	Mental hospital
Occupational	Employed, retired, housewife, or student	Incapacitated due to physical illness	Incapacitated due to mental illness
Psychiatric symptoms	None	Some	Incapacitating

3. Research instruments

In recent years both in American and European psychiatry, in addition to assessing individual psychopathology, increasing attention has been paid to a patient's functioning in society. This is reflected in some newer efforts to standardize psychiatric assessment and diagnosis on both sides of the Atlantic.

Thus the Diagnostic and Statistical Manual III (DSM III) of the American Psychiatric Association (1980), adhering to principles of multi-axial classification, includes an axis (V) about the 'Highest Level of Adaptive Functioning'. It is stressed, that "this axis reflects the level of adaptive functioning and not subjective distress or other psychopathological signs or symptoms". Although the rating is global (on a 7 point scale: 1 = 'superior' = unusually effective functioning in social relations, at work, and in use of leisure time; 7 = 'grossly impaired' = unable to function in almost all areas) and cannot be used as such in an evaluative study (for which it is not intended) the introduction of this axis should have far reaching consequences for psychiatric thinking. Similarly the Present State Examination (PSE) (Wing *et al* 1974), a semi-structured interview for eliciting psychopathological information, contains separate items for rating 'social impairment' on a global 3 point scale. If nothing else, at least the clinician's and researcher's interest is drawn to the field of social adjustment by inclusion of the notion in these important psychiatric tools.

With simple rating scales about marital, residential and occupational status some more specific information about the social functioning of a patient can be obtained in long-term outcome studies of psychiatric disorders. Tsuang *et al* (1979) provide a good example for this type of multidimensional assessment of outcome (see Table 2). As long as psychiatric symptoms are kept separate from the social outcome variables these rather simple indicators seem to be very useful for getting at least some knowledge in a field which is still very dark. Although the authors in fact do not invoke the concept of 'social adjustment' but speak simply of 'outcome variables', this study is an example of a more specific approach to social functioning than the global ratings included in DSM III and in the PSE.

Table 3. Instruments for assessing social adjustment (see Weissman, 1975; Weissman *et al* 1980)

Normative Social Adjustment Scale (Barrabee *et al* 1955)
Social Ineffectiveness Scale (Frank *et al* 1959)
Mandel Social Adjustment Rating Scale (Mandel 1959)
Social Adjustment Inventory Method (Berger *et al* 1964)
Personal Adjustment and Role Skills (PARS III) (Ellsworth 1975)
The Katz Adjustment Scale: Relative's Form (KASR) (Katz & Lyerly 1963)
Personality and Social Network Adjustment Scale (Clark 1968)
Community Adaptation Schedule (CAS) (Roen & Burnes 1968)
The Social Disability Scale (Ruesch 1969)
Social Dysfunction Rating Scale (SDRS) (Linn *et al* 1969)
Psychiatric Status Schedule (PSS) (Spitzer *et al* 1970)
Psychiatric Evaluation Form (PEF) (Endicott & Spitzer 1972)
Current and Past Psychopathological Scales (CAPPS) (Endicott & Spitzer 1972)
Structured and Scaled Interview to Assess Maladjustment (SSIAM) (Gurland *et al* 1972)
Social Adjustment Scale (SAS) (Weissman & Paykel 1974)
KDS-15 Marital Questionnaire (Frank & Kupfer 1974)
Social Adjustment Scale: Self-Report (SAS-SR) (Weissman & Bothwell 1976)
Self-Assessment Guide (Willer & Biggin 1974)
Psychological Adjustment to Illness Scale (PAIS) (Morrow *et al* 1978)
Denver Community Mental Health Questionnaire (DCMHQ) (Ciarlo & Reihman 1977)
Standardized Interview to Assess Social Maladjustment (Clare & Cairns 1978)
Personal Resources Inventory (PRI) (Clayton & Hirschfeld 1977)
Social Role Adjustment Instrument (SRAI) (Cohler *et al* 1974)
Social Behaviour Assessment Schedule (SBAS) (Platt *et al* 1980)
Social Adjustment Scale II (SAS-II) (Schooler *et al* 1979)
Levels of Function Scale (Strauss & Carpenter 1972)
Social Functioning Schedule (SFS) (Remington & Tyrer 1979)
Interview Schedule for Social Interaction (ISSI) (Duncan-Jones & Henderson 1980)
Social Performance Schedule (Stevens 1972, 1973)

A closer look will be given here to those quantitative methods defining themselves as instruments for measuring the 'social adjustment' of an individual. A useful review of 'Social Adjustment Scales' used in psychiatric research is given by Weissman (1975; recently updated by Weissman *et al* 1980). Item content, method of obtaining information, source of information, time period assessed and scoring are among the criteria used for describing these instruments. The compact comparisons of altogether 27 scales for assessing social adjustment are to some extent overwhelming and, although the reviews are most useful, may lead to a certain confusion and helplessness on the part of the reader (see Table 3, which contains also a few scales not mentioned by Weissman). Why so many different instruments? How can results obtained with one scale be compared with those of another scale?

A number of these scales were developed for very specific purposes, such as for assessing circumscribed social areas like marital adjustment (KDS-15), the adjustment to medical illness (PAIS), the impact of illness on other people who are involved (SBAS), or women's adjustment to adult roles (SRAI). A number of instruments, though, claim to assess social adjustment in a more or less comprehensive way. Among the most elaborate of these comprehensive instruments are the Social Adjustment Scale, published both in an interview form (SAS; Weissman & Paykel 1974; Paykel *et al* 1971) and as a self-report scale (SAS-SR; Weissman & Bothwell 1976) and the Standardized Interview to Assess Social Maladjustment and Dysfunction (also referred to as Social Interview Scale = SIS; Clare & Cairns 1978), which will be given a closer look here by way of example.

As far as the items and their organization are concerned, the characteristics of these more elaborate instruments are that not only different life areas like work, marital relationships, leisure activities, etc., are taken into consideration in turn one after the other, but that each of these areas is assessed separately on a number of different dimensions like material conditions, social management and satisfaction (SIS) or observable behaviour and role functioning on the one hand and feelings and satisfaction on the other hand (SAS). These dimensions partly reflect the tendency to separate social adjustment into 'instrumental role performance' (Parsons & Bales 1954) and 'expressive functioning' (Geismar 1964). Unfortunately the division of items into different groups (e.g. areas of life) differs from instrument to instrument so that no comparison is possible of the results of different studies carried out with different instruments. The organization of items in the SIS and SAS along these lines is shown in Tables 4 and 5.

Table 4. Standardized Interview to Assess Social Maladjustment and Dysfunction (Clare & Cairns 1978): examples for items in different categories

| Subject area | Rating category, with each item rated shown below the appropriate category ||||
	Material conditions	Social management	Satisfaction
Housing	Housing conditions	Household care	Satisfaction with housing
Occupational/social role	Occupational stability	Quality of personal interaction with work-mates	Satisfaction with occupation/social role (includes housewives, unemployed, disabled, retired)
Economic situation	Family income	Management of income	Satisfaction with income
Leisure/social activities	Opportunities for leisure and social activities	Extent of leisure and social activities	Satisfaction with leisure and social activities
Family and domestic relationships	Opportunities for interaction with relatives	Quality of interaction with relatives	Satisfaction with interaction with relatives
Marital		Fertility and family planning	Satisfaction with marital harmony

Table 5. Social Adjustment Scale (Paykel et al 1971): item content and organization

Qualitative categories	Role areas					
	Work	Social and leisure	Extended family	Marital as spouse	Parental	Marital family unit	Additional item
Behaviour performance	Time lost; impaired performance	Diminished contact with friends; diminished social interactions; impaired leisure activities; diminished dating		Diminished intercourse; sexual problems	Lack of involvement; impaired communication	Economic inadequacy of family unit	
Interpersonal behaviours		Reticence, hypersensitive behaviour	Reticence; withdrawal; family attachment; rebellion	Reticence; domineering behaviour; dependency; submissiveness			
Friction	Friction	Friction	Friction	Friction	Friction		
Feelings and satisfaction	Distress; disinterest; feelings of inadequacy	Social discomfort; loneliness; boredom; disinterest in dating	Guilt; worry; resentment	Lack of affection; disinterest in sex	Lack of affection;	Guilt; worry; resentment	
Global judgements	Work, global	Social and leisure, global	Extended family, global	Marital as spouse, global	Parental, global		Overall, global

The inclusion of items for 'expressive functioning' or 'satisfaction' in a given scale should be given special scrutiny. Given the independence of social from psychopathological outcome in therapeutic studies (e.g. Weissman et al 1974), scales which contain items reflecting at least partly psychopathological symptoms should be regarded with great caution, especially if these items are analysed simultaneously with the other items of the scale (e.g. in a factor analysis).

Apart from the item content and its organization according to different dimensions, the question of how information is obtained is methodologically relevant. The main data-gathering procedures are interview or self rating, the main sources of information are the patient or a close relative.

Although results from a comparison of the same instrument used both in a self-rating and in an interview format are quite promising (Weissman & Bothwell 1976), caution seems appropriate in several respects with self-rating instruments for social adjustment. First, self-rating procedures are not appropriate for certain types of patients, like deluded or psychotic patients. But, also in a more general sense, self-ratings of social events and social situations tend to be subject to distortion through the patient. Objective social situation and subjective feeling about it — two dimensions which should be kept separate — may be confounded by such procedures. An 'effort after meaning' (Brown 1974) may lead patients to perceive their social situation in a distorted or aggravated way. In the study by Weissman & Bothwell patients considered themselves in fact as more impaired than they were rated by the interviewer. Experiences with the Social Readjustment Rating Scale (Holmes & Rahe 1967) also suggest the need for caution with self-rating procedures in the social field. This instrument (which has nothing to do with the methods for rating social adjustment discussed so far, but is rather a method of rating the psychosocial stress to which an individual has to adapt) has a very low test-retest reliability as far as individual items are concerned (Katschnig 1980). Self-rating, therefore, does not seem to be a reliable method of data gathering in the field of social adjustment, desirable as it might be as a cheap research method for large numbers of cases. In any case an interview seems more appropriate.

As far as the source of information is concerned, a close relative of a patient may seem at first glance to be a good informant. The problem is that close relatives are frequently emotionally over-involved and may distort facts in the same way as patients may do.

The SIS and SAS are both administered as a semi-structured interview (except in the SAS-SR, which is a self-rating scale) and ratings are made on a 4 point (SIS) or 5 point (SAS) scale. It has to be stressed that in these scales (to a lesser degree in the SAS) the scoring refers mainly to dysfunction and does not provide a differentiation of adequate, good, and excellent levels of functioning. Both scales have been shown to be satisfactorily reliable.

To calculate indices reflecting 'social adjustment' of an individual patient who has been given a 'social adjustment scale', different strategies are used in the literature. The two procedures applied most frequently are the calculation of total (or mean) scores or the use of factor analysis or principal component analysis. There are several problems with these two strategies.

A simple arithmetical problem arises from the fact that up to one-third of items contained in social adjustment scales do not apply to all persons studied in a specific research project. Questions concerning a person's functioning in the role of a parent are obviously not meaningful if the subject is not a father or a mother. The calculation of simple total scores thus is usually not possible and mean scores have to be calculated for those items which are relevant for a specific person. This problem left aside, a more principal one emerges: given the fact that social adjustment itself is probably not a homogeneous entity — clinical experience and research result suggest that a person's functioning may well be impaired in some areas of life but not in others — and given the fact that many scales contain items for instrumental role functioning as well as for affective functioning, the calculation of global (mean) scores is not appropriate. On the contrary, the reduction of different pieces of information into one global score would in fact hide structural differences which in reality may exist. The calculation of scores for different life areas or for instrumental role functioning on the one hand and affective functioning on the other seems a way out of this problem. This strategy is chosen in many studies; however, the comparability across different studies is not possible, as the grouping of items into discrete sub-areas of social functioning differs from research instrument to research instrument and from study to study. Data analysis should in any case be carried out item by item in order not to lose important information on defects in specific areas of social adjustment which may be susceptible to change by specific therapeutic methods.

In many studies the authors of social adjustment scales try to reduce the complexity of their data by factor analysis or principal component analysis. However, Clare & Cairns (1978) in studying different populations with the same social adjustment instrument found different factor solutions in all three instances. They concluded that in such a field as social adjustment, factors will always vary according to the composition of the population studied. I would like to join Clare & Cairns in warning against reliance on multivariate analysis with the idea of arriving at simple scoring procedures. It is where 'overquantification' occurs in a field that the conceptual issues and the definition of individual items lag behind the highly developed statistical methods frequently used. What we need is a reliable and operationalized taxonomy of social maladjustment and social handicaps. If we put it briefly: not quantification but 'qualification' seems to be the problem of most social adjustment scales available today.

4. Conclusion

Despite many efforts in the last years to improve the methodology for assessing social adjustment of psychiatric patients and despite the great number of quantitative methods available, a certain degree of caution still seems appropriate.

The main reason for suggesting such a cautious attitude towards social adjustment scales stems from a lack of common conceptual thinking about the notion of 'social adjustment' among the many authors of different scales. This is reflected in a great number of different terms used in this field, of which each represents a somehow different aspect of social adjustment. A clarification of concepts seems urgently necessary, especially in the differentiation between social support, social attachments, social competence, social status and social role performance (Weissman *et al* 1980). Disturbances in these dimensions of 'social adjustment' may have quite different consequences for therapy and management. Social adjustment clearly is an umbrella concept which as such may be of little use, just as the concept of 'mental illness' needs differentiation into subgroups of different diseases if we want to talk in a meaningful way about practical and research problems of mental illness.

I would like to conclude with a recommendation to the European Medical Research Councils. Just as in the field of standardized assessment of psychopathology, it seems necessary that the multitude of instruments available for assessing social adjustment be reduced to a small number of instruments which a large number of researchers in different countries can agree upon. The fact that the Present State Examination pays great attention to an operational definition of its items and is used in many different cultures, will probably contribute much more to the progress of psychiatry than many perhaps more 'quantitative' methods developed here and there which never reach international attention.

The possible role of international organizations in reaching agreement on research instruments is perhaps not yet sufficiently realized. The World Health Organization has successfully promoted the use of the Present State Examination in many countries and has itself stimulated the development of the Disability Assessment Schedule (DAS; Jablensky *et al* 1980;

Schwarz 1981) which is currently being employed in different countries showing that it is possible to assess social maladjustment in schizophrenic patients reliably across cultures.

It may be advisable that a more regional body like the European Medical Research Councils should promote the idea that a common instrument for measuring social adjustment should be developed. It may well be necessary to limit standardization of a variable like social adjustment, which is much more culture-dependent than psychopathology, to a certain geographical area with at least some common social and cultural background. A candidate as starting point for a European-wide accepted instrument for measuring social adjustment could be the Standardized Interview to Assess Social Maladjustment and Dysfunction by Clare & Cairns (1978). This is certainly my personal choice and the race is open for other instruments to become candidates for such a commonly agreed upon instrument. Once experience has accumulated with one widely used instrument improvements can be based on much better data than is possible nowadays.

Given the growing interest in and necessity for applying multiaxial systems of assessment both in psychiatric research and practice, it seems imperative that those axes representing social characteristics of the patient's disturbance should be conceived with the same rigour which has guided the development of standardized assessment of psychopathology. I do hope that it will be possible for the European Medical Research Councils to act as some kind of catalyst in this field.

References

American Psychiatric Association (1980): DSM III: *Diagnostic and Statistical Manual of Mental Disorders,* 3rd ed. APA, Washington, DC.

Barrabee, R., Barrabee, E.L. & Finesinger, J.E.F. (1955): A normative adjustment scale. *Am. J. Psychiatry, 112,* 252-259.

Berger, D.G., Rice, C.E., Sewall, L.G. et al (1964): The post-hospital evolution of psychiatric patients: The social adjustment inventory method. *Psychiatric Stud. Proj. 2,* 1-30.

Brown, G.W. (1974): Meaning, measurement and stress of life events. In Dohrenwend, B.S., Dohrenwend, B.P. (eds.): *Stressful Life Events: Their Nature and Effects.* Wiley, New York, 167ff.

Ciarlo, J.A. & Reihman, J. (1977): The Denver Community Mental Health Questionnaire: Development of a multi-dimensional program evaluation instrument. In Coursey, R., Spector, G., Murrell, S. et al (eds.): *Program Evaluation for Mental Health: Methods, Strategies, and Participants.* Grune & Stratton, New York, 131-167.

Clare, A.W. & Cairns, V.E. (1978): Design development and use of a standardized interview to assess social maladjustment and dysfunction in community studies. *Psychol. Med. 8,* 589-604.

Clark, A.W. (1968): The personality and social network adjustment scale. *Hum. Rel. 21,* 85-96.

Clayton, P. & Hirschfeld, R. (1977): *Personal Resources Inventory (PRI).* Washington University School of Medicine, St. Louis.

Cohler, B., Grunebaum, H., Weiss, J. et al (1974): Social role performance and psychopathology among recently hospitalized mothers. *J. Nerv. Ment. Dis. 159,* 81-90.

Duncan-Jones, P. & Henderson, S. (1978): *Interview Schedule for Social Interaction (ISSI),* 10th ed. Social Psychiatry Research Unit, Australian National University, Canberra, Australia.

Ellsworth, R.B. (1974): Consumer feedback in measuring the effectiveness of mental health programs. In Guttentag, P., Struening, M. (eds.): *Handbook of Evaluation Research.* Sage Publications, Beverly Hills.

Endicott, J. & Spitzer, R.L. (1972a): Current and past psychopathology scales (CAPPS): Rationale, reliability and validity. *Arch. Gen. Psychiatry, 27,* 678-687.

Endicott, J. & Spitzer, R.L. (1972b): What! Another rating scale? The psychiatric evaluation form. *J. Nerv. Ment. Dis. 154,* 88-104.

Frank, E. & Kupfer, D.J. (1974): *The KDS 15: A Marital Questionnaire.* Western Psychiatric Institute and Clinic, University of Pittsburgh, Pittsburgh.

Frank, J.D., Gliedman, L.H., Imber, S.D. et al (1959): Patients' expectancies and relearning as factors determining improvement in psychotherapy. *Am. J. Psychiatry, 115,* 961-968.

Geismar, L.L. (1964): Family functionings as an index of need for welfare services. *Family Process, 3,* 99-113.

Gurland, B.J., Yorkston, N.J., Stone, A.R. et al (1972a): The structured and scaled interview to assess maladjustment (SSIAM): I. Description, rationale and development. *Arch. Gen. Psychiatry, 27,* 259-264.

Gurland, B.J., Yorston, N.J., Goldberg, K. et al (1972b): The structured and scaled interview to assess maladjustment (SSIAM): II. Factor analysis, reliability, and validity. *Arch. Gen. Psychiatry, 27,* 264-267.

Holmes, T.H. & Rahe, R.H (1967): The social readjustment rating scale. *J. Psychosom. Res. 11,* 213-218.

Jablensky, A., Schwarz, R. & Tomov, J. (1980): WHO-Collaborative Study on Impairments and Disabilities Associated with Schizophrenic Disorders. A preliminary communication: objectives and methods. In Strömgren, E., Dupont, A., Nielsen, J.A. (eds.): Epidemiological Research as Basis for the Organization of Extramural Psychiatry. *Acta Psychiatr. Scand. Suppl. 285, 62,* 152-163.

Katschnig, H. (ed.) (1980): *Sozialer Streß und psychische Erkrankung.* Urban & Schwarzenberg, Munich.

Katz, M.M. & Lyerly, S.B. (1963): Methods of measuring adjustment and social behaviour in the community: I. Rationale, description, discriminative validity and scale development. *Psychol. Rep. 13,* 503-535.

Linn, M.W., Schulthorpe, W.B., Evje, M. et al (1969): A social dysfunction rating scale. *J. Psychiatr. Res. 6,* 299-316.

Mandel, N.G. (1959): *Mandel Social Adjustment Scale.* University of Minnesota, Minneapolis.

Morrow, G.R., Chiarello, R.J. & Derogatis, L.R. (1978): A new scale for assessing patients' psychosocial adjustment to medical illness. *Psychol. Med. 8,* 605-610.

Parsons, T. & Bales, R.F. (1954): *Family Socialization and Interaction Process.* Free Press, Glencoe, Illinois.

Paykel, E.S., Weissman, M., Prusoff, B.A. & Tonks, C.M. (1971): Dimensions of social adjustment in depressed women. *J. Nerv. Ment. Dis. 152,* 158-172.

Platt, S., Weyman, A., Hirsch, S. et al (1980): The social behaviour assessment schedule (SBAS): Rationale, contents, scoring and reliability of a new interview schedule. *Soc. Psychiatry, 15,* 43-55.

Remington, M. & Tyrer, P. (1979): The social functioning schedule — a brief semi-structured interview. *Soc. Psychiatry, 14,* 151-157.

Roen, S.R. & Burnes, A.J. (1968): *Community Adaptation Schedule Preliminary Manual.* Behavioural Publ., New York.

Ruesch, J. (1969): The assessment of social disability. *Arch. Gen. Psychiatry, 21,* 655-664.

Schooler, N., Hogarty, G. & Weissman, M.M. (1979): Social Adjustment Scale II (SAS II). In Hargreaves, W.A., Attkisson, C.C., Sorenson, J.E. (eds.): *Resource Materials for Community Mental Health Program Evaluators.* U.S. Dept. of Health, Education & Welfare, publ. No. (ADM) 79-328, 290-330.

Schwarz, R. (1981): *Behinderungseinschätzung bei schizophrenen Patienten: Eine WHO-Mehrländeruntersuchung.* Verlauf und Ergebnisse in Mannheim. Unpublished manuscript.

Spitzer, R.L., Endicott, J., Fleiss, J.L. et al (1970): The psychiatric status schedule: A technique for evaluating psychopathology and impairment in role functioning. *Arch. Gen. Psychiatry, 23,* 41-55.

Stevens, B.C. (1972): Dependence of schizophrenic patients on elderly relatives. *Psychol. Med., 2,* 17-32.

Stevens, B.C. (1973): Role of fluphenazine decanoate in lessening the burden of chronic schizophrenics on the community. *Psychol. Med., 3,* 141-158.

Strauss, J.S. & Carpenter, W.T. Jr. (1972): The prediction of outcome in schizophrenia: I. Characteristics of outcome. *Arch. Gen. Psychiatry, 27,* 739-746.

Tsuang, M.T., Woolson, R.F. & Fleming, J.A. (1979): Long-term outcome of major psychoses. *Arch. Gen. Psychiatry, 36,* 1295-1301.

Weissman, M.M., Klerman, G.L., Paykel, E.S., Prusoff, B. & Hanson, B. (1974): Treatment effects on the social adjustment of depressed patients. *Arch. Gen. Psychiatry, 30,* 771-778.

Weissman, M.M. & Paykel, E.S. (1974): *The Depressed Woman: A Study of Social Relationships.* University of Chicago Press, Chicago.

Weissman, M.M. (1975): The assessment of social adjustment. *Arch. Gen. Psychiatry, 32,* 357-365.

Weissman, M.M. & Bothwell, S. (1976): The assessment of social adjustment by patient self-report. *Arch. Gen. Psychiatry, 33,* 1111-1115.

Weissman, M.M., Sholomskas, D. & John, K. (1981): The assessment of social adjustment. An update. *Arch. Gen. Psychiatry, 38,* 1250-1258.

Willer, B. & Biggin, P. (1974): *Self-Assessment Guide: Rationale, Development, and Evaluation.* Lakeshore Psychiatric Hospital, Toronto.

Wing, J.K., Cooper, J.E. & Sartorius, N. (1974): *The Measurement and Classification of Psychiatric Symptoms.* Cambridge University Press, London.

Wing, J.K. (1976): Impairments in schizophrenia: A rational basis for social treatment. In Wirt, R.D., Winokur, C., Roff, M. (eds.): *Life History Research in Psychopathology.* University of Minnesota Press, Minneapolis.

IV: OTHER QUANTITATIVE METHODS OF EVALUATION OF TREATMENT

Psychophysiological Criteria

M. LADER

1. Introduction

Darrow (1964) defined psychophysiology as "the science which concerns those physiological activities which underlie or relate to psychic functions". This wide definition could be construed to refer to a very comprehensive range of central nervous system functions but in practice a particular experimental approach using certain physiological measures is accepted as that of psychophysiology. The position of psychophysiology has been an uneasy one, spanning the area between human physiology and psychology and yet developing concepts and principles which are peculiar to itself. Nevertheless, certain fundamental principles have to be upheld. Firstly, the functions that are recorded are basically physiological and, therefore, must be measured under strictly physiological conditions. For example, cardiovascular variables must be recorded under carefully controlled conditions. Secondly, the measures have to be shown to have some psychological validity. The heart pumps blood round the body and its rate is primarily governed by this need. In times of stress an increase in heart-rate may occur but this may reflect increased bodily activity rather than psychological arousal. There is no easy solution to this problem of apportioning bodily changes into the physiological and psychophysiological. However, two measures have come over the years to be regarded as particularly useful because their physiological element is minor. These are skin conductance (sweat-gland activity) and the electroencephalogram (EEG) analysed mathematically.

Psychophysiological techniques have been used mainly to aid in the diagnosis of psychiatric patients, to elucidate central mechanisms of mental illness and to monitor response to treatment. In this presentation, the last application will be outlined with particular emphasis on the practical value of these complex techniques. Firstly, the relevant techniques will be briefly outlined.

2. Psychophysiological techniques

2.1 Peripheral autonomic

The most commonly used measure is the palmar skin conductance which provides an indirect measure of non-thermo-regulatory sweating on the palms of the hands. The responses to stimuli, an increase in conductance, are termed galvanic skin responses (GSR) or electrodermal responses. Useful information can be obtained from the changes in skin conductance level, the responses, and 'spontaneous' fluctuations in level. Skin potential is a related but more complex measure.

Several cardiovascular measures are in use of which heart-rate is the most popular. This can be recorded from the ECG or from a pulse detector. Variations in beat-to-beat interval rate are of interest. Blood flow through the forearm (muscle blood flow) or the finger (skin blood flow) can be measured plethysmographically. Blood-pressure is difficult to measure on a continuous basis without arterial catheterization and the pulse transit time has been evaluated as an alternative (Geddes *et al* 1981).

Pupil size is another autonomic measure, occasionally used. It can be measured in a variety of ways ranging from disc comparison to a scanning infra-red pupillometer. Salivation can be assessed by placing suction cups over the salivary ducts and weighing the aspirate over a fixed interval. Whole mouth salivation can be quantified by placing pre-weighed dental rolls in the floor of the mouth for a specified interval and re-weighing them.

2.2 Peripheral somatic

The electromyogram, recorded under isometric conditions, provides a useful estimate of muscle tension. The technique comprises the attachment of two surface electrodes to the skin over the muscles of interest. The spiky discharges are usually integrated electronically to give a smoothed record.

Tremor of the extremities can be quantified using an accelerometer attached to a finger tip. Analysis of the signal usually requires mathematical calculations using a computer.

Respiration is difficult to measure as it is a complex of thoracic and abdominal movements. Changes in the girth of the trunk can be monitored or a temperature-sensitive device inserted in the nostril. A semi-quantitative estimate only is obtained.

2.3 Central measures

The electroencephalogram (EEG) is a complex electrical signal varying with the psychological state of the individual. The best-known example of this is the development of alpha rhythms in the relaxing person. Modern EEG evaluation comprises sophisticated frequency analyses of the waveform or even more complex techniques when more than one channel is involved. The measure remains empirical as the neurophysiological basis for the EEG is not known in detail. EEG responses evoked by auditory or visual stimuli can be quantified using computer techniques and comprise complex waveforms related to several psychological variables such as attention, arousal and novelty of stimulus.

2.4 Neuroendocrine measures

Plasma and urinary corticosteroids and catecholamines can also be used in a psychophysiological context. However, they are more useful in providing estimates of effects over periods of time rather than a continuous record as with the physiological techniques. Plasma cortisol estimates are now routine and radioenzymatic methods have greatly improved the precision of catecholamine assays.

2.5 Current developments

As the above outline intimates, the development of the EEG and the EEG-evoked responses as measures of great psychophysiological importance has depended on the wide availability of small on-line laboratory computers. The autonomic and somatic measures can also be conveniently recorded on a computer which enables sophisticated and complex analyses to be carried out rapidly. Although such computers were expensive, the advent of the microcomputer has meant that powerful computer capabilities are available at the same sort of cost as the classical pen-writing polygraph.

Another development has been the use of telemetry or portable monitoring equipment. This has enabled studies to be conducted outside the constraints of the psychophysiology laboratory with its cumbersome equipment and its tethered subjects. For example, we use the Oxford Medilog system and can record heart-rate, skin conductance, EEG and EMG for several hours on a miniature tape-cassette. The tapes are speeded up 60-fold for computer analysis.

3. Psychophysiological measures and central state

The above outline has confined itself to those measures generally regarded as psychophysiological. These measures occupy an area between more basically physiological measures on the one side and more clearly psychological variables on the other. The former group includes measures such as the photopalpebral reflex (Tanaka et al 1978), the H-reflex of the spinal cord (Metz et al 1980), and sleep recording. These measures provide no information about central state except in a very indirect way. Psychological measures include the whole gamut of cognitive, psychomotor, perceptual tests, etc., which provide more direct behavioural data but little about bodily functioning. However, these distinctions are not always clearcut: critical flicker fusion can be interpreted as a psychophysiological measure.

If psychophysiology is the use of physiological measures for their behavioural connotations, what sort of information can they convey? The vast body of psychophysiological literature is devoted to this question. The physiological correlates of information input, attention, conditioning processes, motivation, level of arousal, etc., have all been studied in depth in normal subjects. The psychological significance of changes in the waveform of the cerebral evoked response, or heart-rate variability or amplitude of the GSR are becoming clearer. However, work in psychiatric patients has been more problematical.

Two areas have been extensively researched: symptom mechanisms and anxiety and phobic states. In the former case, the physiological changes underlying such symptoms as palpitations and tension headache have been delineated. In the latter conditions — anxiety and phobic states — clear evidence of heightened physiological activity has been obtained in study after study (Lader 1980). The psychophysiological approach has allowed a more precise quantification of the severity of such symptoms and conditions.

However, in the case of schizophrenia and the major affective disorders, the position is much more confused. The observations on psychophysiological measures are not consistent and it will be some time before a consensus can emerge concerning psychophysiological abnormalities in schizophrenia, depression and mania (Öhman 1981; Venables 1980; Saletu 1980; Christie et al 1980; Perris 1980).

4. Psychophysiological measures and treatment response

It is against this background of physiological technicality, psychological complexity and psychiatric limitations that the use of psychophysiological measures to monitor treatment must be set. But there is yet another factor which militates against the facile use of such measures as precise indicators of central state. This problem arises from the multiple pharmacology of many psychotropic drugs.

The use of psychophysiological measures in monitoring treatment can be conveniently divided under four headings. Each will be briefly reviewed with a few illustrations from the recent literature. A comprehensive review is not attempted.

4.1 Peripheral effects of psychotropic drugs

Many psychotropic drugs, in particular the three major classes of antipsychotics, tricyclic antidepressants and monoamine oxidase inhibitors (MAOIs) have marked autonomic effects. For example, chlorpromazine is an antagonist to dopamine, alpha-adrenaline, 5 hydroxytryptamine, acetylcholine and histamine receptors. Amitriptyline blocks acetylcholine receptors and potentiates adrenergic mechanisms. Several MAOIs are useful hypotensive agents, and so on. Consequently, marked peripheral actions are caused by these drugs and this will affect many psychophysiological measures. The practical outcome is that these measures, such as heart-rate, blood-pressure, salivation and pupil size, can be used to detect and to quantify such peripheral effects, and correlations can be sought with subjective side-effects (e.g. Szabadi *et al* 1980).

An example concerns the anticholinergic effects of tricyclic and related antidepressants. The first generation of such drugs, typically imipramine and amitriptyline, are associated with troublesome anticholinergic effects, to the point that some patients cease taking the medication. Animal studies, using receptor binding techniques and standard physiological preparations, predicted that newer antidepressants such as mianserin, nomifensine and trazodone should be virtually devoid of such effects. Normal subjects and patients have been given acute and chronic dosage of these drugs and anticholinergic effects sought by measuring salivation, for example with ciclazindol (Oh *et al* 1979). No measurable diminution in salivary flow rate was detected and the lack of anticholinergic side-effects has been confirmed in practice.

However, it could be argued that this use of standard psychophysiological measures is not strictly speaking a psychophysiological one. Because the measures are affected by the peripheral effects of the drug, no inferences can be made concerning the central effects. For example, sweat-gland activity is diminished by single doses of imipramine. This might be construed as indicating a drop in arousal following imipramine. However, the diminution in sweating is due, at least in part, to peripheral anticholinergic effects as it follows the local administration of atropine. The problem is that it is impossible to apportion the central and peripheral effects of psychotropic drugs with autonomic effects. Consequently, the psychophysiological measures which are affected peripherally must be interpreted cautiously.

A further complication regarding this use relates to the finding mentioned earlier that some important groups of psychiatric patients differ from normal values. For example, in normal subjects, single doses of imipramine produce dose- and time-related diminutions in palmar skin conductance (sweat-gland activity) due to the anticholinergic actions of the drug. In patients treated with imipramine, say, 150 mg/day in divided doses for 4 weeks, a similar drop in skin conductance occurs over the first week to be followed by a steady recovery almost to pre-treatment levels (Bhanji & Lader 1977). One explanation might be that the sweat-glands have become 'tolerant' to the anticholinergic effects of imipramine: perhaps, cholinergic receptors have increased in number or in affinity in order to overcome the blockade. But many depressives, especially the clinically retarded, have abnormal physiological responses; for example, the dexamethasone suppression test gives abnormal results (Greden *et al* 1980). Among these changes, glandular function such as salivation and sweat-gland activity is diminished. Thus, skin conductance levels are low as an association of the illness. Imipramine depresses skin conductance even more but effects a clinical improvement which, in turn, is associated with an increase in glandular function. Thus, the levels in the fourth week of treatment represent the opposing effects of imipramine lowering and clinical improvement increasing skin conductance.

4.2 Peripheral measures of central effects

It is obvious that the use of peripheral psychophysiological measures to assess central psychotropic effects must be restricted to those drugs devoid of peripheral effects and to patients suffering from conditions which do not affect the peripheral mechanisms of the psychophysiological measures (Gruzelier *et al* 1981). There is still plenty of scope for this approach: the anxiolytics and hypnotics, among the most widely used of all drugs, have nugatory peripheral effects. Some stimulants also act centrally.

An example concerns the use of skin conductance and heart-rate measures in the evaluation of anxiolytics (e.g. Lader & Wing 1966). Three skin conductance variables were found to distinguish anxious patients from control subjects, to yield linear dose-effect curves with single doses of a barbiturate in normal subjects and to distinguish treatment with amylobarbitone sodium from that with a placebo in patients. These variables were change in conductance level over the period of recording (30 minutes), the number of fluctuations in that level, and the rate of habituation of the skin conductance responses. All these variables were, therefore, presumed to reflect some general factor of alertness or arousal, the anxious patients being overaroused and returned towards normal by the sedative drug. From a preliminary pilot 'staircase assay' to establish rough comparative dosage, a trial of chlordiazepoxide and amylobarbitone sodium, each given for one week with double-blind procedures, was undertaken. Two doses of chlordiazepoxide (22.5 and 45 mg/day), two doses of amylobarbitone sodium (150 and 300 mg/day) and a placebo were administered using an incomplete block design. In this 2 + 2 + 1 assay, the three variables showed appreciable drug effects, allowing a fairly precise dose comparison of the two drugs. An important finding was that clinical ratings were several times less precise. Thus, the psychophysiological measures provided an empirical precision in contrast to the less precise but directly relevant clinical measures.

Peripheral measures are also useful when non-drug treatments are being assessed and are much less limited in their applicability. An example concerns measurement of heart-rate in chronic psychotic patients being treated by behavioural methods of milieu therapy, token economies and social involvement (Kay 1981). Early morning resting pulse rate was the psychophysiological measure. Treatment was associated with a rise in pulse rate, suggesting an increase in arousal rather than a fall. Kay (1981) elaborates the theoretical implications and suggests that schizophrenia has two components of arousal, a treatment-resistant component monitored by autonomic arousal and a treatment-responsive component associated with central arousal.

These two examples contrast sharply. In the former, precise and fairly easily interpretable measures were devised but at the cost of elaborate techniques. It is not surprising that few laboratories have taken up the GSR skin conductance techniques for drug assessments (Lapierre 1975; Johnstone *et al* 1981). In Kay's (1981) study, simple measures were taken but interpretation is somewhat speculative.

4.3 Central measures

The EEG and, to a lesser extent, its responses have become increasingly popular in assessing drug effects. A large body of data has been built up cataloguing the effects of drugs on the various wavebands of the EEG. The EEG can be used to predict the potential anxiolytic, antidepressant or antipsychotic properties of a new compound (Fink 1975). These methods seem to be reliable (Itil *et al* 1981).

The EEG techniques can also be used to detect a drug's activity. For example, hypnotic drugs may persist into the next day and can be detected by quantitative electroencephalography. This is particularly useful when techniques to measure plasma levels of a drug are not yet available, or are complex and expensive. Furthermore, the EEG reflects a drug's effects and not merely its presence.

Despite the sensitivity and precision of the EEG measures, there are limitations. The first is the technical one — the EEG must be recorded and then analysed quantitatively usually by computer. The advent of cheap, consumer-oriented microcomputers has lessened this difficulty but carefully trained staff are necessary and this becomes expensive.

The second problem concerns the interpretation of the EEG changes. Firstly, changes in mental alertness, arousal, are accompanied by well-known changes in the EEG pattern. Drowsiness is associated with lessened fast-wave activity, increased alpha and then increased theta. Drugs produce their own changes in the EEG directly but also may change the level of alertness. For example, a barbiturate will increase drowsiness which would normally be reflected by less fast-wave activity and more alpha. However, barbiturates directly increase fast-wave activity and this outweighs the alertness-related changes so that the EEG actually contains much fast-wave activity. The outcome is that the EEG provides an empirical measure of a drug's effects but interpretations concerning central psychological influences must be cautious. These caveats apply also to the EEG evoked responses.

5. Monitoring behavioural treatments

Behavioural treatments involve relatively clear-cut stimulus parameters in patients suffering from affective disturbances either as a primary symptom or an accompaniment to a behavioural abnormality. In a typical study, phobic patients were subjected to six sessions of flooding treatment with intense fear-inducing stimuli and to six sessions of systematic desensitization in a cross-over design (Boulougouris *et al* 1971). Heart rate and skin conductance during phobic and neutral fantasies were recorded before and after each treatment session. Before the course of treatment was begun, heart rate and skin conductance activity increased sharply from neutral to phobic fantasy scenes. After the course of flooding treatment, the heart rate no longer increased during phobic imagery and the change in skin conductance was much less. No such changes accompanied desensitization treatment. Measures of subjective anxiety paralleled the skin conductance measure. Thus, psychophysiological measures provided independent confirmation of the subjective and behavioural responses.

6. Prognostic indicators

Finally, psychophysiological measures can be used as prognostic indicators. Frith and his co-workers (1979) measured skin conductance responses (SCR) to a series of tones in 41 patients during an acute episode of schizophrenia before they received treatment and after 4 weeks of treatment with an antipsychotic drug or a placebo. Patients who showed no habituation of the SCRs to the tones tended not to improve symptomatically during the treatment. Patients who habituated and who also had an acute onset to their current episode improved markedly even without active medication. Thus, type of onset plus habituation pattern were quite useful predictors of outcome.

This approach can be purely arbitrary with prognostic indicators being developed on an empirical basis. Interpretation of these relationships is much more problematical and raises all the factors which are outlined above.

7. Conclusions

Psychophysiological measures can be used in a variety of ways ranging from elucidation of symptom measures to the monitoring of behavioural treatments. Nonetheless, despite their lure of providing precision in measurement, their use must be hedged about with a long series of caveats. The techniques are complex, physiological needs must be met, many drugs have peripheral or direct central actions which affect autonomic measures and the EEG respectively, some psychiatric conditions are associated with psychophysiological abnormalities, and so on. But within their limitations, these measures can provide useful insights into the way treatments might act as well as increasing the precision of measurement. Technical advances including ambulant monitoring and analysis by microcomputers, together with increasing understanding of the measures themselves, should lead to a continuing albeit limited use of the psychophysiological approach to the evaluation of psychiatric treatments.

References

Bhanji, S. & Lader, M. (1977): The electroencephalographic and psychological effects of imipramine in depressed patients. *Euro. J. Clin. Pharmacol.*, 12, 349-354.

Boulougouris, J.C., Marks, I.M. & Marset, P. (1971): Superiority of flooding (implosion) to desensitization for reducing pathological fear. *Behav. Res. Ther.*, 9, 7-16.

Christie, M.J., Little, B.C. & Gordon, A.M. (1980): Peripheral indices of depressive states. In van Praag, H.M., Lader, M.H., Rafaelsen, O.J. & Sachar, E.J. (eds.): *Handbook of Biological Psychiatry, Part II: Psychophysiology.* Marcel Dekker, New York, pp.145-182.

Darrow, C.W. (1964): Psychophysiology, yesterday, today, and tomorrow. *Psychophysiology*, 1, 4-7.

Fink, M. (1975): Prediction of clinical activity of psychoactive drugs: application of cerebral electrometry in Phase I studies. In Sudilovsky, A., Gershon, S. & Beer, B. (eds.): *Predictability in Psychopharmacology: Preclinical and Clinical Correlations*. Raven Press, New York, pp.65-82.

Frith, C.D., Stevens, M., Johnstone, E.C. & Crow, T.J. (1979): Skin conductance responsivity during acute episodes of schizophrenia as a predictor of symptomatic improvement. *Psychol. Med., 9,* 101-106.

Geddes, L.A., Voelz, M.H., Babbs, C.F., Bourland, J.D. & Tacker, W.A. (1981): Pulse transit time as an indicator of arterial blood pressure. *Psychophysiology, 18,* 71-74.

Greden, J.F., Albala, A.A., Haskett, R.F., James, N.McI., Goodman, L., Steiner, M. & Carroll, B.J. (1980): Normalization of dexamethasone suppression test: a laboratory index of recovery from endogenous depression. *Biol. Psychiatry, 15,* 449-458.

Gruzelier, J., Connolly, J., Eves, F., Hirsch, S., Zaki, S., Weller, M. & Yorkston, N. (1981): Effect of propranolol and phenothiazines on electrodermal orienting and habituation in schizophrenia. *Psychol. Med., 11,* 93-108.

Itil, T.M., Schneider, S.J. & Fredrickson, J.W. (1981): The replicability of the psychophysiological effects of diazepam. *Biol. Psychiatry, 16,* 65-70.

Johnstone, E.C. *et al* (1981): The relationships between clinical response, psychophysiological variables and plasma levels of amitriptyline and diazepam in neurotic outpatients. *Psychopharmacology, 72,* 233-240.

Kay, S.R. (1981): Disjunctive arousal changes as a consequence of non-drug clinical intervention. *Biol. Psychiatry, 16,* 35-46.

Lader, M.H. & Wing, L. (1966): *Physiological Measures, Sedative Drugs, and Morbid Anxiety.* Oxford University Press, London.

Lader, M.H. (1980): Psychophysiological studies in anxiety. In Burrows, G.D. & Davies, B. (eds.): *Handbook of Studies on Anxiety.* Elsevier, Amsterdam, pp.59-88.

Lapierre, Y.D. (1975): Clinical and physiological assessment of clorazepate, diazepam and placebo in anxious neurotics. *Int. J. Clin. Pharmacol., 11,* 315-322.

Metz, J., Goode, D.J. & Meltzer, H.Y. (1980): Descriptive studies of H-reflex recovery curves in psychiatric patients. *Psychol. Med., 10,* 541-548.

Oh, V.M.S., Ehsanullah, R.S.B., Leighton, M. & Kirby, M.J. (1979): Influence of ciclazindol on monoamine uptake and CNS function in normal subjects. *Psychopharmacology, 60,* 177-181.

Öhman, A. (1981): Electrodermal activity in schizophrenia: a review. *Biol. Psychol.* (in press).

Perris, C. (1980): Central measures of depression. In van Praag, H.M., Lader, M.H., Rafaelsen, O.J. & Sachar, E.J. (eds.): *Handbook of Biological Psychiatry. Part II: Psychophysiology.* Marcel Dekker, New York, pp.183-224.

Saletu, B. (1980): Central measures in schizophrenia. In van Praag, H.M., Lader, M.H., Rafaelsen, O.J. & Sachar, E.J. (eds.): *Handbook of Biological Psychiatry. Part II: Psychophysiology.* Marcel Dekker, New York, pp.97-144.

Szabadi, E., Bradshaw, C.M. & Gaszner, P. (1980): The comparison of the effects of DL-308, a potential new neuroleptic agent, and thioridazine on some psychological and physiological functions in healthy volunteers. *Psychopharmacology, 68,* 125-134.

Tanaka, M., Isozaki, H., Inanaga, K. & Ogawa, N. (1978): The effects of a new benzodiazepine derivative, ID-540, on the averaged photopalpebral reflex in man. *Psychopharmacology, 58,* 217-222.

Venables, P.H. (1980): Peripheral measures of schizophrenia. In van Praag, H.M., Lader, M.H., Rafaelsen, O.J. & Sachar, E.J. (eds.): *Handbook of Biological Psychiatry. Part II. Psychophysiology.* Marcel Dekker, New York, pp.79-96.

Biological Quantitative Methods in the Evaluation of Psychiatric Treatment: Some Biochemical Criteria

P. UYTDENHOEF, P. LINKOWSKI and
J. MENDLEWICZ

1. Introduction

Different biological approaches (genetic, biochemical, neuroendocrine, neurophysiological) are used for studying psychiatric disorders. Some studies have attempted to find biological predictors of the response to various treatments. Although this field is a relatively new one, the results being sometimes controversial, its impact on research and treatment is of great importance.

We shall attempt to review some of the promising areas of research into biochemical predictors in relation to treatment response mainly in affective illnesses, as little data is available for schizophrenia and other psychiatric disorders. Table 1 shows the main biochemical predictors of treatment response in affective disorders.

2. Response to tricyclic antidepressants

2.1 3-Methoxy-4-hydroxyphenyl glycol (MHPG) studies

MHPG, the major metabolite of central norepinephrine (NE), may provide a useful index of brain NE turnover when measured in 24-hour urine tests (Schildkraut *et al* 1978). Maas *et al* (1972) reported low (<900 mg MHPG/g creatinine) pre-treatment urinary MHPG concentration in depressed patients who responded to imipramine and desipramine and high (>1350 mg MHPG/g creatinine) MHPG concentration in imipramine and desipramine non-responders. In the same study, Maas *et al* also reported that other NE metabolites (vanillyl mandelic acid, normetanephrine and metanephrine) did not predict response to imipramine in the same patients.

Schildkraut (1973) found high urinary MHPG excretion in amitriptyline-responders and low pre-treatment urinary MHPG levels in amitriptyline non-responders.

Table 1. Potential biochemical parameters predicting treatment response in affective disorders

1. Response to tricyclic antidepressants
   Urinary MHPG
   CSF 5-HIAA
   Red blood cell COMT
   Plasma levels of tricyclics

2. Response to MAO inhibitors
   Acetylation rate
   Platelet MAO inhibition

3. Response to lithium
   Plasma levels
   Lithium excretion test
   Platelet MAO activity
   CSF 5-HIAA
   Urinary MHPG
   Red blood cell lithium ratio
   Ca^{2+}/Mg^{2+} ratio

4. Response to ECT
   TSH response to TRH
   Dexamethasone suppression test

Beckman & Goodwin (1975) reported the mean urinary excretion of MHPG to be high (2,170 µg/24h) in the imipramine responders. A low urinary MHPG excretion rate was also found by Hollister *et al* (1980) in patients responding to nortriptyline.

In a recent study, Cobbin *et al* (1979) applied these observations to clinical practice. The authors found a significantly better drug response in the group of patients when treatment was chosen by biochemical criteria (pre-treatment MHPG urinary level) than in those where treatment was decided on the basis of clinical criteria.

An interesting finding is the prediction of good response to imipramine and desipramine by the D-amphetamine test. When given D-amphetamine orally for two days, some depressed patients show a transitory enhancement of mood. In the study of Fawcett & Siomopoulos (1971), D-amphetamine responders showed a good response to imipramine and desimipramine and had low pre-treatment urinary MHPG levels.

This procedure, confirmed by Van Kammen & Murphy in a larger study (1978), could be of considerable predictive value. For Maas (1975), low MHPG urinary excretion could characterize a biochemical subgroup of depression with a noradrenergic deficit.

Nevertheless, these MHPG studies were not universally confirmed (Schildkraut 1978) and, although they are encouraging, "they need prospective studies with larger numbers of patients and with concurrent measurement of tricyclic plasma levels to verify the usefulness of this technique" (Stern *et al* 1980).

2.2 5-Hydroxyindol acetic acid (5-HIAA) studies

Several authors, mainly van Praag and Åsberg, have studied CSF 5-HIAA, the major metabolite of serotonin (5-HT). Some depressed patients seem to have a central deficiency of serotonin. In these patients, several studies showed a decreased baseline concentration of 5-HIAA (Åsberg *et al* 1976) and a decreased 5-HIAA accumulation after probenecid administration (van Praag & Korf 1974). Probenecid inhibits transport of 5-HIAA from the central nervous system to the blood stream. The resulting 5-HIAA accumulation seems to be an indication of central serotonin turnover.

Van Praag (1981) has reported that depressed patients with low CSF 5-HIAA accumulation respond to 5-hydroxytryptophan much better than those with normal or high CSF 5-HIAA accumulation. This author has also found in the patients with low CSF 5-HIAA a good response to clomipramine (van Praag 1977a) and an optimal response to clomipramine in association with 5-hydroxytryptophan (van Praag *et al* 1974). These depressed patients are believed to have a tryptophan depletion or a serotoninergic deficit, which can be improved by the administration of serotonin precursors or drugs known for their blocking action on serotonin reuptake.

Having found that in most patients with low CSF 5-HIAA accumulation, the level of this metabolite stayed low even when the symptomatology had disappeared (van Praag 1977b), van Praag recently reported a good prophylactic efficacy of 5-hydroxytryptophan in those patients with low CSF 5-HIAA accumulation (van Praag & de Haan 1980).

In the study of Åsberg *et al* (1973), depressed patients with high CSF 5-HIAA responded to nortriptyline while patients with low CSF 5-HIAA did not seem to benefit from nortriptyline.

In the study of Zis & Goodwin (1979) patients with low CSF 5-HIAA showed a poor response to imipramine, while in another study (Goodwin *et al* 1978), patients with high CSF 5-HIAA were imipramine responders. In the same study, Goodwin *et al* found amitriptyline responders to have low CSF 5-HIAA.

A bimodal distribution of CSF 5-HIAA and urinary MHPG levels in depressed patients was reported in some studies (Åsberg *et al* 1976; Maas 1978). According to these studies and the monoamines hypothesis of depression, Maas (1975) has suggested a biochemical classification of depression in two subgroups. Table 2 shows the characteristics of these two subgroups. On the basis of this biochemical classification, the clinician can prescribe more selective antidepressants (see Table 3).

Table 2. Two biochemical groups in depression

	Urinary MHPG	CSF 5-HIAA	Response to:	No or poor response to:
Type A: NE deficit	Low	Normal or raised	Imipramine Desipramine Nortriptyline Amphetamine	Amitriptyline Clomipramine
Type B: 5-HT deficit	Normal or raised	Low	Amitriptyline Clomipramine 5-Hydroxytryptophan	Imipramine Desipramine Nortriptyline

Table 3. Selective action of antidepressants

Drug	Biogenic amines		
	5-HT	NE	DA
Amitriptyline	+ + + +	±	0
Nortriptyline	+	+ + +	0
Imipramine	+ + +	+ +	0
Desipramine	0	+ + + +	0
Clomipramine	+ + + +	0	0
Des-methyl-chlorimipramine	+	+ +	0

As shown in Table 3, amitriptyline and clomipramine have a more selective action on serotonin reuptake while nortriptyline and desipramine seem to block norepinephrine reuptake more specifically.

Although the monoamines studies are encouraging, they are not universally confirmed (Bielski & Friedel 1976; Coppen & Wood 1979; Pickar et al 1978).

The controversies in this field could be explained at least partially by the technical problems of obtaining valid urine or CSF samples and comparing standardized values. For instance, CSF 5-HIAA values vary with age, circadian rhythms, physical activity and volume of the samples (because of the existence of a ventriculo-lumbar gradient for HIAA), so the results of these studies must be interpreted with caution.

2.3 Red blood cell catechol-O-methyltransferase (COMT) studies

COMT is an important enzyme in the degradation of catecholamines. Davidson *et al* (1976) have reported, in a series of 15 unipolar depressed women, that good response to imipramine was correlated with a low red blood cell COMT activity. This study requires confirmation before it can be applied in clinical practice.

2.4 Sleep EEG studies

The sleep EEG studies could be an approach of considerable predictive value in the treatment of affective disorders. In a series of 18 unipolar depressed patients, Kupfer *et al* (1976) found REM changes (a decrease in percentage of REM sleep and an increase of REM latency) to be predictive of the clinical response to imipramine.

2.5 Determination of optimal dosage by monitoring plasma levels of tricyclics

Plasma levels of tricyclics have been correlated with the response to antidepressants. The plasma levels are usually measured at the steady-state (usually after 10-20 days of constant dosage).

For *nortriptyline* (the demethylated metabolite of amitriptyline), a curvilinear relationship between steady-state plasma levels of the drug and clinical response has been found by most authors (Kragh-Sørensen *et al* 1976; Åsberg *et al* 1971; Ziegler *et al* 1976). The range of plasma levels within which a patient is most likely to respond (the 'therapeutic window') seems to be between 50 and 200 ng/ml for nortriptyline.

For *desipramine* (the demethylated metabolite of imipramine), the relationship is probably also curvilinear (Friedel *et al* 1979), but this is still a subject of controversy (Khalid *et al* 1978; Amin *et al* 1978).

For *imipramine,* four studies reported a positive correlation between combined plasma levels of imipramine and desipramine at a certain threshold, but no evidence of a therapeutic window (Reisby *et al* 1977; Olivier-Martin *et al* 1975; Muscettola *et al* 1978). The threshold seems to be around 200 ng/ml or above and the usual dosage of 150 mg/day may be too low for many patients (Glassman *et al* 1977; Simpson *et al* 1976).

For *amitriptyline,* several groups have reported a linear relationship between therapeutic response and combined plasma levels of amitriptyline and nortriptyline (Braithwaite *et al* 1972; Ziegler *et al* 1976; Kupfer *et al* 1977); other reports suggest the existence of a therapeutic window (Montgomery *et al* 1979). However, other authors (Coppen *et al* 1978; Mendlewicz *et al* 1980) have found no relationship between plasma levels and therapeutic response to amitriptyline. Fig. 1 shows the shape of the curves relating the clinical response to plasma levels for nortriptyline and imipramine. Table 4 shows the therapeutic plasma levels of some tricyclics.

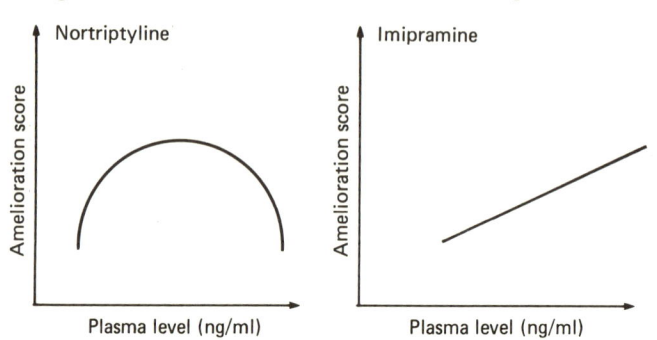

Fig. 1. Plasma levels of tricyclics and clinical response.

Table 4. Therapeutic plasma levels of some antidepressants

	Usual dosage (mg)	Half-life (hours)	Therapeutic plasma levels (ng/ml)
Amitriptyline	75-400	17-75	>200
Nortriptyline	50-150	12-93	50-200
Imipramine	100-400	9-24	>200
Desipramine	50-150	12-77	50-150?

When measuring plasma levels of tricyclics, one can sometimes find very low plasma levels in some patients, although they receive the usual dosage of tricyclics. This monitoring makes it possible to increase the daily dosage of the same antidepressant before changing the treatment.

A pharmacological action of the hydroxylated metabolites of tricyclics has been reported in recent studies (Potter *et al* in press; Potter *et al* 1980). These metabolites could thus contribute to the antidepressant effect of the tricyclics.

Cooper & Simpson (1978) have reported a test which predicts the daily dosage for obtaining optimal plasma levels of nortriptyline by measuring plasma levels 24 hours after a single dose of the drug. Brunswick *et al* (1979) used a similar approach for predicting the optimal dosage of imipramine. The preliminary results are encouraging, but this test needs prospective confirmation.

3. Response to MAO inhibitors
3.1 Rate of acetylation
Acetylation is an important way of degradation and inactivation

for phenelzine (Price Evans *et al* 1965). The rate of phenelzine acetylation can be tested by sulphapyridine acetylation. Using this test, Johnstone & March (1973; 1976) reported a significantly greater response to phenelzine in slow acetylators than in fast acetylators, so that this procedure could predict whether a patient would respond to phenelzine. Unfortunately, other authors failed to confirm these findings (Davidson *et al* 1978).

3.2 Platelet MAO inhibition

Robinson *et al* (1978) have studied the relationship between clinical response to phenelzine (at the dosage of 60 mg/day) and the degree of platelet MAO inhibition; they found a 40 per cent response when platelet MAO inhibition was less than 80 per cent, a 68 per cent response when platelet MAO inhibition was above 80 per cent, and a 79 per cent response when platelet MAO inhibition was more than 90 per cent. So platelet MAO inhibition should be at least 80 per cent for phenelzine to be effective in the treatment of depression.

In a study of the antidepressant potentiation of 5-hydroxytryptophan by L-deprenil, a selective MAO-B inhibitor, Mendlewicz & Youdim (1980) found a correlation between the degree of platelet MAO inhibition and clinical response in the group of 5-hydroxytryptophan-deprenil responders. As shown in Figs. 2 and 3, the percentage inhibition of MAO activity was considerably lower (<85 per cent) in the non-responders than in the patients who responded.

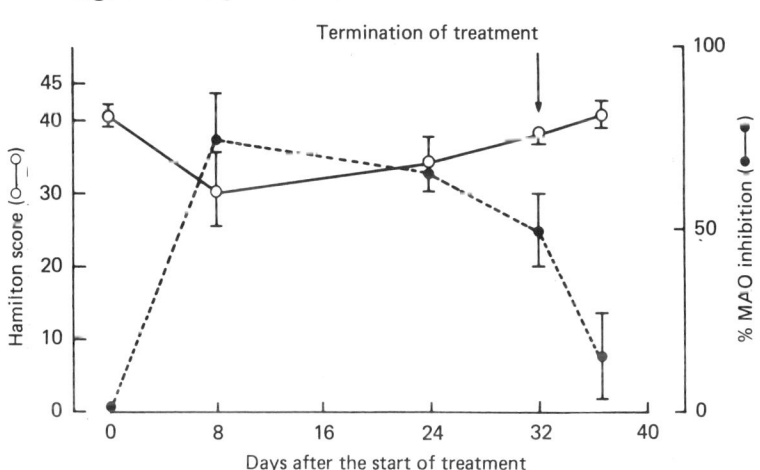

Fig. 2. Non-responders. For details see text.

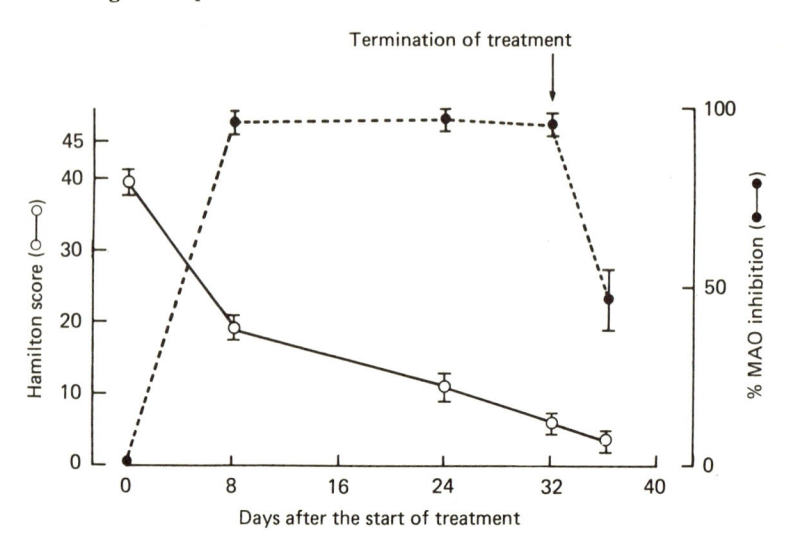

Fig. 3. Responders. For details see text.

4. Response to lithium

4.1 Mania

In 1968, Serry (Serry 1969; Serry & Andrews 1969), suggested a lithium excretion text; in his series, he had found a bimodal lithium excretion in manic patients: the lithium excreting manics had poor response to lithium, and lithium retainers showed a good response to lithium. Unfortunately, other studies failed to replicate these results (Stokes et al 1972). In any case, adequate plasma levels are needed for a good response in mania, but very high plasma levels (above 1.5 mEq/l) — as recommended earlier — may not be necessary in all patients.

Fyrö et al (1975) observed that lithium increased CSF 5-HIAA levels and lowered CSF HVA levels but found no relationship between these biochemical effects and the antimanic response.

Sullivan et al (1977) found that low platelet MAO activity was associated with poor response to lithium in mania.

4.2 Depression

Many authors (Carroll 1979; Mendels 1976; Goodwin et al 1969) believe that lithium acts as an antidepressant in some patients.

Mendels linked low platelet MAO activity with an antidepressant response to lithium (1975) but this report is no longer considered valid (Mendels; personal communication, 1978). Beckman et al (1975) found an association between bipolarity, low pre-treatment MHPG urinary excretion, and good response to lithium. They also reported the increase of urinary MHPG excretion during lithium therapy in these patients. Goodwin *et al* (1973) reported that depressed patients with lowered CSF 5-HIAA accumulation by the probenecid test showed a good response to lithium, but this was not confirmed by Bowers & Heninger (1977).

Carmen *et al* (1974) reported that a higher Ca^{2+}/Mg^{2+} plasma ratio tended to predict a good response to lithium, but Mendels *et al* (1978) failed to confirm these results.

4.3 Prophylactic treatment
4.3.1. Plasma levels

A lithium plasma level between 0.8 and 1.2 mEq/l is generally recommended. Prien & Caffey (1976) found 80 per cent response in patients with lithium levels above 0.8 mEq/l and only 45 per cent response when lithium levels were below 0.7 mEq/l. Another study (Jerram & McDonald 1978) reported the same efficacy for levels below 0.5 mEq/l, between 0.5 and 0.7 mEq/l, and above 0.7 mEq/l.

4.3.2. Red blood cell lithium ratio

Mendels & Frazer (1973) reported that a high red blood cell lithium ratio predicts a good response to lithium, but this is a subject of controversy. The same authors on larger samples (Frazer *et al* 1978) as well as other investigators (Carroll & Feinberg 1977; Mendlewicz *et al* 1978) were unable to confirm these results. Rybakowski *et al* (1974) found no correlation between red blood cell lithium ratio and the duration of successful lithium prophylaxis in 37 patients.

Some studies have reported *genetic factors* predicting long-term lithium response. Bipolar patients with a positive family history of bipolar illness seem to have a better long-term lithium response than patients without family history (Mendlewicz *et al* 1973; Stallone *et al* 1973).

No similar association was observed for the presence of unipolar illness in relatives of bipolar patients (Mendlewicz *et al* 1973; Stallone *et al* 1973). In twin studies a higher concordance rate for affective illness was found in twin pairs when the subject had experienced good long-term response to lithium (Mendlewicz *et al* 1973; Stallone *et al* 1973). The histocompatibility antigenic system has also been studied to find immunogenetic markers of lithium prophylaxis. Perris *et al* (1979) reported that long-term lithium responders showed a reduction in the HLA-B18 antigen. This interesting observation needs further replication.

5. Response to electroconvulsive therapy (ECT)

Although several authors have studied the biochemical effects of

ECT (Essman 1973; Ilaria & Prange 1975; van Praag 1977c), showing an increase of norepinephrine, serotonin and dopamine in the central nervous system and of plasma tyrosine hydroxylase and MAO activity, none of these has been shown to be predictive in the treatment of depression. Funkenstein (Funkenstein et al 1952) had suggested a predictor test using methacholine (a cholinergic stimulator) and epinephrine (an adrenergic stimulator): a chill after methacholine was linked with 97 per cent response to ECT and an increase of blood pressure (>50 mmHg) after epinephrine with 89 per cent ECT response.

Nevertheless, other authors questioned this test (Feinberg 1958; Rose 1962). Neuroendocrine studies seem to be of great interest in the prediction of ECT response. In the studies of Kirkegaard et al (1978), the thyroid-stimulating hormone (TSH) response to thyrotropin-releasing hormone (TRH), reduced in some depressed patients, returned to normal in patients who responded to ECT but not in patients who relapsed. The administration of dexamethasone fails to suppress the cortisol secretion in endogenous depressed patients (Stokes 1972). The abnormal response to the 'dexamethasone suppression test' (DST) gradually returns to normal before complete clinical recovery, as an indication of good long-term prognosis to ECT (Carroll et al 1981).

6. Biochemical predictors of antipsychotic treatment

As for the antidepressant drugs, interest is growing in the study of biological correlates of antipsychotic response in schizophrenic patients, considering the variable rate of response to antipsychotics.

6.1 Biochemical variables

A significant correlation between clinical improvement and CSF HVA increase has been reported for chlorpromazine as well as for haloperidol, perphenazine and thiothixene (van Praag 1978; Sedvall et al 1978). The greater the increment in CSF HVA, the more the patients tended to improve. Chlorpromazine treatment also resulted in a marked reduction of the MHPG and the HIAA concentration in CSF (Wode-Helgodt et al 1978).

6.2 Neuroendocrine studies

Enhanced growth hormone response to apomorphine (suggesting hypersensitivity of dopamine systems in schizophrenia) predicts a poor response to neuroleptic treatment (Rotrosen et al 1978). These results have been questioned by other authors (Meltzer et al 1976) who reported normal growth hormone response to apomorphine in chronic and acute schizophrenic patients.

Radioimmunoassayable activity for prolactin can be found in cerebrospinal fluid of psychotic patients; Sedvall et al (1978) found a significant elevation of the prolactin-like material in the CSF of schizophrenic patients during treatment with chlorpromazine and a positive correlation was found between the elevation of the prolactin level and the clinical change. According to their 'prolactin model', Langer & Puhringer (1980) studied the relationship between neuroleptic treatment (haloperidol and droperidol), plasma prolactin response and psychopathological changes. Their preliminary observations suggest a relationship between prolactin response and therapeutic response to a neuroleptic, a blunted response being associated with less effective therapeutic response.

6.3 Plasma levels studies

In several studies, non-responding schizophrenic patients undergoing chronic treatment with chlorpromazine had high plasma levels of chlorpromazine sulphoxide whereas responders had high concentrations of 7-hydroxy-chlorpromazine or unchanged chlorpromazine (Sakalis et al 1973; MacKay et al 1974). Another study has reported that poor responders to chlorpromazine showed very high levels of chlorpromazine sulphoxide in their CSF (Rotrosen et al 1978). Recently, Sakurai et al (1981) reported that predictability of response to chlorpromazine in schizophrenic patients could be assessed by a single oral 50 mg chlorpromazine test and the subsequent determinations of chlorpromazine metabolites in plasma.

Sedvall et al (1980) reported significant correlation between antipsychotic effect and drug concentration at the second week of treatment but not at the fourth, suggesting that inductive changes occur during long-term treatment with chlorpromazine. Plasma levels of haloperidol measured by radioimmunoassay have been less studied although this substance is particularly interesting in view of the fact that there is only one active metabolite (reduced haloperidol) for this drug. Plasma levels of less than 6 ng/ml were associated with a poor therapeutic response (Mendlewicz et al 1981) whereas Magliozzi et al (1981) reported the existence of a therapeutic window (between 8 and 18 ng/ml) for this substance. Studying serum neuroleptic levels by radioreceptor assay based on competition of these drugs for the binding of ^{3}H-spiroperidol or ^{3}H-haloperidol to dopamine receptors, Tune et al (1980) reported that poor therapeutic responses were associated with serum levels under 50 ng/ml of chlorpromazine equivalents.

7. Conclusion

The different studies reviewed in this paper are encouraging. However, the determination of biological predictors of treatment response depends on our knowledge of the biological etiologies of mental disorders and of the mechanisms of action of the various biological treatments. We must admit that our knowledge is still fragmentary in both of these fields.

Studies in neurochemistry, neuroendocrinology, pharmacology and electrophysiology should be integrated in the same patients in order to provide a multidisciplinary approach to the problems. Clinical studies should be supported by basic research in animal models.

Finally, the evaluation of treatment response requires better clinical-biological diagnostic criteria as well as an improvement in the psychometric rating scales used today in biological psychiatry research.

References

Amin, N.M., Cooper, R., Khalid, R. et al (1978): A comparison of desipramine and amitriptyline plasma levels and therapeutic response. *Psychopharmacol. Bull. 14* (1), 45-46.

Åsberg, M., Cronholm, B., Sjöqvist, F. et al (1971): Relationship between plasma level and therapeutic effect of nortriptyline. *Br. Med. J., 3,* 331-334.

Åsberg, M., Bertilsson, L., Tuck, D., Cronholm, B. & Sjöqvist, F. (1973): Indoleamine metabolites in the cerebrospinal fluid of depressed patients before and during treatment with nortriptyline. *Clin. Pharmacol. Ther., 14,* 277-286.

Åsberg, M., Thorén, P., Träskman, L., Bertilsson, L. & Ringberger, V. (1976): Serotonin depression. A biochemical subgroup within the affective disorders. *Science, 191,* 478-480.

Axelson, S., Jonsson, S. & Nordgrem, L. (1975): Cerebrospinal fluid levels of chlorpromazine and its metabolites in schizophrenia. *Arch. Psychiatr. Nervenkr. 221,* 167-170.

Beckman, H. & Goodwin, F.K. (1975): Antidepressant response to tricyclics and urinary MHPG in unipolar patients: clinical response to imipramine and amitriptyline. *Arch. Gen. Psychiatry, 32,* 17-21.

Beckman, H., St-Laurent, J. & Goodwin, F.K. (1975): The effect of lithium on urinary MHPG in unipolar and bipolar depressed patients. *Psychopharmacology, 42,* 277-282.

Bielski, A.J. & Friedel, R.O. (1976): Prediction of antidepressant response. *Arch. Gen. Psychiatry, 33,* 1479-1489.

Bowers, M.G. & Heninger, G.R. (1977): Lithium clinical effects and cerebrospinal fluid acid monoamine metabolites. *Commun. Psychopharmacol. 1,* 135-145.

Braithwaite, R.A., Goulding, R. & Thenao, G. (1972): Plasma concentration of amitriptyline and clinical response. *Lancet 1,* 1297-1300.

Brunswick, D.J., Amsterdam, J.D., Mendels, J. et al (1979): Prediction of steady-state imipramine and desmethylimipramine plasma concentrations from single-dose data. *Clin. Pharmacol. Ther. 25,* 605-610.

Carman, J.S., Post, R.M., Teplitz, T.A. et al (1974): Divalent cations in predicting antidepressant response to lithium (ltr to ed.). *Lancet 2,* 1454.

Carroll, B.J. & Feinberg, M.P. (1977): Intracellular lithium abstracted. *Neuropharmacology, 16,* 527.

Carroll, B.J. (1979): Prediction of treatment outcome with lithium. *Arch. Gen. Psychiatry, 36,* 870-878.

Carroll, B.J., Feinberg, M., Greden, J. et al (1981): A specific laboratory test for the diagnosis of melancholia. Standardization, validation and clinical utility. *Arch. Gen. Psychiatry, 38,* 15-22.

Cobbin, D.M., Requin-Blow, B., Williams, L.R. & Williams, W.O. (1979): Urinary MHPG levels and tricyclic antidepressant drug selection. A preliminary communication on improved drug selection in clinical practice. *Arch. Gen. Psychiatry, 36,* 1111-1115.

Cooper, T.B. & Simpson, G.M. (1978): Prediction of individual dosage of nortriptyline. *Am. J. Psychiatry, 135,* 333-335.

Coppen, A., Montgomery, S., Ghose, K. et al (1978): Amitriptyline plasma concentration and clinical effect: a World Health Organization collaborative study. *Lancet 1,* 63-66.

Coppen, A. & Wood, K. (1979): Etudes cliniques et biologiques du L-tryptophane dans la dépression. *Encéphale 5* (5), 627-632.

Davidson, J.R.T., McLeod, M.N., White, H.L. & Raft, D. (1976): Red blood cell catechol-O-methyl transferase and response to imipramine in unipolar depressed women. *Am. J. Psychiatry, 133,* 952-955.

Davidson, J., McLeod, M.N. & Blum, M.R. (1978): Acetylation phenotype, platelet monoamine oxidase inhibition, and the effectiveness of phenelzine in depression. *Am. J. Psychiatry, 135,* 467-469.

Essman, W.B. (1973): *Neurochemistry of Cerebral Electroshock.* Spectrum Publications, New York, pp.181.

Fawsett, J. & Siomopoulos, V. (1971): Dextroamphetamine response as a possible predictor of improvement with tricyclic therapy in depression. *Arch. Gen. Psychiatry, 25,* 247-255.

Feinberg, I. (1958): Current status of the Funkenstein test. *Arch. Gen. Psychiatry, 80,* 488-501.

Frazer, A., Mendels, J., Brunswick, E. et al (1978): Erythrocyte concentrations of the lithium ion: clinical correlates and mechanism of action. *Am. J. Psychiatry, 135,* 1005-1019.

Friedel, R.O., Veith, R.C., Bloom, V. et al (1979): Desipramine plasma levels and clinical response in depressed out-patients. *Commun. Psychopharmacol., 3,* 81-87.

Funkenstein, D.H., Greenblatt, M. & Salomon, H.C. (1952): An autonomic nervous system test of prognostic significance in relation to electroshock treatment. *Psychosom. Med., 14,* 347-362.

Fyrö, B., Petterson, U. & Sedvall, G. (1975): The effect of lithium treatment on manic symptoms and levels of monoamine metabolites in cerebrospinal fluid of manic patients. *Psychopharmacology, 44,* 99-103.

Glassman, A.H., Perel, J.M., Shostak, M. et al (1977): Clinical implications of imipramine plasma levels for depressive illness. *Arch. Gen. Psychiatry, 34,* 197-204.

Goodwin, F.K., Murphy, D.L. & Bunney, W.E. Jr. (1969): Lithium carbonate in depression and mania. *Arch. Gen. Psychiatry, 21,* 486-496.

Goodwin, F.K., Post, R.M., Dunner, D.L. et al (1973): Cerebrospinal fluid amines metabolites in affective illness. The probenecid technique. *Am. J. Psychiatry, 130,* 73-79.

Goodwin, F.K., Cowdry, R.W. & Webster, M.H. (1978): Predictors of drug response in the affective disorders: towards an integrated approach. In Lipton, M.A., Di Mascio, A. & Killam, F. (eds.): *Psychopharmacology: a generation of progress.* Raven Press, New York, pp.1277-1288.

Hollister, L.E., Kenneth, L.D. & Berger, P.A. (1980): Subtypes of depression based on excretion of MHPG and response to nortriptyline. *Arch. Gen. Psychiatry, 37,* 1107-1110.

Ilaria, R. & Prange, A.J. (1975): Convulsive therapy and other biological treatments. In Flack, F.F. & Draghi, S.S. (eds.): *The Nature and Treatment of Depression.* John Wiley & Sons, New York, pp.271-308.

Jerram, T.C. & McDonald, R. (1978): Plasma lithium control with particular reference to minimum effective levels. In Johnson, F.N., Johnson, S. (eds.): *Lithium in Medical Practice.* University Park Press, Baltimore, pp.407-413.

Johnstone, E.C. & March, W. (1973): Acetylator status and response to phenelzine in depressed patients. *Lancet 1,* 567-570.

Johnstone, E.C. (1976): The relationship between acetylator status and inhibition of monoamine oxidase, excretion of free drug and antidepressant response in depressed patients on phenelzine. *Psychopharmacology, 46,* 289-294.

Kammen, D.P. van & Murphy, D.L. (1978): Prediction of imipramine antidepressant response by a one-day D-amphetamine trial. *Am. J. Psychiatry, 135,* 1179-1184.

Khalid, R., Amin, M.N. & Ban, T.A. (1978): Desipramine plasma levels and therapeutic response. *Psychopharmacol. Bull. 14* (1), 43-44.

Kirkegaard, C., Nörlem, N., Cohn, D. & Lauridsen, V.B. (1978): Thyrotropin releasing hormone (TRH) stimulation test in manic-depressive illness. *Arch. Gen. Psychiatry, 35,* 1017-1021.

Kragh-Sörensen, P., Hansen, C.E. & Baastrup, P.C. (1976): Relationship between antidepressant effect and plasma level of nortriptyline: clinical studies. *Pharmakopsychiatr. Neuropsychopharmakol. 9,* 27-32.

Kupfer, D.J., Foster, F.G., Reich, L. *et al* (1976): EEG sleep changes as predictors in depression. *Am. J. Psychiatry, 133,* 622-626.

Kupfer, D.J., Hanin, I., Spiker, D.G. *et al* (1977): Amitriptyline plasma levels and clinical response in primary depression. *Clin. Pharmacol. Ther. 22,* 904-911.

Langer G. & Puhringer, W. (1980): Haloperidol and droperidol treatment in schizophrenics. Clinical application of the 'prolactin model'. *Acta Psychiatr. Belg. 80* (5), 574-584.

Maas, J.W., Fawcett, J.A. & Dekirmenjian, H. (1972): Catecholamine metabolism, depressive illness and drug response. *Arch. Gen. Psychiatry, 26,* 252-262.

Maas, J.W. (1975): Biogenic amines and depression. *Arch. Gen. Psychiatry, 32,* 1357-1361.

Maas, J.W. (1978): Clinical and biochemical heterogeneity of depressive disorders. *Ann. Intern. Med. 88* (4), 556-563.

MacKay, A.V.P., Healey, A.F. & Baker, J. (1974): The relationship of plasma chlorpromazine to its 7-hydroxy and sulphozide metabolites in a large population of chronic schizophrenics. *Br. J. Clin. Pharmacol. 1,* 425-430.

Magliozzi, Y.R., Hollister, L., Arnold, K. & Earle, G. (1981): Relationship of serum haloperidol levels to clinical response in schizophrenic patients. *Am. J. Psychiatry, 133,* 365-367.

Meltzer, A.Y., Goode, D.J., Fang, V.S. *et al* (1976): Dopamine and schizophrenia. *Lancet 2,* 1142.

Mendels, J. & Frazer, A. (1973): Intracellular lithium concentration and clinical response: towards a membrane theory of depression. *J. Psychiatr. Res. 10,* 9-18.

Mendels, J. (1975): Lithium in the acute treatment of depressive states. In Johnson, F.N. (ed.): *Lithium Research and Therapy.* Academic Press, London, pp.43-62.

Mendels, J. (1976): Lithium in the treatment of depression. *Am. J. Psychiatry, 133,* 373-378.

Mendels, J., Ramsey, T.A., Dyson, W.L. *et al* (June 5-9, 1978): Lithium as an antidepressant. Presented at the International Lithium Conference: Controversies and Unresolved Issues. New York, N.Y.

Mendlewicz, J., Fieve, R.R. & Stallone, F. (1973): Relationship between the effectiveness of lithium therapy and family history. *Am. J. Psychiatry, 130,* 1011-1013.

Mendlewicz, J., Verbanck, P., Linkowski, P. *et al* (1978): Lithium accumulation in erythrocytes of manic depressive patients: an in vivo twin study. *Br. J. Psychiatry, 133,* 436-444.

Mendlewicz, J. & Youdim, M.B.H. (1980): Antidepressant potentiation of 5-hydroxytryptophan by L-deprenil in affective illness. *J. Affect. Disorders, 2,* 137-146.

Mendlewicz, J., Linkowski, P. & Rees, J.A. (1980): A double-blind comparison of dothiepin and amitriptyline in patients with primary affective disorder: serum levels and clinical response. *Br. J. Psychiatry, 136,* 154-160.
Mendlewicz, J., Linkowski, P., Alexandre, J. & Schoutens, A. (1981): Haloperidol plasma levels and clinical response in schizophrenia. In: *Clinical pharmacology in psychiatry: Neuroleptic and antidepressant research.* MacMillan, New York.
Montgomery, S.A., McAuley, R., Rani, S.J. et al (1979): Amitriptyline plasma concentration and clinical response. *Br. Med. J. 1,* 230-231.
Muscettola, G., Goodwin, F.K., Potter, W.Z. et al (1978): Imipramine and desipramine in plasma and spinal fluid: relationship to clinical response and serotonin metabolism. *Arch. Gen. Psychiatry, 35,* 621-625.
Olivier-Martin, R., Marzin, D., Buschsenschutz, E. et al (1975): Concentrations plasmatiques de l'imipramine et de la desmethylimipramine et effect antidépresseur au cours d'un traitement contrôlé. *Psychopharmacology, 41,* 187-195.
Perris, C., Strandman, E. & Wahlby, L. (1979): *HLA antigens and the response to prophylactic lithium.* XIth CINP Congress, Vienna, 1978, pp.9-14.
Pickar, D., Sweeney, D.R., Maas, J.W. & Heninger, G.R. (1978): Primary affective disorder, clinical state change and MHPG excretion. *Arch. Gen. Psychiatry, 35,* 1378-1383.
Potter, W.C., Calil, H.M., Manian, A.A. et al. Hydroxylated metabolites of tricyclic antidepressants: preclinical assessment of activity. *Biol. Psychiatry* (in press).
Potter, W.C., Calil, H.M., Zavadil, A.P. et al. (1980): Steady-state concentrations of hydroxylated metabolites of tricyclic antidepressants in patients: relationship to clinical effect. *Psychopharmacol. Bull., 16,* 32-34.
Praag, H.M. van & Korf, J. (1974): Serotonin metabolism in depression: clinical application of the probenecid test. *Int. Pharmacopsychiatry, 9,* 35-51.
Praag, H.M. van, Burg, W. van den, Bos, E.R.H. & Dols, I.C.W. (1974): 5-Hydroxytryptophan in combination with clomipramine in 'therapy-resistant' depression. *Psychopharmacology, 38,* 267.
Praag, H.M. van (1977a): New evidence of serotonin-deficient depression. *Neuropsychobiology, 3,* 56.
Praag, H.M. van (1977b): Significance of biochemical parameters in the diagnosis, treatment and prevention of depressive disorders. *Biol. Psychiatry, 12,* 101.
Praag, H.M. van (1977c): *Depression and Schizophrenia. A contribution on their chemical pathologies.* Spectrum Publications, New York, pp.260.
Praag, H.M. van (1978): The significance of central dopamine metabolism in the pathogenesis and treatment of psychotic disorders. In Gershon, E.S., Belmaker, R.H., Ketty, S.S. & Rosenblum, M. (eds.): *The Impact of Biology on Modern Psychiatry.* Plenum Press, New York, pp.1-27.
Praag, H.M. van & Haan, S. de (1980): Depression vulnerability and 5-hydroxytryptophan prophylaxis. *Psychiatry Res. 3,* 75-83.
Praag, H.M. van (1981): Management of depression with serotonin precursors. *Biol. Psychiatry, 16,* 291-310.
Price Evans, D.A., Davison, K. & Pratt, R.T.C. (1965): The influence of acetylator phenotype on the effects of treating depression with phenelzine. *Clin. Pharmacol. Ther. 6,* 430-435.
Prien, R.F. & Caffey, E.M. (1976): Relationship between dosage and response to lithium prophylaxis in recurrent depression. *Am. J. Psychiatry, 133,* 567-570.
Reisby, N., Gram, L.F., Beck, P. et al (1977): Imipramine: clinical effects and pharmacokinetic variability. *Psychopharmacology, 54,* 263-272.

Robinson, D.S., Nies, A., Ravaris, C.L., Ives, J.O. & Barlett, D. (1978): Clinical psychopharmacology of phenelzine: activity and clinical response. In Lipton, M.A., Di Mascio, A. & Killam, K.F. (eds.): *Psychopharmacology: A generation of progress.* Raven Press, New York, pp.961-973.

Rose, J.T. (1962): The Funkenstein test. A review of literature. *Acta Psychiatr. Scand. 38,* 124-153.

Rotrosen, J., Angrist, B.M. & Gershon, S. (1978): Dopamine receptor alteration in schizophrenia: neuroendocrine evidence. *Psychopharmacology* (Berlin), *51,* 1-7.

Rybakowski, J., Chlopocka, M., Kapelski, Z. *et al* (1974): Red blood cell lithium index in patients with affective disorders in the course of lithium prophylaxis. *Int. Pharmacopsychiatry, 9,* 166-171.

Sakalis, G., Chan, T.L. & Gershon, S. (1973): The possible role of metabolites in therapeutic response to chlorpromazine treatment. *Psychopharmacology* (Berlin), *32,* 279-284.

Sakurai, Y., Takahashi, R., Nakahara, T. & Ikenaga, H. (1980): Prediction of response to and actual outcome of chlorpromazine treatment in schizophrenic patients. *Arch. Gen. Psychiatry, 37,* 1057-1062.

Schildkraut, J.J. (1973): Norepinephrine metabolites as biochemical criteria for classifying depressive disorders and predicting responses to treatment. Preliminary findings. *Am. J. Psychiatry, 130,* 695-699.

Schildkraut, J.J., Orsulak, P.J., Schatzberg, A.F., Gudeman, J.E., Cole, J.O., Rohde, W.A. & La Brie, R.A. (1978): Toward a biochemical classification of depressive disorders. I. Differences in urinary excretion of MHPG and other catecholamine metabolites in clinically defined subtypes of depressions. *Arch. Gen. Psychiatry, 35,* 1427-1433.

Schildkraut, J.J. (1978): Current status of the catecholamine hypothesis of affective disorders. In Lipton, M.A., Di Mascio, A. & Killam, K.F. (eds.): *Psychopharmacology: A generation of progress.* Raven Press, New York, pp.1223-1234.

Sedvall, G., Alfredson, G., Bjerkenstedt, L., Eneroth, P., Fyrö, B., Hanzyd, C. & Wode-Helgodt, B. (1978): Central biochemical correlates to antipsychotic drug action in man. In Gershon, E.S., Belmaker, R.H., Kety, S.S. & Rosenblum, M. (eds.): *The Impact of Biology on Modern Psychiatry.* Plenum Press, New York, pp.41-55.

Sedvall, G. (1980): Relationship among biochemical, clinical and pharmacokinetic variables in neuroleptic treated schizophrenic patients. In: *Adv. Biochem. Psychopharmacology, 24,* 521-528.

Serry, M. (1969): The lithium excretion test. I. Clinical application and interpretation. *Aust. N.Z. J. Psychiatry, 3,* 390-394.

Serry, M. & Andrews, S. (1969): The lithium excretion test. II. Practical and biochemical aspects. *Aust. N.Z. J. Psychiatry, 3,* 395-397.

Simpson, G.M., Lee, J.H., Cerulic, Z. *et al* (1976): Two dosages of imipramine in hospitalized endogenous and neurotic depressives. *Arch. Gen. Psychiatry, 33,* 1093-1102.

Stallone, F., Shelley, E. & Mendlewicz, J. (1973): The use of lithium in affective disorders. III. A double-blind study of prophylaxis in bipolar illness. *Am. J. Psychiatry, 130,* 1006-1010.

Stern, S.L., Rush, A.J. & Mendels, J. (1980): Toward a rational pharmacotherapy of depression. *Am. J. Psychiatry, 137,* 545-552.

Stokes, J.W., Mendels, J., Secunda, S.K. *et al* (1972): Lithium excretion and therapeutic response. *J. Nerv. Ment. Dis. 154,* 43-48.

Stokes, P.E. (1972): Studies on the control of adrenocortical function in depression. In Williams, T.A., Katz, M. & Shields, J.A. (eds.): *Recent Advances in the Psychobiology of the Depressive Illnesses.* U.S. Govt. Printing Office, Washington D.C., pp.199-220.

Sullivan, J.L., Cavenar, J.O., Maltbie, A. *et al* (1977): Platelet monoamine oxidase activity predicts response to lithium in manic-depressive illness. *Lancet 2,* 1325-1327.

Tune, L.E., Creese, I., De Paulo, R., Slavney, P.R., Coyle, J.T. & Snyder, S.H. (1980): Clinical state and serum neuroleptic levels measured by radioreceptor assay in schizophrenia. *Am. J. Psychiatry, 137,* 187-190.

Tyrer, P. & Gardner, M. (1978): Acetylator status and response to phenelzine. *Lancet 2,* 994-995.

Wode-Helgodt, B., Borg, S., Fyrö, B. & Sedvall, G. (1978): Clinical effect and drug concentrations in plasma and cerebrospinal fluid in psychotic patients treated with fixed doses of chlorpromazine. *Acta Psychiatr. Scand. 58,* 149-173.

Ziegler, V.E., Clayton, P.J., Taylor, J.R. *et al* (1976): Nortriptyline plasma levels and therapeutic response. *Clin. Pharmacol. Ther 20,* 458 463.

Ziegler, V.E., Co, B.T., Taylor, J.R. *et al* (1976): Amitriptyline plasma levels and therapeutic response. *Clin. Pharmacol. Ther. 19,* 795-801.

Zis, A.P. & Goodwin, F.K. (1979): Novel antidepressants and the biogenic amine hypothesis of depression. *Arch. Gen. Psychiatry, 36,* 1097-1107.

V: ETHICAL AND PRACTICAL PROBLEMS

Ethical and Practical Problems in Therapeutic Research in Psychiatry

H. HELMCHEN

1. Basic statements

Therapeutic research in psychiatry cannot be done without patients. The main reason is that therapeutic effects can be established only against diseases, but adequate disease models of most human specific psychiatric diseases do not exist. Furthermore, knowledge gained from pre- or extra-clinical investigations can be applied only to a rather limited extent to psychiatric patients, particularly to those with more severe psychiatric diseases. This is valid not only for the results of animal pharmacology (Helmchen & Müller-Oerlinghausen 1978), but also for observations with psychological procedures, called psychotherapy, on non-psychiatric people — for example, psychoanalytic experiences in healthy persons, or results of behaviour modification in smokers or obese clients (!) (Helmchen et al 1982) or even for sociological hypotheses such as the labelling theory, the irrelevance of which has been shown for some psychiatric diseases (van Praag 1978).

But the validity of results from investigations with psychiatric patients is limited too. The more the scope of a piece of research is narrowed, for example by a high selection of patients, by quasi-experimental standardization of the setting, or by short duration of controlled clinical trials, the less general will be the application of its results, and the more clearly the question must be answered whether such trials are ethically justified. From this comes the demand for developing research methods that will be less difficult ethically and yet justified scientifically. Examples are methods for research in 'natural' settings or with out-patients or over long periods (Helmchen 1978; Lasagna 1974; Linden & Schüssler 1981; Rüther et al 1980; Wing 1981). However, it should be added that of course for different research questions, different methods and designs have to be applied, and their ethical implications must be considered separately in any project.

Insofar as therapeutic research in psychiatry cannot be done without patients it is related to therapeutic practice. Its framework can be defined by three statements:

1.1 Therapy

Therapy in a broad sense includes techniques and attitudes. The term is used here for all procedures that prevent or remove a disease or shorten or attenuate the natural course of it and disease-related handicaps in the individual. By therapeutic attitude is meant the ability to assist the patient not only to overcome the illness by himself but also to endure it. It is the background for an adequate application of the therapeutic knowledge.

1.2 Therapeutic techniques and attitudes

Techniques depend on knowledge, attitudes on values. The former is the main area of research, the latter is rather a question of education. Ethical research cannot be done without a firm ethical attitude. It must be built up continuously by continuing clinical education which is sensitive to ethical problems. Regulations may help to define ethical norms but they alone do not ensure ethical behaviour. Thus, for example, criminal experiments with humans were performed by German physicians between 1933 and 1945 in spite of valid guidelines for therapeutic and medical research with humans which had been in existence since 1931 when they were published by the German Government. These guidelines were as clear as the declaration of Helsinki (Mitscherlich & Mielke 1960).

1.3 Psychiatric research

The following general statements are especially valid for therapy in psychiatry. Psychiatric diseases involve the personality of the ill more than other medical diseases. Furthermore, the personality of the physician may exert a much greater and even therapeutic influence on the patient than in other doctor-patient relationships. The stronger individuality of this special human relationship means that both the psychiatrist's image of the patient as a person and the selective aims of research become more relevant in psychiatric research. The researcher has to be aware that the selective approach of research may be dangerous for the patient as well as for himself: the patient may lose personal values, the researcher may be tempted to generalize from partial observations (Heimann 1978). In this respect the scientific obligation to resist this temptation and the ethical obligation to preserve the personal dignity of the patient may and should parallel each other.

Clinical research should not be separated too much from clinical practice. In that case it could be difficult to translate the results of research into practice, the principal identity of ethical problems could be concealed and the work of different clinical practitioners and researchers with the same patients could cause psychological and organizational problems and irritate the therapeutic process.

2. The basic problem
2.1 Outline

As stated in the Hippocratic oath it is the basic obligation of each physician to give his patient the best therapy available. But what is the best therapy available? Ideally it is the therapy with the highest, most specific and most speedy efficacy and with no side-effects, risks or disadvantages. Unfortunately, in most cases such an ideal therapy does not exist. Therefore, the physician has to strike a balance between the benefits and ill-effects of therapies in general (the so-called pharmacologically therapeutic range) and furthermore he has to balance the possible benefits and ill-effects of therapy in respect of the individual patient, his own personal therapeutic experience and abilities, and the particular situation. Almost never will he have an unequivocal and sound knowledge of all these elements and their weight in the special case to influence his choice of therapy. Therefore, each therapeutic decision and its outcome involves an element of guess-work. In this respect it can be said that each therapeutic decision is an experiment (Helmchen & Müller-Oerlinghausen 1978). From this can be deduced the following:

(a) Every therapeutic decision implies the ethical obligation to keep a balance between benefits and ill-effects.
(b) Every such balance is uncertain to some degree.
(c) This uncertainty depends on the knowledge as well as the clinical and personal competence of the physician.
(d) Thus it is an ethical obligation for the physician to keep abreast of current knowledge in order to make the best choice of treatment, i.e. to maximize the benefits and to minimize the damage in each individual case. And it is also an ethical demand to improve one's general knowledge.

It is the aim of therapeutic research to improve and extend knowledge on the absolute and relative efficacy and safety of therapy. Such knowledge is supra-individual in nature: i.e. it is gained from more than one patient and it surmounts the experience of each individual physician. Owing to the comparability of individual observations, this kind of scientifically gained knowledge implies stereotyping (systematization, standardization, operationalization) of observations and of therapeutic measures, and for testing hypotheses an experimental design often is necessary — as in controlled clinical trials, a major tool in modern therapy research (Report on the Scientific and Ethical Basis of the Clinical Evaluation of Medicines 1980). All these measures, obligatory from a methodological point of view, may bring inconvenience, disadvantages or risks to the research patient.

This seems to oppose the ethical obligation of the physician to minimize the possible harm caused by therapy in the individual case. But this in turn opposes the ethical demand for scientifically based improvement of therapy for all ill people. We called this the paradox of the clinical trial (Helmchen & Müller-Oerlinghausen 1975a,b). Wing explained that it is really not a paradox but rather a complication of the everyday therapeutic decision based on balancing between good and harm (Wing 1981). Factors of this complication are as follows:

(a) The degree of uncertainty is higher: the risk of investigational or experimental therapies is often unknown or less clear than with established standard therapies, although this is by no means true in every case.

(b) The patient's burden of inconvenience or even harmful effects is perhaps higher or not necessary.

(c) The concern is not exclusively the individual patient here and now but also other patients.

2.2 Solutions

Thoughts for overcoming these complications are as follows:

(a) The only reasons for an investigational therapy are that there is no efficient therapy for a particular disease, or that the range of standard therapies needs to be improved. Therefore, the higher degree of uncertainty and perhaps disadvantage may be counterbalanced by the chance that the patient under investigation will receive a therapy which is better than the existing ones. From this it follows that the balance between advantage and disadvantage has to be more explicit than in the everyday therapeutic decision.

(b) Although it is ethical to give the individual patient the best therapy available as well as to improve therapy by research there is a difference: the first is an unconditional obligation, the second is an obligatory demand. From this order of priorities it follows that the requirements of information and consent must be stricter with research therapy than in the everyday therapeutic decision.

Thus ethically there is no principal difference between therapeutic decisions in clinical practice and in research. But there are differences of degree in the need both for accurate balancing between benefits and harm, and for informed consent. These are the ethical norms as stated in the declaration of Helsinki/Tokyo 1964/75.

2.3 Comments

It seems desirable to differentiate this outline a little more by three further comments:
(a) The reason for giving the benefit of the individual patient the highest priority is that this in general will be more unequivocal, more stable in time, and less open to misuse. Besides, this is not a question of 'individual' versus 'collective' ethics as mentioned in a report on the scientific and ethical basis of the clinical evaluation of medicines but a question of ranking the individual versus society as a whole (Report . . ., 1980). Nowadays in the Western European societies, this question is answered in favour of the individual.
(b) The informed consent should not be misunderstood as a purely technical measure in order to minimize risks. It should rather give the patient the opportunity of choice and self-determination in order to make his dignity as a person a basic element of the therapeutic relationship (Lebacqz & Levine 1978). But even in this respect there are some problems in psychiatry.
(c) The uncertainty mentioned above of each individual therapeutic decision may create innovations. This brings up the question of where clinical practice becomes research. The answer must be threefold: In respect to the *ethical* dimension there is no difference in principle between an innovative variation of a standard therapy or even a new therapy and an investigational therapy in the framework of a research project. But *methodologically* there is a difference insofar as the former is based on individual observations, thoughts, or inferences alone or on serendipity, whereas the latter tries to answer a question in a controllable way. (It may be added that the two ways are by no means mutually exclusive but rather complementary: for example, unusual effects of a variation of a standard therapy should provoke a question for research.) And especially from a *practical* point of view there seems to be a rather big difference: in Western European countries an investigational therapy declared as research is more or less under the control of the scientific community and ethical committees whereas this is often not the case with 'innovative' therapies, which

may be introduced or accepted before having been tested because of the suggestive power of personal experience, ideology or a persuasive, warmhearted and engaged initiator.

The British social psychiatrist John Wing states: "There is nowadays a fairly general acceptance of the view that new drugs should not be introduced without being tested. There is no similar consensus in respect of social treatments, most of which become firmly adopted before they have been thoroughly examined. The harm that may come from the application of misguided social theories, or the misapplication of sensible theories, is at least as great as any harm that can follow the prescription of a harmful drug or an unnecessary course of psychotherapy. In fact, it can be much greater, since harmful social practices can become institutionalized into the structure of a complete psychiatric service."

3. Psychiatric specifications
3.1 Informed consent

The declaration of Helsinki/Tokyo requires the patient to be given sufficient information on the aim, the mode, the expected benefits, risks and possible inconveniences of the trial. But what does 'sufficient' mean with a psychiatric patient? The validity and extent of his informed consent may be restricted either by the patient's reduced ability to understand or to consent, by a therapeutic privilege in respect of a patient's limited endurance capacity, or by methodological necessities, for example, the use of a placebo.

Informing the patient will be insufficient or even impossible with patients with severe psychiatric disorders such as delirious states or dementias; the same will be true for the consent of patients with states of excitation, anxiety, dependency, aggressiveness, or suicidality. However, for just such patients there is a strong need to improve existing therapies by research. This problem cannot be solved by the appointment of a legal guardian because the possible negative social consequences of such a procedure may score rather high in considerations of the risk-benefit ratio.

Not only in everyday practice but also in clinical therapy research it is necessary to balance the risks and benefits of informed consent. Thus it seems to be unethical to increase the anxiety of patients by detailed information on possible inconveniences or complications or to get informed consent from patients with retarded depressions who could also develop feelings of guilt after having consented or not (Loftus & Fries 1979). According to the German Drug Law this so-called therapeutic privilege can be used only as a very rare exception under special conditions. In such cases it is appropriate to get a comment from an ethical committee.

In Denmark all research protocols have to be referred to the committee. "But a committee statement is necessary before the scientists can start their experiment or trial only if informed consent cannot be obtained (or is omitted) in the interests of the patient" (Riis 1980).

Informing the patient on details of blind or placebo designs may both increase his subjective suffering and contradict the purpose of the study. It may cause not only a high drop-out rate (Verstraete 1971) but may be considered as a scientific absurdity (Davidson 1969) because the exclusion of a subjective bias is the purpose of keeping the patient (and the doctor) ignorant of the application of such techniques (Martini 1947). Bobon in Belgium "successfully supported the view that, in psychiatry, the informed consent . . . is contrary to research neutrality, inducing uncontrollable placebo or nocebo effects" (Bobon 1981). Others, however, argue that not giving full information to the patient on the use of a blind technique or a placebo is a fraud that will destroy a trusting doctor-patient relationship (Simmons 1978). In any case it can be said that "recognizing the existence of ethical dilemmas is a necessary prelude to the quest for objective solutions" (Howard & Friedman 1981). With respect to research it must be made very clear that empirical knowledge on the consequences of informed consent is rather lacking (Helmchen 1981a; Leff 1973). Research should answer at least the following questions:

(a) What are the consequences of information and consent on therapy, for example, on compliance or outcome?
(b) What role does informed consent play as a selection factor, particularly in a psychiatric population? If it does play a role, what are the consequences for the comparability and validity of research results? (Guelfi-Sozzi; Helmchen 1981b).

3.2 Controlled trials

Control groups, randomization, blind techniques and the use of placebos are the major elements of controlled clinical trials carried out with the aim of eliminating unspecific known or unknown, objective or subjective influences. Especially in psychiatry the elimination of the latter is essential because of the high level of unspecific personality-dependent influences on the therapeutic outcome with respect to both the experience of the patient and the observation and interpretation of phenomena by the physician.

The use of blind techniques and placebos poses not only the already discussed contradictive methodological difficulty of informing the patient of techniques in a way which will keep him ignorant. In the case of placebos there is also the problem of giving a supposedly inefficient therapy. But it is a misunderstanding that placebo treatment has no efficacy. The up to 40 per cent positive placebo response is an argument against this view. This is, of course, an unspecific but nevertheless a therapeutic effect. Therefore, it seems ethical to use a placebo where a specific therapy with an evident efficacy does not exist or where the disease has no dangerous or life-threatening intensity or acuteness. It may be mentioned that there is a rather broad variety of views on the ethical admissibility of placebos (Angst 1969; Guelfi-Sozzi; Pichot 1979). An example: placebo-controlled investigations on the relapse prophylactic efficacy of lithium were already considered unethical in the Scandinavian countries in the late 1960s whereas at the same time in England they were still called for (Rafaelsen 1977).

Practical problems may arise from the formalized structure of the research design, for example, the restriction of individual or additional therapies or their randomization. Sometimes the care personnel may exert a subliminal pre-screening of patients, if they are not well informed of the aims and justification of the investigation and if they are unconvinced that there will be no real disadvantages for the patient. Therefore, information on aims, procedures, and results of research and corresponding training of all personnel involved in clinical research is an often neglected but nevertheless important task (Guelfi-Sozzi).

3.3 Confidentiality

Nowadays in clinical practice the necessary and unavoidable time-sharing teamwork calls for an exchange of patient data among the immediate members of the team (Wing). Particularly in psychiatry this exchange often will include very personal and, therefore, confidential information. This extended confidence is generally accepted and its misuse is apparently rather unlikely and not to be feared by the public.

But clinical research seems to complicate the situation. The number of informed persons increases owing to both the research personnel and the persons concerned with ethical control. Therefore, the likelihood of a leak in confidentiality may arise. However, this is a minor problem compared with a rather comprehensive public mistrust of the current possibilities of linking electronically stored personal data.

Some types of research such as epidemiological investigations, cohort studies, evaluations of health services, etc., which are particularly relevant to long-term psychiatric diseases, cannot be done without data linkage and case registers. In some countries new laws for the security of privacy tend to curtail such necessary psychiatric research. The only way not to destroy either these research facilities or the public trust in the strict confidentiality of each patient's details is to implement strictly controlled rules for defined personal responsibility, restricted access to data, and security of codes for personal identification, storage and data transfer. British proposals in this field seem to be the most elaborate and best balanced ones (Wing). And it seems necessary to inform the public on the need for and the safety of clinical research.

4. Questions of control

As discussed before, the validity and extent of informed consent may be restricted. The less valid informed consent is, the more it seems justified to control the ethical admissibility of a research investigation. The control may concern the design, performance and results of research including the sufficiency of informed consent and the confidentiality of personal data of patients. But by whom, how and when will or should ethical control be performed?

According to an inquiry in Western European countries everyone seems to have adopted in general the principles of the declaration of Helsinki/Tokyo.* (For legislation see Guelfi *et al* 1978; Guelfi-Sozzi.) But there are rather big differences in the implementation or even system of controlling whether or not a research project follows that declaration: formal control declines from north to south in Western Europe.

4.1 Levels of control

Control generally operates on two or three levels: on a local and/or on a regional level as well as on a national level. On the local level there seems in all cases to be control by the head of the department, who is ultimately responsible for the care of the patients; besides this, there may be experienced colleagues especially appointed (e.g. Finland), or research conferences with members of the hospital (e.g. in Austria or in the Federal Republic of Germany).

These conferences do not deal with ethical questions alone but with all the questions of a research project as, for example, its scientific aim and value, the necessary methodology, and the organizational problems with its realization. Therefore, not only the researchers but also the doctors and nurses of the involved patients participate in such conferences. Apparently these conferences are not formalized very strongly. On the regional level formal committees operate for a hospital (e.g. in Austria, Belgium,

---

*This impression is based on information which I requested from the following colleagues: K.A. Achté, Finland; J. Angst, Switzerland; P. Berner, Austria; J. Bobon, Belgium; G.B. Cassano, Italy; J.J. Lopez-Ibor-Alino, Spain; J.-O. Ottosson, Sweden; P. Pichot, France; H.M. van Praag, Netherlands; O.J. Rafaelsen, Denmark; N. Retterstöl, Norway; J. Wing, Great Britain.

Sweden), a region (e.g. in Denmark) or a special research area (e.g. in the Federal Republic of Germany). Central or national ethical committees are established in a few countries such as Belgium, Denmark, Norway. Mostly they are affiliated with national research foundations or councils. The national committees will mainly be asked by regional committees for help in difficult problems or by authorities for advice on basic problems. (In Finland psychopharmacological research projects can be started only with the permission of the health administration.)

4.2 Composition of ethical committees

Composition varies broadly. There are committees with medical doctors alone (e.g. in Belgium), particularly pharmacologists, anaesthesiologists, psychiatrists, specialists in internal and in forensic medicine. Other committees (as in Denmark) have parity between scientific and non-scientific members; the latter will be nominated by the local county boards. Others have one representative of the nurses (e.g. in Finland) or one lay member (e.g. a lawyer in the Federal Republic of Germany) (Deutsch 1981).

4.3 Access and competence

Access to and competence of the committees are rather different, too. Some committees seem to evaluate only ethical questions, others comment on scientific as well as on ethical aspects of research projects. In some countries (e.g. in Denmark, Norway) there is an obligation to send notification of all research projects involving patients or human volunteers to such a committee. In others (e.g. in Austria, Federal Republic of Germany) the committee can be asked for advice if a researcher is in doubt. It is not clear whether some committees have the competence to decide in principle on research projects or whether the competence of all committees is limited to commentary on a research project and to counselling the researcher. In fact such comment may exert an effective control where financial support depends on it. In the German Research Association each reviewer of an application for a research grant has to evaluate it along the principles of the declaration of Helsinki/Tokyo.

4.4 Benefits and risks

It seems necessary to evaluate the benefits and possible harm of these procedures. There is a good opportunity for a comparative evaluation because of the rather different stages of development in different countries of Western Europe. Thus the risks and difficulties expected in countries with a more traditional approach to clinical research may be contrasted with the experiences of the countries which have implemented such controls during the last years. National abilities to deal with these problems in different ways should not be forgotten in such a study.

Benefits of control by committees seem to be:
- (a) to make the researcher more sensitive to ethical questions by forcing him to make explicit the problems involved and the criteria used for decisions;
- (b) to meet the need of the public to be protected against misuse as a guinea pig and to diminish the public distrust against research by giving evidence of an efficient control, and — at least in the case of lay members of the committee — to develop an understanding for the aims, methods, and results of clinical research.

Risks of such control procedures are as follows:
- (a) The more they leave the area of counselling and enter that of decision-making the more the risks develop that
  (i) the responsibility will shift from the researcher to the control body, and
  (ii) the control body itself becomes liable (Bar & Fischer 1980).
- (b) The more perfect, institutionalized and formalized the control mechanisms become, the more
  (i) bureaucracy may restrict innovative research, and
  (ii) innovative research may be done under other terms without any control.

4.5 General control

Besides the control by immediate senior colleagues and by review committees there exists a further control mechanism by the scientific and perhaps the public community. They may discuss critically the published results of scientific work. But a supposition is that, of course, all results will be published. From this point of view the recommendation I.8 of the Helsinki/Tokyo declaration is a questionable one. Its strict application would have made impossible the most sensitive evaluation of Beecher in 1966 (Beecher 1966) and it is possible that it would not have prevented the performance of research, the ethical aspects of which were at least doubtful.

4.6 Task oriented modes of control

From a patient-oriented and realistic point of view, the different procedures of ethical control should be restricted to certain aspects or phases of clinical research.

A review committee may be helpful in commenting on a research design and perhaps the regulations for the confidentiality of patient data; it is the responsibility of both the scientific and the public community to discuss the results of research, but the control of the ethical performance of research (and the validity of informed consent) seems to be an obligation among colleagues.

4.7 Education for ethical self-control

This is the place to repeat that therapeutic research must be related to clinical practice more than has been the case. The development of the ethical conscience of the researcher and his ability to deal with ethical problems must be integrated into his education in clinical practice. Ethical control may be a help for the clinical researcher, but his ethical education will make it safer for the patient.

5. Conclusions

The ethical problems of therapeutic research are, in principle, the same as those of therapeutic practice. They concern mainly the appropriate balance between expected benefits and possible harm. In research this balance is complicated by greater uncertainty over the decisive factors and perhaps more inconvenience for the patient. But this may be counterbalanced by the opportunity for the patient to receive better therapy, by weighing benefits and risks more explicitly than in everyday practice, and by the stronger obligation to receive fully informed consent from the patient.

In psychiatry, the effects of therapy as well as the evaluation of such effects are more personality-dependent and, therefore, more open to bias than in other medical disciplines. Therefore it is a methodological need to apply the currently available techniques for the elimination of such biases (because to produce doubtful or non-interpretable results would be unethical in itself). But techniques such as randomization, blind or placebo designs as well as the informed consent or the confidentiality of electronically stored and processed data of patients pose difficult problems especially for the doctor-patient relationship in psychiatry. Answers with general validity cannot be given and sufficient empirical knowledge on the consequences of such answers does not exist. Therefore, risk-benefit considerations must be weighed carefully in every particular case. Also empirical research is needed on the effects of all these procedures, the aim of which is to secure both the scientific value of research results and the personal values of the involved patients.

Control of the ethical admissibility of psychiatric research will be helpful for the researcher, but his ethical training will offer greater security to the patient. Ethical sensitization of the researcher may be a benefit of ethical committees. At the same time the risks must be considered that increasing formalization of clinical research may impair the doctor-patient relationship and bureaucracy may diminish innovative therapeutic research in psychiatry.

Acknowledgement

The author's thanks are due to Jane Helmchen, M.A., for help in translation.

References

Angst, J. (1969): Leerpräparate in Therapie und Forschung. *Prakt. Psychiatr., 48,* 1-12.
Bar, C.V. & Fischer, G. (1980): Haftung bei der Planung und Förderung medizinischer Forschungsvorhaben. *Neue Jurisil. Wochensche., 33,* 2734-2740.
Beecher, H.K. (1966): Ethics and clinical research. *N. Engl. J. Med., 274,* 1354-1360.
Bobon, J. (1981): Personal communication.
Davidson, H.A. (1969): Legal and ethical aspects of psychiatric research. *Am. J. Psychiatry, 126,* 237-240.
Deutsch, E. (1981): Ethik-Kommissionen für medizinische Versuche am Menschen: Einrichtung, Funktion, Verfahren. *Neue Juristl. Wochensche., 34,* 614-617.
Guelfi, J.D., Dreyfus, J.F. & Pull, C.-B. (1978): *Les essais thérapeutiques en psychiatrie; méthodologie, éthique et législation.* Masson, Paris, p.235.
Guelfi-Sozzi, C.: Problèmes éthiques et législatifs des essais thérapeutiques en psychiatrie. In Roche: *Cahiers d'information du practicien, o.J.*
Heimann, H. (1978): Ärztlich-ethische Fragen in der psychiatrischen Forschung Entwurf einer allgemeinen Grundlagung. In Helmchen, H., Müller-Oerlinghausen, B. (eds.): *Psychiatrische Therapieforschung, Ethische und juristische Probleme.* Springer-Verlag, Berlin, p.126-134.
Helmchen, H. & Müller-Oerlinghausen, B. (1975a): Ethische und juristische Schwierigkeiten bei der Effizienzprüfung psychiatrischer Therapieverfahren. *Nervenarzt, 46,* 397-403.
Helmchen, H. & Müller-Oerlinghausen, B. (1975b): The inherent paradox of clinical trials in psychiatry. *J. Med. Ethics, 1,* 168-173.
Helmchen, H. & Müller-Oerlinghausen, B. (eds.) (1978): *Psychiatrische Therapieforschung. Ethische und juristische Probleme.* Springer-Verlag, Berlin, p.179.
Helmchen, H. (1978): Forschungsaufgaben bei psychiatrischer Langzeitmedikation. *Nervenarzt, 49,* 534-538.
Helmchen, H. (1981a): Aufklärung und Einwilligung bei psychisch Kranken. In Bergener, M. (ed.): *Psychiatrie und Rechtsstaat.* Luchterhand-Verlag, Neuwied, pp.79-96.
Helmchen, H. (1981b): Problems of informed consent for clinical trials in psychiatry. *Controlled Clinical Trials, 1,* 435-440.
Helmchen, H., Linden, M. & Rüger, U. (eds.) (1982): *Psychotherapie in der Psychiatrie.* Springer-Verlag, Berlin.
Howard, J. & Friedman, L. (1981): Protecting the scientific integrity of a clinical trial: some ethical dilemmas. *Clin. Pharmacol. Ther., 29,* 561-569.
Lasagna, L. (1974): A plea for the 'naturalistic' study of medicines. *Europ. J. Clin. Pharmacol., 7,* 153-154.
Lebacqz, R. & Levine, R.J. (1978): Informed consent. II. In Reich, W.T. (ed.): *Encyclopedia of Bioethics* Vol. 2. New York, pp.755, 760f.

Leff, J.P. (1973): Influence of selection of patients on results of clinical trials. *Br. Med. J. IV,* 156-158.

Linden, M. & Schüssler, G. (1981): Collaborative studies with psychiatric practitioners. In Sartorius, N., Helmchen, H. (eds.): *Multicentre Trials.* Karger, Basel.

Loftus, E.F. & Fries, J.F. (1979): Informed consent may be hazardous to health. *Science, 204,* 11.

Martini, P. (1947): *Methodenlehre der therapeutisch-klinischen Forschung.* Springer-Verlag, Berlin, Göttingen, Heidelberg.

Mitscherlich, A. & Mielke, F. (1960): *Medizin ohne Menschlichkeit.* S. Fischer-Verlag, Frankfurt/M.

Pichot, P. (1979): Les essais thérapeutiques. *Rev. Trav. Acad. Sci. morales pol. 139,* 29-51.

Praag, H.M.van (1978): The scientific foundation of anti-psychiatry. *Acta Psychiat. Scand., 58,* 113-141.

Rafaelsen, O.J. (1977): Ethics of psychopharmacological research. Vortrag auf dem internationalen Symposium 'Perspectives in Psychopharmacotherapy', Florence, April 6-8.

Report on the Scientific and Ethical Basis of the Clinical Evaluation of Medicines (1980): *Europ. J. Clin. Pharmacol., 18,* 129-134.

Riss, P. (1980): Personal communication.

Rüther, E., Benkert, O., Eckmann, F., Eckmann, I., Grohmann, R., Helmchen, H., Hippius, H., Müller-Oerlinghausen, B., Poser, W., Schmidt, L., Stille, G., Strauss, A. & Überla, K. (1980): Drug monitoring in psychiatrischen Kliniken. *Arzneim.-Forsch./Drug Res. 30,* 1181-1183.

Simmons, B. (1978): Problems in deceptive medical procedures: an ethical and legal analysis of the administration of placebos. *J. Med. Ethics, 4,* 172-185.

Verstraete, M. (1971): General aspects of clinical pharmacology. *Arch. Int. Pharmacodyn. Suppl., 192,* 17-19.

Wing, J. (1981): Ethical aspects of psychiatric research. In: Bloch, S., Chodoff, P. (eds.): *Psychiatric Ethics.* Oxford University Press.

Index

acetylation rate and phenelzine response, 236-7
ACTH and dexamethasone suppression test, 108-9
adrenaline, *see* epinephrine
affective disorders (*see also* individual disorders)
  biochemical predictors of treatment response in, 231-40 (Table 1)
  classification of, 7, 77-8
  and life expectancy, 45-6
  rating scales for (*see also* rating scales), 171-9
agoraphobia, development of, 43-4
alcoholic hallucinosis, 87
alcoholism, chronic
  and antisocial behaviour, 48
  treatment for, 50, 129
algorithms for classification systems, 85-6
  and hierarchy of symptoms, 89-90
AMDP, *see* Association for Methodology and Documentation in Psychiatry
American Psychiatric Association, *see Diagnostic and Statistical Manual of Mental Disorders*
amitriptyline
  autonomic effects of, 225
  prediction of response to, 234 (Tables 2 and 3; and 5-HIAA levels, 233; using plasma levels, 235-6 (Table 4); and renal MHPG excretion, 99-100, 231
  treatment, self-rating and, 193-4 (Figs. 2 and 3)
D-amphetamine
  growth hormone secretion after, 116 (Table 2)
  and prediction of response to antidepressants, 232, 234 (Table 2)

amylobarbitone sodium, psychophysiological evaluation of, 226-7
Anafranil, *see* clomipramine
anticholinergic drug effects, 225-6
antidepressant(s) (*see also* individual agents)
  autonomic effects of, 225-6
  long-term therapy with, 35-6
  monoamine metabolism after, 22, 94
  prediction of response to, 102-4 (Table 1), 116 (Table 2), 231-9 (Tables 1, 2, 3 and 4); and dexamethasone suppression test, 111; and growth hormone responses, 116; and 5-HIAA levels, 95-7, 233-4; and homovanillic acid levels, 101-2, 238; using plasma drug levels, 22, 235-6 (Fig. 1 and Table 4), 239; and platelet MAO activity, 237-8 (Figs. 2 and 3); and renal MHPG excretion, 99-100, 231-3; and tryptophan/competing amino acids ratio, 98, 103; and TSH response to TRH, 114-15
  psychotherapy versus 35-6
  self-rating scales and, 188, 192-5 (Figs. 2 and 3)
  and suicide attempts, 35-6
  TRH as an, 113
antigen markers in lithium responders, 239
antipsychotic drugs (*see also* individual agents)
  long-term therapy and, 40-1
  peripheral effects of, 225
  prediction of response to, 22, 240-1
  self-rating of side-effects of, 195-7 (Table 5)

anxiety
  and 'flooding' therapy, 4, 228
  and mortality rates, 46
  physiological parameters of, 19–20, 224, 226–7
  rating scales for, 15–16, 174–5
anxiolytics, evaluation of, 19, 226–7
apomorphine, growth hormone secretion after
  in depressions, 115–16
  in schizophrenia, 240–1
arrhythmias, cardiac, and emotional disorders, 46
Association for Methodology and Documentation in Psychiatry (AMDP, formerly AMP) rating systems, 12, 86, 151–60, 179
  compared with other rating scales, 158–60
  development of, 151–2
  reliability of, 154–6
  second order scales in, 155–8 (Tables 3 and 4)
  symptoms and signs for, 152 (Tables 1 and 2)
  validity of, 155–7
autonomic function
  and biofeedback, 4–5
  measurement of, 222, 223; in chronic schizophrenia, 227; in evaluation of anxiolytics, 226–7; in phobic patients, 228; prognostic value of, 229
  after psychotropic drugs, 225–6

barbiturates, psychophysiological evaluation of, 226–7, 228
Bech–Rafaelsen Mania Scale (MAS), 174 (Table 1)
Bech–Rafaelsen Melancholia Scale (MES), 173–4 (Table 1)
Beck Depression Inventory (D-I), 14, 189 (Table 1), 198
behavioural disorders, see personality disorders
behaviour therapy
  aims of, 6, 53
  and analysis of personality disorders, 48–9
  for neuroses, 42–3
  for neurotic depression, 198
  psychophysiological evaluation of, 227, 228
  and psychosomatic disease, 45–7
  types of, 4–5, 124–5
Beigel Mania State Scale, 174
Benton Visual Retention Test, 18

biochemical methods, (see also hypophyseal hormones and psychophysiological measures), 21–2
  in diagnosis of depressions, 93–104 (Table 1), 233–4 (Tables 2 and 3); dopamine metabolism, 101–2; noradrenaline metabolism, 98–101; serotonin metabolism, 94–8
  and prediction of response to treatment, 104 (Table 1), 231–42 (Table 1); antipsychotics, 240–1; dopamine-potentiating agents, 101–2; electroconvulsive therapy, 239–40; 5-hydroxytryptophan, 95; lithium, 238–9; monoamine oxidase inhibitors, 236–8 (Figs. 2 and 3); tricyclic antidepressants, 95–7, 99–100, 231–6 (Tables 2, 3 and 4, Fig. 1)
  and prognosis of depression, 97–8, 104 (Table 1)
biofeedback techniques, 4–5, 46–7
blood flow, measurement of, 222
blood pressure and autonomic function, 222, 225
Bourdon tests, 17
Brief Psychiatric Rating Scale (BPRS), 12
  compared with AMDP rating scales, 156, 158–9
Buss anxiety rating scale, 15–16

calcium/magnesium plasma ratio and lithium response, 239
carbidopa and renal MHPG excretion, 99
cardiac arrhythmias and emotional disorders, 46
case reports, single, 8–9
case studies, single, 25
catecholamines (see also adrenaline, dopamine, noradrenaline and individual metabolites), 223
catechol-O-methyltransferase (COMT) in red blood cells, 235
childhood history and personality disorders, 49–51
chlordiazepoxide, psychophysiological evaluation of, 227
chlorpromazine
  autonomic effects of, 225
  prediction of response to, 240, 241
ciclazindol, anticholinergic side-effects of, 225
classification systems, standardized (see also diagnosis and rating scales), 6–8, 81–91
  advantages of, 81–5

Index

methodology and, 53-5, 85-91
multiaxial, 54-5, 71-9, 85-9, 208
multidimensional, 74-5, 175, 184, 208-9 (Table 2)
World Health Organization (WHO) and, 63-7
Clinical Self-Rating Scales (Klinische Selbstbeurteilungs-Skalen) (KSb-S)
application of, in drug trials, 192-9 (Figs. 2, 3 and 4, Table 5)
compared with other self-rating scales, 189 (Table 1), 192-3 (Table 4)
contents of, 188-90 (Table 1)
factorial analysis of, 190-2 (Tables 2 and 3)
clomipramine, prediction of response to, 95-6, 233-4 (Tables 2 and 3)
Clyde Mood Scale, 188
cognitive therapy
compared with pharmacotherapy, 126
for neurotic depression, 198
Comprehensive Psychopathological Rating Scale (CPRS), 12-13, 163-9 (Table 1)
compared with AMDP rating system, 159-60
depression scale developed from, 13-14
confidentiality of patient data, 258-9
consent, informed see informed consent
controlled trials
ethics of, 257-8
and methodology, 24-5, 53-5
for milieu therapy, 145-6
corticotropin-releasing factor (CRF) and dexamethasone suppression test, 108-9
cortisol levels, 223
and dexamethasone suppression test, 108-12 (Fig. 1)
and TSH response to TRH, 114
cost-benefit analysis of psychiatric methods, 25-7, 127-32
of self-rating scales, 187
cost-effectiveness of psychotherapy, 127-9
criminal behaviour and personality disorders, 48-9
Critical Flicker Fusion Frequency (CFFF), 19, 224
Cronholm-Ottosson Depression Scale, 173
culture
and evaluation of psychiatric therapy, 64-6
and milieu therapy, 139-40
and recognition of mental disorder, 34, 61
'cyclothymic axial syndrome', 77 (Table 1)

data, patient, see patient data

decision-trees (see also network analysis)
in diagnosis, 175-6
in rating of AMDP symptoms, 154 (Fig. 1)
delinquency and social maladjustment, 50-1
L-deprenil potentiation of 5-hydroxytryptophan, 237-8 (Figs. 2 and 3)
depression
diagnosis of, biological variables in, 7-8, 93-118, 233-4 (Table 2); dexamethasone suppression test, 108-12 (Fig. 1 and Table 1); growth hormone responses, 115-116; 5-HIAA in cerebrospinal fluid, 8, 94-8; homovanillic acid, 101-2; imipramine binding sites, 103; renal MHPG excretion, 98-101; tryptophan/competing amino acids ratio, 98, 103; TSH response to TRH, 112-15 (Figs. 2 and 3)
multinational study of, 65
neurotic, 35-6, 52, 198-9
pharmacogenic, after neuroleptics, 195-7 (Table 5)
and physical disease, 46
psychophysiological changes in, 226
rating of, 13-14, 172-4 (Table 1), 176-8 (Table 2); in AMDP system, 155-9 (Table 3); and anxiety, 174-5; self-, 189 (Table 1), 198-9; as a symptom, 165-6
social factors in, 36-9
therapy for (see also antidepressants, electroconvulsive therapy and lithium), 34-6; cognitive, 126, 198
design, experimental, see experimental design
desipramine
growth hormone response to, 116
prediction of response to, 234 (Tables 2 and 3); and D-amphetamine response, 232; using plasma levels, 235, 236 (Table 4); and renal MHPG excretion, 99-100, 231-2
desmethylclomipramine and monoamine metabolism, 96, 234 (Table 3)
dexamethasone suppression test (DST), 108-12 (Fig. 1 and Table 1), 116 (Table 2)
and response to ECT, 240
and TSH response to TRH, 114
diagnosis (see also rating scales and classification systems)

268 Index

diagnosis (*cont.*)
  of depression: biochemical variables in, 7-8, 93-104, 233-4 (Table 2); hormonal variables in, 107-18
  poly-diagnostic approach to, 75-9 (Table 1)
  standardized clinical, 6-8, 53-5, 81-91; advantages of, 81-5; methodology and, 85-91, 175-9 (Tables 2 and 3); World Health Organization (WHO) and, 63-7, 91
Diagnostic and Statistical Manual of Mental Disorders (DSM III) (American Psychiatric Association), 54
  algorithms for, 85-6
  and diagnosis of schizophrenia, 83-4
  poly-diagnostic approach of, 75-6
  and social adjustment, 208
Diagnostic Interview Schedule, 86, 91
diary, for self-monitoring, 133-4
Digit Symbol Test, 17-18
disability, *see* physical disability and disease *and* social adjustment
Disability Assessment Schedule (DAS), 65-6, 215-16
dopamine metabolism
  in depression: and growth hormone levels, 115-16; and homovanillic acid levels, 101-2, 104 (Table 1)
  in schizophrenia, and therapeutic response, 22, 240-1
droperidol and the 'prolactin model', 241
drug dependence
  cost-effectiveness of therapy for, 129
  and personality disorders, 48-50
drug therapy, *see* pharmacotherapy

Early Clinical Drug Evaluation Unit System (ECDEU), 188
electroconvulsive therapy (ECT)
  memory dysfunction after, 18
  prediction of response to, 232 (Table 1), 239-40
electroencephalogram (EEG), 223
  to measure drug effects, 227-8
  sleep, and response to imipramine, 235
electromyogram for muscle tension, 222
emotion, expressed, and relapse in schizophrenia, 41
epinephrine and ECT response, 240
ethical committees and psychiatric research, 256-7, 259-62
ethical problems in psychiatric research, 251-63
European Medical Research Councils, 215-16
·experimental design in psychiatric research, 22-5, 53-5

ethics of, 256-9
  in milieu therapy, 139-46
  and self-rating scales, 199-200
  and Type II statistical errors, 175
expressed emotion (EE) and relapse in schizophrenia, 41
Eysenck's Psychoticism Scale (*see also* Maudsley Personality Inventory), 192 (Table 4)

family
  environment and schizophrenic relapse, 41
  factors in depressive illness, 37-9
  factors in personality disorders, 48-51
  history, *see* genetic factors
  rating by, 213
  and stigma of mental illness, 61
Fear Survey Schedule (FSS-III), 189 (Table 1)
Feighner's diagnostic criteria, *see* St. Louis Diagnostic Criteria

galvanic skin responses (GSR), *see* sweat gland activity
general practice, rating of depression in, 173, 177-8 (Table 2)
genetic factors
  in personality disorders, 49
  in response to lithium, 239
growth hormone (GH) responses
  in depression, 115-16 (Table 2)
  in schizophrenia, 240-1
'guessing' methods of rating, 16

haloperidol, prediction of response to, 240, 241
Hamilton Anxiety Scale (HAS), 174-5
Hamilton Depression Scale (HDS), 13
  compared with AMDP scales, 156, 158
  compared with self-rating scales, 192-3 (Fig. 2)
  statistical analysis of, 172-3
heart disease, coronary, behaviour predisposing to, 133
heart rate, measurement of, 222
  after behavioural therapy, 227, 228
heredity, *see* genetics
heroin addiction, cost-effective therapy for, 129
HLA antigens in lithium responders, 239
homovanillic acid (HVA)
  after antipsychotics, 22, 240
  in depression, 101-2
  after lithium, 238
Hopkins Symptom Checklist, 188
hormones, *see* catecholamines, hypophyseal hormones, hypothalamus *and* individual hormones

Index

hospital staff and milieu therapy, 140–1, 142, 146–7
hospital ward atmosphere and milieu therapy, 141–2
hostility, rating scale for, 16
5-hydroxyindol acetic acid (5-HIAA) levels in cerebrospinal fluid, 94–5
  after chlorpromazine, 240
  and dexamethasone suppression test, 111
  and prediction of response to treatment, 102, 104 (Table 1); with 5-hydroxytryptophan, 95, 233; with lithium, 238, 239; with tricyclic antidepressants, 22, 95–7, 233–4 (Tables 2 and 3)
  and prognosis of depression, 8, 97–8
  and TSH response to TRH, 114
5-hydroxytryptamine (5-HT), *see* serotonin
5-hydroxytryptophan (5-HTP)
  antidepressant effect of, 95, 233
  potentiation with L deprenil, 237–8 (Figs. 2 and 3)
  prophylactic effect of, 97, 233
hypnotic drugs and EEG changes, 227–8
hypophyseal hormones, anterior, and monoamine metabolism (*see also* individual hormones), 102–3, 107–18
hypothalamus and control of hypophyseal hormones, 22, 108–9, 112–15

imipramine
  anticholinergic side-effects of, 225–6
  binding sites, 103, 104 (Table 1)
  compared with psychotherapy, 126
  prediction of response to, 234 (Tables 2 and 3); D-amphetamine test, 232; COMT activity in red blood cells, 235; 5-HIAA levels in cerebrospinal fluid, 233; plasma levels, 235–6 (Fig. 1 and Table 4); renal MHPG excretion, 99–100, 231–2; sleep REM changes, 235
immunogenetic predictors of lithium response, 239
informed consent in psychiatric research, 256–7, 259
In-patient Multidimensional Psychiatric Scale (IMPS)
  compared with AMDP scales, 156, 158–9
  used with self-rating scales, 188
insulin, growth hormone response to, 115, 116 (Table 2)
intelligence tests (*see also* memory tests)
  in 'multi-area' classifications, 74–5 (Fig. 1)
  and self-rating scales, 184, 190–1 (Tables 3 and 4), 200
  validity of, 23

International Classification of Diseases 9th revision (ICD 9) (WHO 1978), 83, 85
  development of, 63–4
  and poly-diagnostic approach, 75, 77–8
International Pilot Study of Schizophrenia (WHO 1973), 83
'interrupted time series', 145–6

Klinische Selbstbeurteilungs-Skalen (KSb-S), *see* Clinical Self-Rating Scales
Krakau Visual Acuity Test (KVAT), 19

L-DOPA
  growth hormone secretion after, 115–16
  response to, and homovanillic acid levels, 101
life events, adverse
  and depression, 37–8
  and neuroses, 44
  and physical illness, 46
life expectancy and affective disorders, 45–6
lithium
  prediction of response to, 232 (Table 1), 238–9
  prophylactic effect of, 24–5, 239
logical decision-trees, *see* decision-trees

Mania-Depression Scale (previously Manic-Depressive Syndrome), 155–7 (Table 3)
manic states
  lithium for, 24–5, 238
  rating of, 155–7 (Table 3), 174 (Table 1)
maprotiline, clinical trial of, 193–5 (Fig. 3)
Maudsley Personality Inventory (MPI) (Eysenck), 185, 187–9 (Table 1)
melancholia, *see* depression
memory tests (*see also* intelligence tests), 18
  validation of, 23–4
menstrual cycle and growth hormone secretion, 115
mental health
  care programmes (*see also* milieu therapy *and* psychiatric treatment), 59–67; collection of data for, 61–3; World Health Organization (WHO) and, 63–7; services involved in, 59–61
  definitions of, 33
'meta-analysis' for evaluation of psychotherapy, 131–2
metanephrine, 231
methacholine and ECT response, 240
3-methoxy-4-hydroxyphenol glycol (*cont.*) (MHPG)
  in cerebrospinal fluid: after

3-methoxy-4-hydroxyphenol glycol (*cont.*)
  chlorpromazine, 240; in depression, 101
  renal excretion of, 98–101, 103, 104 (Table 1); and lithium response, 238–9; and tricyclic antidepressant response, 22, 99–100, 231–3, 234 (Table 2)
mianserin, clinical trial of, 193–5 (Fig. 3)
milieu therapy, evaluation of, 137–47
  control groups for, 145–6
  hospital and patient variables in, 139–43
  outcome criteria for, 143–5
  psychophysiological measures for, 227
Minnesota Multiphasic Personality Inventory (MMPI), 187
monoamine(s) (*see also* individual amines *and* metabolites)
  control of anterior hypophyseal hormones, 107–8
  metabolism: and pathogenesis of depression, 103–4 (Table 1), 117, 233–4; and response to antidepressants, 94, 234 (Tables 2 and 3); and response to ECT, 240
monoamine oxidase (MAO) activity in platelets
  and response to lithium, 238
  and response to MAO inhibitors, 237–8 (Figs. 2 and 3)
monoamine oxidase (MAO) inhibitors
  autonomic effects of, 225
  and monoamine metabolism, 94
  prediction of response to, 232 (Table 1), 236–8 (Figs. 2 and 3)
mortality and affective disorders, 45–6
'multi-area' classification (MAC), 74–5, 76
multiaxial (*see also* multidimensional) classification systems, 54–5, 71–9
  alternative terminology for, 74–5
  methodological problems in, 85–9
  and poly-diagnostic approach, 75–9 (Table 1)
multicategorical classification systems, 74
multidimensional (*see also* multiaxial) classification systems
  alternative terminology for, 74–5
  self-rating, 184
  sensitivity of, 175
  and social adjustment, 208–9 (Table 2)
Multiple Affect Adjective Check List, 188
multivariate analysis in diagnosis of depression, 176–7, 179 (Table 3)
muscle tension, measurement of, 222
network analysis models for cost-effectiveness, 129
neuroendocrinology, *see* catecholamines, hypophyseal hormones, hypothalamus *and* monoamines

neuroleptic drugs (*see also* individual agents)
  long-term therapy with, 40–1
  peripheral effects of, 225
  prediction of response to, 240–1
  self-rating of side-effects of, 195–7 (Table 5)
neuropsychological tests (*see also* psychophysiological measures), 18–19
neuroses
  biofeedback for, 4–5
  and personality disorders, 47
  rating of symptoms in, 16
  treatment for, 42–5, 52–3, 123–4
neurotic depression, 35–6, 52, 198–9
neurotic personality traits and depression, 178 (Table 2), 198–9
neurotransmitters, *see* monoamines
Newcastle Scales for depression, 176–7
nomifensine and dopamine metabolism, 101–2
noradrenaline (NA, or norepinephrine NE) metabolism in depression (*see also* 3-methoxy-4-hydroxyphenyl glycol *and* vanillylmandelic acid), 98–101, 104 (Table 1)
  and dexamethasone suppression test, 109, 111
  and growth hormone responses, 115–16
  and response to tricyclic antidepressants, 95–6, 99–100, 231–3, 234 (Tables 2 and 3)
  and TSH response to TRH, 112, 114
norepinephrine, *see* noradrenaline
normetanephrine, 231
nortriptyline, therapeutic effect of
  and biochemical variables, 95–6, 232, 233, 234 (Tables 2 and 3)
  and plasma levels, 22, 235–6 (Fig. 1 and Table 4)
Nurses' Observation Scale for In-patient Evaluation (NOSIE), 12

oestrogens and growth hormone levels, 115
Opinions About Mental Illness Scale (OMI), 140–1
Oxford Medilog system, 223

patient data (*see also* statistical analysis *and* symptoms)
  accuracy of, in self-reporting, 9, 132–4, 213
  confidentiality of, 258–9
  for evaluation of milieu therapy, 139–42
  sources of, 59–63
  standardization of, *see* classification systems
Perception of Ward Scales (POW), 141
perphenazine, therapeutic response to, 240

Index

Personal Adjustment and Role-Skill Scale (PARS III), 144
personality disorders, 47–51, 53
personality inventories, 187–8, 197–9
personality traits
  and development of neuroses, 43–4
  neurotic, and depression, 178 (Table 2), 198–9
pharmacotherapy (*see also* antidepressants, antipsychotics *and* individual agents)
  plasma drug levels and, 22, 235–6 (Fig. 1 and Table 4), 238, 239, 241
  psychotherapy versus, 35–6, 126
  side-effects of: evaluation of, 185, 195–8 (Table 5 and Fig. 4); of long-term therapy, 35–6, 40–1; peripheral, 225–6
phenelzine, prediction of response to, 236–8
phobias
  behavioural therapies for, 4, 228
  development of, 43–4
  psychophysiological measures in, 224, 228
  self-rating of, 189 (Table 1)
physical disability and disease (*see also* psychosomatic disease)
  assessment of, 65–6
  and mental health, 6, 45–6, 60, 131–2
piribedil, therapeutic effect of, 101
pituitary hormones, *see* hypophyseal hormones
placebos (*see also* controlled trials)
  ethics of, 257–8
  and pain relief, 22
platelets
  imipramine binding sites in, 103, 104 (Table 1)
  monoamine oxidase activity in, 237–8 (Figs. 2 and 3)
poly-diagnostic approach (PDA), 75–9
pregnancy, self-reporting of smoking in, 9, 132–3
Present State Examination (PSE), 54, 64, 86, 90–1
  -CATEGO system, 87, 91
  in poly-diagnostic approach, 76
  for social adjustment, 65, 208, 215
probabilistic transition models of treatment, 129
probenecid test
  and dopamine turnover, 101–2
  and serotonin turnover, 95, 233
projective tests, 20–1
prolactin
  after antipsychotics, 22, 241
  response to TRH, 113, 114
psychiatric treatment (*see also* electroconvulsive therapy, milieu therapy, pharmacotherapy *and* psychotherapy)
  aims of, 5–6, 33–55
  evaluation of: classification systems for, *see* classification systems; data for, *see* patient data; ethical and practical problems in, 251–63; experimental design in, *see* experimental design; methods for (*see also* biochemical methods, psychophysiological measures, rating scales *and* statistical analysis), 6–22; World Health Organization (WHO) and, 63–7
psychoanalysis, 3–4, 43
  cost-benefits of, 4, 130–1
psychodynamic therapies, 3–4, 43, 124
psychogenic illness, *see* psychosomatic disease
Psychological Impairments Rating Schedule (PIRS), 65–6
psychological tests, 16–19, 224
psychometric 'paper and pencil' tests, 17–18, 23
psychophysiological measures, 19–20, 221–9
  and central state, 223–4
  and treatment response, 224–9
psychoses, diagnostic hierarchy of, 175–6
psychosomatic disease, 45–7
  and biofeedback, 4–5, 46–7
  after female sterilization, 65
  psychotherapy to prevent, 129–32
psychotherapy (*see also* milieu therapy *and* individual methods), 123–35
  accuracy of data for evaluation of, 132–4
  cost-benefit analysis of, 26–7, 127–32
  definition of, 123
  experimental design and evaluation of, 53–5, 125–6
  Eysenck's views of, 123–4
  methods of, 3–5, 124–5
  and neuroses, 42–5, 53
  and neurotic depression, 35–6, 52, 198–9
  and personality disorders, 48–50
  pharmacotherapy versus, 35–6, 126
  self-monitoring as, 133–4
  single case reports of, 8–9
  utilization of medical services after, 129–31
Psychoticism Scale, Eysenck's, 192 (Table 4)
pulse rate, *see* heart rate
pupil size and autonomic function, 222, 225

Rasch model for analysis of rating scales, 173, 179 (Table 3)

rating scales (*see also* classification systems *and* individual scales)
  for affective disorders, 171–9
  AMDP and AMP, 151–60
  Comprehensive Psychopathological Rating Scale, 163–9
  and raters: diagnostic prejudices of, 165–6; opinions of different scales, 158–60; training of, 11, 153, 177
  self-, 14, 183–200
  for social adjustment, 208–15
  statistical analysis of, *see* statistical analysis
  types of, 9–18
Reaction Times, tests of, 19
red blood cell catechol-*O*-methyltransferase (COMT), 235
red blood cell lithium ratio, 239
rehabilitation, *see* social adjustment
reliability of evaluation methods, 23
  of AMDP rating system, 154–5
  and comparability in clinical research, 82–3
  of Comprehensive Psychopathological Rating Scale, 166, 169
  of depression rating scales, 173, 176
  of self-rating scales, 185–6 (Fig. 1), 213
Research Diagnostic Criteria (RDC), 54, 77 (Table 1), 85
Rorschach test, 20–1

St Louis Diagnostic Criteria (Feighner *et al*), 74, 77 (Table 1), 85
salivation, measurement of, 222, 225–6
Schedule for Affective Disorders and Schizophrenia (SADS), 7
schizo-affective psychoses and monoamines, 99, 102
schizophrenia (*see also* antipsychotic drugs)
  biochemical predictors of therapeutic response in, 240–1
  chronic, and social adjustment, 39–42, 88–9, 207, 215–16
  diagnosis of: and decision-trees, 176; discrepancies in, 83–4; polydiagnostic approach to, 76–8 (Table 1)
  international studies on, 64–5, 83–4
  psychophysiological measures and, 224, 229
  rating scales for, 12, 14–15, 16, 77 (Table 1), 155–8 (Table 4)
Schizophrenia Syndrome Scale (previously Schizophrenic Scale), 155–8 (Table 4)
'schizophrenic axial syndrome', 77 (Table 1)
self-evaluation of antidepressants (McNair), 188
self-monitoring as psychotherapy, 133–4

Self-Rating Anxiety Scale (SAS) (Zung), 189 (Table 1), 192 (Table 4)
Self-Rating Depression Scale (SDS) (Zung), 14, 189 (Table 1), 192 (Table 4)
  in clinical drug trials, 192–3 (Fig. 2)
self-rating scales (*see also* self-reporting), 14, 183–200
  applications of, in drug trials, 192–9 (Figs. 2, 3 and 4, Table 5)
  comparisons of, 187–92 (Tables 1, 2 and 3)
  criteria required of, 185–7 (Fig. 1)
  limitations of, 184–5, 199–200, 213
  recommendations for use of, 199–200
  for social adjustment, 213
self-reporting, accuracy of, 9, 132–3, 213
Self-Report Symptom Inventory, 188
serotonin (5-hydroxytryptamine, 5-HT)
  metabolism in depression (*see also* 5-hydroxyindol acetic acid), 94–8, 104 (Table 1)
  and 5-hydroxytryptophan response, 95, 97, 233
  and imipramine binding sites, 103
  and prognosis, 8, 97–8
  and tricyclic antidepressant response, 95–6, 100, 233–4 (Tables 2 and 3)
  and tryptophan/competing amino acids ratio, 98, 103
  and TSH response to TRH, 114
skin conductance, *see* sweat gland activity
sleep EEG studies, 235
smoking in pregnancy, self-reporting of, 9, 132–3
social adjustment (*see also* social maladjustment), 205–16
  in chronic schizophrenics, 39–42, 88–9, 207, 215–16
  in multiaxial classifications, 75 (Fig. 1), 88–9, 208–9
  scales, 209 (Table 3): analysis of, 214; comparison of, 208–15 (Tables 2, 4 and 5); development of standardized, 65–6, 215–16; after milieu therapy, 143–5
  terminology of, 205–7 (Table 1), 215
Social Adjustment Scale, 143, 210, 212 (Table 5)
social factors (*see also* life events, adverse)
  in depression, 36–9, 52
  in personality disorders, 48–51
Social Interview Scale (SIS, or Standardized Interview to Assess Social Maladjustment and Dysfunction), 210–14 (Table 4)
social maladjustment (*see also* social adjustment)
  causes of, 207
  and personality disorders, 47–51, 53

Index

Social Re-adjustment Rating Scale, 213
spiroperidol, for radioreceptor assay, 241
Staff–Resident Interaction Chronograph, 142
Standardized Interview to Assess Social Maladjustment and Dysfunction (or Social Interview Scale, SIS), 210–14 (Table 4)
statistical analysis (*see also* cost-benefit analysis, reliability *and* validity)
  and classification systems, 54–5; for development of AMDP subscales, 154–6; for diagnosis of depression, 176–7, 179 (Table 3)
  in 'interrupted time series', 145–6
  methods of, 23–5
  of scores: for Comprehensive Psychopathological Rating Scale, 168; for depression scales, 172–5; for social adjustment scales, 214–15
  of self rating scales, 188–92 (Tables 2, 3 and 4)
  Type II errors in, 175
Subject's Treatment Emergent Symptom Scale (STESS), 188
suicide, risk of
  and availability of antidepressants, 35
  and personality disorders, 48, 50
  in 'serotonin-deficient' depression, 8, 97–8
Süllwold Scale for schizophrenic basic symptoms, 76–7
sulphapyridine acetylation and phenelzine response, 236–7
surgery, psychological intervention and, 131–2
sweat gland activity (galvanic skin resistance and skin conductance), 19, 222
  in phobics after behaviour therapy, 228
  and therapeutic response, 225–7, 229
symptom(s) (*see also* patient data)
  drug-induced (*see also* pharmacotherapy), 197–8 (Fig. 4)
  hierarchy of, 78, 89, 176
  mechanisms and physiological changes, 224
  rating of, 9–16; in AMDP system, 12, 152–4 (Tables 1 and 2, Fig. 1); in Comprehensive Psychopathological Rating Scale, 12–13, 164–8 (Table 1); in depression, 13–14, 177–8 (Table 2); self-, 184

tardive dyskinesia after neuroleptics, 40
Taylor Manifest Anxiety Scale (MAS), 15
tetracyclic antidepressants, trials of, 193–5 (Fig. 3)
Thematic Apperception Test (TAT), 21

thiothixene, therapeutic response to, 240
thyroid-stimulating hormone (TSH) response to TRH
  in depression, 112–15 (Figs. 2 and 3), 116 (Table 2)
  in ECT responders, 240
thyrotropin-releasing hormone (TRH)
  growth hormone response to, 115
  prolactin response to, 113
  TSH response to: in depression, 112–15 (Figs. 2 and 3), 116 (Table 2); in ECT responders, 240
trazodone compared with amitriptyline, 192–3 (Fig. 2)
tricyclic antidepressants (*see also* antidepressants *and* individual agents)
  autonomic effects of, 225–6
  long-term therapy with, 35
  and monoamine metabolism, 22, 94
  prediction of response to, 102–4 (Table 1), 231–6 (Tables 1, 2 and 3); and dexamethasone suppression test, 111; and 5-HIAA levels, 95–7, 233–4 (Tables 2 and 3); using plasma drug levels, 22, 235–6 (Fig. 1 and Table 4); and renal MHPG excretion, 99–100, 231–3
tryptophan/competing amino acids ratio, 98, 103, 104 (Table 1)

USA–UK Diagnostic Project, 84

validity of evaluation methods, 23–4
  of AMDP rating system, 155–6
  of depression scales, 172, 176
  of self-rating scales, 186–7
vanillylmandelic acid (VMA), 98, 231
Visual Analogue Scale (VAS), 189 (Table 1)

Ward Atmosphere Scale, 141–2
Wechsler Memory Scale, 18, 191 (Tables 2 and 3), 200
World Health Organization (WHO) (*see also International Classification of Diseases*)
  Depression Scale, 65, 176–9
  development of standardized classifications by, 63–7, 91
  and measures of social adjustment, 65–6, 215–16

Zung self-rating scales, *see* Self-Rating Anxiety Scale *and* Self-Rating Depression Scale